Social Media for Nurses

Educating Practitioners and Patients in a Networked World

Ramona Nelson, PhD, RN-BC, ANEF, FAAN

Irene Joos, PhD, MSIS, MSN, RN

Debra M. Wolf, PhD, MSN, BSN, RN

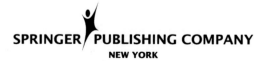
SPRINGER PUBLISHING COMPANY
NEW YORK

Springer Publishing Company, LLC
11 West 42nd Street
New York, NY 10036
www.springerpub.com

Acquisitions Editor: Allan Graubard
Project Manager: Michael O'Connor
Composition: diacriTech, India

ISBN: 978-0-8261-9588-3
E-book ISBN: 978-0-8261-9589-0

12 13 14 15/ 5 4 3 2 1

The authors and the publisher of this work have made every effort to use sources believed to be reliable to provide information that is accurate and compatible with the standards generally accepted at the time of publication. Because medical and informatics science is continually advancing, our knowledge base continues to expand. Therefore, as new information becomes available, changes in protocols and procedures become necessary. We recommend that the reader always consult current research, specific institutional policies, and current drug references before providing patient care including any clinical procedure or administering any drug. The author and publisher shall not be liable for any special, consequential, or exemplary damages resulting, in whole or in part, from the readers' use of, or reliance on, the information contained in this book. The publisher has no responsibility for the persistence or accuracy of URLs for external or third-party Internet Web sites referred to in this publication and does not guarantee that any content on such websites is, or will remain, accurate or appropriate.

Library of Congress Cataloging-in-Publication Data

CIP data is available from the Library of Congress.

Special discounts on bulk quantities of our books are available to corporations, professional associations, pharmaceutical companies, health care organizations, and other qualifying groups.

If you are interested in a custom book, including chapters from more than one of our titles, we can provide that service as well.

For details, please contact:
Special Sales Department,
Springer Publishing Company, LLC
11 West 42nd Street, 15th Floor,
New York, NY 10036-8002s
Phone: 877-687-7476 or 212-431-4370; Fax: 212-941-7842
Email: sales@springerpub.com

Printed in the United States of America by Gasch Printing.

The value of Health 2.0 is created by nurses, other health care providers, patients, families, and significant others through their telepresence and information sharing. This book is dedicated to these contributors as they shape the next generations of Health 3.0, 4.0, and so on.

Co-Authors

As one of the co-authors of this book, I also dedicate this book to my grandchildren: Mackenzie Elizabeth and Hope Elizabeth Hollis. They are today's joy and tomorrow's hope.

Ramona Nelson

I dedicate this book to my husband, Brian, for his understanding and support in all I do and for his hours of editing work, and to our son, Brian, for his editing work (I knew his writing degrees would be helpful) and for his critique of the social media concepts and exercises.

Irene Joos

As a reflection of the love and support my family has given me, I dedicate this book to them. To my husband, Ken, for his patience and support throughout my professional career, to my children, Carrie, Stephanie, Colin, Jeff, and Matt, who inspire me daily, and, lastly, to my father Angelo, who has always taught me to be loving, caring, considerate, and aware of those around me who are in need.

Debra M. Wolf

Contents

Preface

The use of Web 2.0 applications in the delivery of health care is creating an online health care delivery world where nurses and other health care professionals must establish a telepresence if they are to meet the health-related needs of the community. By understanding and using Health 2.0 applications and technology, nurses have the opportunity to extend their services and professional practice to this new online environment with the goal of improving the health of individuals, families, significant others, and communities.

The authors of this book believe nurses and other health care professionals are responsible for educating patients and consumers to effectively use Health 2.0 tools in managing their health and health care. This belief stimulated us to write a text that would assist nurses in maximizing the use of social media, the Internet, and electronic devices to inform, support, and empower the consumer in adhering to a healthier lifestyle. Just imagine the extent to which a nurse working in all settings can support patients through online educational sessions, blogs, wikis, or telehealth services by sharing accurate and pertinent information that further empowers those patients to play an active and informed role in addressing their health care needs. Just imagine the number of health care consumers that can be reached, assessed, treated, or supported using the technology that is currently available. Just imagine what we can learn from our patients by partnering with them in working to improve health and health care.

Patients are more likely to experience positive health outcomes if they have the opportunity to be informed, engaged, and serve as a true partner in working with their health care team. Consumers are more likely to avoid health care problems and experience good health if they are informed and actively engaged in managing their health. Health care professionals are more likely to achieve excellence in the delivery of health care if they are continuously engaged in the improvement of their knowledge and skills. Web 2.0 and, in turn, Health 2.0 provide a new range of tools and applications for achieving these goals. However, with this opportunity comes responsibility. Health care providers are responsible for the effective and professional use of these applications in the delivery of health care.

This book introduces health care professionals to the knowledge and skills needed to effectively and professionally use Health 2.0 applications. Each chapter begins with clear and concise learning objectives and a list of related terms that may be new to the reader. Each term is discussed in the chapter and defined in the Glossary. Each chapter then provides a theoretical foundation for understanding the concepts presented in that chapter. The reader is presented with resources that support additional in-depth learning through URLs or website names. Each chapter incorporates discussion questions that stimulate the use of critical thinking skills in dealing with the issues presented. This content is followed by exercises that reinforce the development of Health 2.0-related knowledge and skills presented in the chapter. The book concludes with an Appendix that lists several additional resources that can be used to further support the needs of nurses, other health care professionals, and consumers.

Ramona Nelson
Irene Joos
Debra M. Wolf

Acknowledgments

The authors of this book could never have completed the manuscript without the support and guidance of several people. First we would like to recognize the support of our families. Each of us is married and has children, so there is a long list of people who "kept the home fires burning" and the process moving forward. Some of those names have been included in the dedication. In addition, Dr. Nelson would like to acknowledge her husband, Glenn M. Nelson, who was unwavering in his belief that this book needed to be written. Dr. Joos would like to acknowledge LaVerne Collins and Jackie Bolte, research librarians, whose excellent research and retrieval skills have consistently ensured that references included the latest information. Dr. Wolf would like to acknowledge Bonnie Anton, MN, RN, whose mentoring has been key to her professional advancement.

We also gratefully acknowledge the support of our publisher and the support of Allan Graubard, our Acquisitions Editor at Springer Publishing Company. In addition we would like to thank Michael O'Connor for following up on each and every question and detail related to the publication of this book.

CHAPTER 1

An Introduction
Social Media and the Transitioning Roles and Relationships in Health Care

Ramona Nelson and Irene Joos

LEARNING OBJECTIVES

At the completion of this chapter the reader will be able to:

1. Analyze historical trends and driving forces impacting the utilization of social media in health care.
2. Define social media related literacies and explain their interrelationships.
3. Apply appropriate criteria to assess the credibility of health information on social media websites.
4. Analyze social media and the transitioning role of nurses and other health care professionals.

TERMS

Computer literacy/fluency
Consumer health informatics
Consumer informatics
Crowd-sourcing
Criteria
Digital literacy
Digital native
eHealth
Engaged consumer gray literature
Health 2.0

Health literacy
Health care consumer
Informatics for consumer health (ICH)
Information literacy
Patient Empowerment 2.0
Social media
Web 1.0
Web 2.0
Wisdom of crowds

*I*n April 2012 the PricewaterhouseCoopers Health Research Institute reported that one-third of consumers are using social media sites to seek medical information, discuss symptoms and express their opinions about doctors, drugs and health insurers. When these same consumers were asked how the information they found within these sites could affect their health-related decisions:

- 45 % said it would affect their decision to get a second opinion;
- 41 % said it would affect their choice of a specific doctor, hospital or medical facility;
- 34 % said it would affect their decision about taking a certain medication; and
- 32 % said it would affect their choice of a health insurance plan (PriceWaterhouse-Coopers Health Research Institute, 2012).

As these statistics demonstrate social media is changing the conversation between health care systems and the communities they serve. Web 1.0 opened up the world of health-related information to provider and patient alike by providing open, easy and rapid access to a wealth of new information. In 1997, free online Medline searching was opened to the public. For the first time both the patient and the health care provider had access to the same health care literature. Information found on the web or via the Internet can be invaluable or inaccurate or even dangerous. For example, a patient can find detailed information on options for treating back pain from top academic medical centers as well as options for "snake oil" that online scams may offer. The challenge for health professionals is to teach patients how to determine the difference.

Web 1.0 refers to static websites that the user views without interactive involvement between the user and the website. Communication is in one direction, meaning Web 1.0 does not offer a dialog with a person who actually tried different treatments for back pain. Social media are web-based and mobile technologies that turn this one-way communication into interactive dialogues. "The engaged consumer is seeking an ongoing dialog on health—not a one-way, 30-second broadcast" (Sarasohn-Kahn, 2008, p. 10). Changing the knowledge base and the communication patterns among individuals as well as between groups changes not only the content of the dialog, but also changes the relationships of the people and groups involved in that communication. In other words, social media will forever change the patient-provider relationship.

This book explores the opportunities and challenges nurses and other health care providers may experience when using social media to dialog with colleagues, patients/consumers, friends and families. The various types of social media are examined while analyzing the impact of social media on the practice of health care delivery. This chapter begins by examining the historical events and driving forces that are impacting how social media is now being used in health care.

HISTORICAL EVENTS AND DRIVING FORCES

Over the last several decades, the role of the patient has been evolving from passive recipient of health care to informed, empowered, and engaged patient/consumer. Underlying and paralleling this changing role of the patient has been the development of communication technologies. These new technologies have increased the opportunities for individuals to function as cohesive groups as well as provide increased access to information and knowledge. The ongoing development of an informed, empowered and engaged patient/consumer is part of a larger movement creating an informed and engaged citizen participating in all aspects of society and not just health care. Table 1.1 demonstrates this process through examining highlights in the history of *Consumer Reports*. It demonstrate emerging trends within the larger consumer movement (Consumers Union of U.S., 2012) as well as health care.

Several parallel, interrelated, and overlapping themes from health care can be identified within this larger consumer movement. These include efforts to control and shift health care costs; the evolution of the empowered health care consumer and the emergence of well-informed, empowered, and engaged patients; the establishment of consumer informatics as a branch of health care informatics and the development of Web 2.0.

Table 1.1 *Highlights and Implications of the History of* **Consumer Reports**

Year	History of *Consumer Reports* (Consumers Union of U.S., 2012)	Consumer Trends	Implications for Health 2.0
1936	Colston Warne, an Amherst College economics professor, announced the founding of Consumers Union during a speech with the statement, "There is in New York City now a consumers' laboratory which tests products, and rates them as to their quality. It is owned and controlled by organized consumers." Warne, one of the founders of Consumers Union, chaired its board from 1936 to 1979. The first *Consumers Union Reports* was published with articles on Grade A and Grade B milk, breakfast cereals, soap, and stockings.	Consumers are in control. A research method is used to determine the quality of products with experts directing the process of determining quality. Information is easily available to the public.	The patient as consumer is in control. This approach is consistent with using the credentials of an individual or organization to evaluate the quality health care information posted on the web. To be empowered, a patient/health care consumer must have full access to information.
1940	*Consumers Union Reports* starts asking its readers about their experiences with various products on its Annual Questionnaire.	Consumers as individuals share valuable information on the quality of products they have used.	Using crowd-sourcing patients can create valuable knowledge that is not available from other sources. Experiential knowledge is as valuable and informative as theoretical knowledge.
1942	Consumers Union changes the name of its magazine to *Consumer Reports* to make it clear that it serves all consumers, not just union members.	Emphasizes the importance of easily available information for all consumers.	Demands access to one's personal health information as well as information about health that is stored in resources such as MEDLINE.
1953	*Consumer Reports* publishes a series of reports on the tar and nicotine content of cigarette smoke and health hazards of smoking. "Information on exactly what cigarettes contained was available from no other source at the time."	Health care and health-related information is a product that can be evaluated.	Changing the health of a population requires that health-related lifestyle information is easily available to the public.

(Continued)

Table 1.1 *Highlights and Implications of the History of* **Consumer Reports** *(Continued)*

Year	History of *Consumer Reports* (Consumers Union of U.S., 2012)	Consumer Trends	Implications for Health 2.0
1970	With the recommendation of *Consumer Reports*, The National Commission on Product Safety is established, in part because of all the products that were unsafe.	Federal policy and, in turn, federal agencies support the consumer movement.	Health policy and government agencies must support the development of and provide regulation for Health 2.0 if the full benefit of this movement and related technology is to be achieved.
1987	*Consumer Reports* becomes available online.	Consumer information is available by Internet, thereby increasing access to this information.	Health care information is available via mobile electronic devices through Wi-Fi connections, thereby increasing access to this information for consumers on the move.
1989	First *Consumer Reports* health newsletter is published.	Health care is increasingly seen as a product requiring a quality type assessment that is available to the public.	Health care is increasingly seen as a product requiring a quality type assessment that is available to the public.
2007	ConsumerReportsHealth and the Consumer Reports Health Ratings Center are launched to meet consumers' demand for health information from a trusted source.	Increased emphasis on the quality of health-related information on the Internet.	Increased emphasis on the quality of health-related information and applications available through a variety of technologies.
Future?	A number of online stores now include reviews from consumers. As the number of reviews for each product offered via the web increases, how will access to this information impact the current role and activities of non-profit independent organizations such as Consumer Reports or government agencies such as the U.S. Consumer Product Safety Commission (http://www.cpsc.gov/about/about.html)?		

Source: Information for columns 1 and 2 from Consumers Union of U.S., Inc. (2012).

Efforts to Control and Shift Health Care Costs

The label "patient" and the label "consumer" carry very different connotations. A patient is someone who receives care that is provided by a health care provider. The phrase "patient–health care provider relationship" indicates that professional services are being provided in a caring manner by the health care provider to the patient and there is a special type of relationship between the receiver and the giver of the services. Evidence of this relationship is the tendency for a patient to say thank you at the end of an office visit with their health care provider. Even though the patient pays for the service either directly or indirectly, the emphasis is on the service. A review of several dictionaries demonstrates that the definition of the word patient does not include the word "cost" or suggest that money is exchanged for this service.

In contrast, a consumer is someone who purchases or takes in a product. The product may be a health care–related service, but the emphasis with the label consumer is on the fact that the service is not free. It is not a gift. The consumer pays for the service directly as an out-of-pocket cost or indirectly through a third party, such as their insurance company. Sometimes a non-profit agency or government program such as Medicare assumes the cost. In each case, cost is implied in the term "health care consumer." A health care consumer is defined as anyone who receives or has the potential to receive health care services, regardless of whether the individual pays for those services directly or indirectly (Guo, 2010). With this definition, the consumer of health care services can be identified as the key to controlling the ever expanding cost of health care for a number of reasons, including:

- Third-party payers for health care services isolate patients from information about actual costs and provide little to no motivation for controlling that cost.
- Providers and institutions paid on a fee-for-service basis have no motivation to provide fewer services. The more service provided, the more income produced with a fee-for-service model.
- Insurance companies that control cost by limiting access to health care services function in a conflict of interest environment. One can question if their decisions are in the best interest of the patient or are based on their profit margin.
- A significant proportion of health care costs are driven by chronic disease, which can be prevented or at least limited by lifestyle choices (Thompson & Cutler, 2010).

By providing health care consumers with larger financial incentives to control cost as well as information on prices, quality, and treatment alternatives, they can take more responsibility for their health by deciding what health care services to purchase. One particular approach to designing health benefits based on this definition of consumerism is called consumer-directed health plans (CDHPs), which include large deductibles and a tax-preferred savings account (Guo, 2010). With this model the consumer is encouraged to save money for future health-related costs and to decide if and when those savings might be spent. "However, there are still many gaps in the typical consumer models" (Thompson & Cutler, 2010, p. 26). The ideal situation is that patients/consumers would become more involved in controlling both their health and their health care costs, thereby improving the health of the community while creating a cost effective health care system. However, there are a number of factors that limit this ideal situation.

- Health care information is complex. Consumers may have difficulty understanding their options when faced with a health-related decision. In 2003, approximately 36% of the adult population in the United States demonstrated limited health literacy. These rates were higher in certain population subgroups (Berkman et al., 2011). In many cases, there is no one right or wrong answer for treating a specific health problem, but rather several options. This reality is demonstrated when patients are encouraged to get second or even third opinions. Questions of cost versus quality adds to the complexity. A recent study by Hibbard, Greene, Sofaer, Firminger, and Hirsh (2012) demonstrated that consumers are more interested in the quality of health care than in its cost, even when paying the cost out of pocket. In addition, a substantial minority of the respondents associated increased cost with increased quality. Interestingly, the researchers did find that "presenting cost data alongside easy-to-interpret quality information and highlighting high-value options improved the likelihood that consumers would choose those options" (p. 843). However, this kind of information is not often available.
- Funding prevention is a long-term investment. It is easy to delay these interventions if money and/or time are limited and there are no signs of impending health problems. Changing lifestyle choices across a population can take years and require a variety of approaches. For example, adult smoking prevalence declined from 42.4% in 1965 to 20.6% in 2009 (CDC, n.d.) as a result of multiple approaches. However, a

survey of employers conducted by PricewaterhouseCoopers found that 70% of surveyed employers include wellness initiatives in their personnel and benefit strategy, but only 15% of their employees participated (2012). In addition, many individuals, for a number of reasons, change their insurance companies several times over their lifetime. For example, some employers change their health insurance company options and some individuals change jobs, retire, or relocate. This reality does not encourage the insurance companies to fund preventative care since they are unlikely to be the insurer years later when illnesses develop.

- Some employees do not participate in prevention programs because they fear that completing a health risk appraisal, thereby revealing their poor health habits to the insurance company, will influence their job status or insurance premiums.
- Both patients and providers often avoid discussions of quality and cost. Many patients are uncomfortable questioning a highly educated health care professional. A feeling that the health care provider is rushed, as well as cultural, age and gender differences can accentuate this discomfort. For example, patients will often not mention to a physician that they would like a second opinion, because they do not want to leave the impression that they would doubt or question in any way the opinion of the first physician. In addition, health care professionals may not be knowledgeable or comfortable discussing health care options in terms of their costs. In many cases, both the patient and the provider would prefer to consider health care in terms of the caring relationship between them and not as a business decision between a consumer and a seller.

The Emergence of the Empowered Health Care Consumer

A search of the OVID Medline literature database (1946 to 2012) for articles that included *consumer* in the title returned 5,511 results (articles). A review of these results demonstrated that the term consumer began to be included in the title of articles during the 1960s. For example, in 1967, the *Journal of the American Dental Association* published an article titled "Consumer Attitudes Toward Prepaid Dentistry" (Simons, 1967). However, a search of this database using the same time period found only two articles that included the phrase "empowered consumer" in the title of the article (Anonymous, 1999; Weber, 1997). Both articles suggested that with the introduction of the Internet patients are becoming consumers with demands. Use of the term "empowered consumer" as a keyword in this same database produced a total of 4 results. In contrast, an Internet search using the search strategies ("empowered consumer" and "health care") in Google resulted in about 50,000 hits. This would suggest the concept that the empowered health care consumer is developing outside the traditional health care literature and maybe even outside the world of many health care providers.

The concept of an empowered consumer, in contrast to the concept of consumer as buyer, suggests that the consumer is not just making choices from predetermined options, but is in the driver's seat and in *control* of his or her health care decisions. The concept of the empowered consumer also suggests that by working in groups the consumer is able to impact and change the health care system.

A significant force in the development of the empowered consumer concept is the mental health consumer movement beginning in the 1960s and 1970s. During this time period, social change movements were part of the American culture. Mental health consumers were inspired by the African American civil rights movement, women, gays and lesbians, and people with disabilities who organized for social change. Large state hospitals across the country closed and new laws limiting involuntary commitment were being instituted. Former patients began meeting together in groups. Initially, these groups expressed anger at their treatment and demanded change. In 1978, the landmark book *On Our Own: Patient Controlled Alternatives to the Mental Health System* was authored by Judi Chamberlin, a psychiatric survivor and a long time activist. Over the next decades, the tone of this movement changed from a confrontational approach demanding change to collaboration and mutual respect as each side continues to work toward improving mental health services for all (Zinman, Budd, & Bluebird, 2009).

The Evolution of Well-Informed, Empowered, and Engaged Patients

Several key individuals, along with the development of the web, played a major role in leading the empowered consumer movement forward to the well-informed, empowered, and engaged patient movement. Table 1.2 provides a sample of health care professionals who are leading this movement on a national and international level. Selected accomplishments demonstrate how these leaders are using social media to change both the patient and provider roles in the health care system.

One of the earliest and most effective leaders was Tom Ferguson, MD. "Dr. Ferguson virtually led the movement to advocate informed self-care as the starting point for good health, and to promote a new kind of relationship between knowledgeable medical consumers and medical professionals. His goal was to encourage medical professionals to treat clients as equal partners in achieving better outcomes and change the entrenched practices of the traditional top-down hierarchy of the doctor-patient relationship. With the advent of broad access to the Internet, Dr. Ferguson's long history of advocacy of information-empowered medical consumers positioned him to be a leading proponent of online health information resources" (Austin American-Statesman, 2006, para. 4).

Table 1.2 *Select Leaders in the Health 2.0 Movement*

Leaders	Examples of Achievements
"e-Patient Dave" Dave deBronkart (http://epatientdave.com/about-dave/#bios)	Diagnosed with stage IV cancer in 2007, Dave went on to become a well-known advocate to e-patient, who takes an active role in managing his own health. He is a blogger, keynote speaker, and health policy advisor.
Daniel Z. Sands, MD, MPH (http://www.linkedin.com/in/dannysands)	Wrote the first official guidelines for physicians using email with patients. He is the President and a founder of the Society for Participatory Medicine.
Matthew Holt (http://www.matthewholt.net/)	Established the Health care blog (http://thehealthcare-blog.com/about/) and co-established the Health 2.0 Conferences (http://www.health2con.com/).
Patricia Flatley Brennan, PhD, RN (http://www.projecthealthdesign.org/about/npo/brennan)	Established *ComputerLink* in the 1980's, one of the earliest online network of patients and caregivers. She is program director of Project HealthDesign, a Robert Wood Johnson Foundation program for personal health records.
Susannah Fox (http://pewinternet.org/Experts/Susannah-Fox.aspx)	Her research conducted as part of the Pew Internet & American Life Project has become a major resource for understanding how society is using the Internet in managing their health care challenges and problems.
Gunther Eysenbach, MD, MPH (http://www.linkedin.com/in/gunthereysenbach)	He founded one of the first research groups on cybermedicine and eHealth at the University of Heidelberg. He is Editor-in-Chief of the *Journal of Medical Internet Research* and established the Medicine 2.0 Conference series.

Tom Ferguson, MD, died April 14, 2006 while undergoing treatment for multiple myeloma, an illness he had battled for 15 years. But the impact of his advocacy continues today. In 2007, his final publication and a classic paper in this field titled *e-patients: how they can help us heal health care* was posted on the Internet at http://e-patients.net/e-Patients_White_Paper.pdf (Ferguson, 2007). This publication was co-authored by a group he called the e-Patient Scholars Working Group. This group, along with other leaders in this field, went on to establish the Society for Participatory Medicine in 2009. Additional information about the Society for Participatory Medicine and their current work in leading Health 2.0 can be viewed at http://participatorymedicine.org.

The Establishment of Consumer Health Informatics

Overlapping the evolution of the well informed, empowered, and engaged patient is the development of consumer health informatics as a branch or sub-specialization within the discipline of health care informatics. The phrases "consumer health informatics" "consumer informatics," and "informatics for consumer health" (ICH) are often used interchangeably in the literature. Health care informatics, which began in the late 1960s, initially focused on using computers and a variety of automated applications to assist in the management of data and information within the health care system. However, in 1990, well before the development of the first graphic interface browser, Patricia Brennan demonstrated that patients and caregivers would use a computer to access information and peer support. She did this by placing a computer terminal in the patient's home, where they could communicate via the mainframe (Brennan, Moore, & Smyth, 1991).

The term "consumer health informatics" was first used in the professional literature indexed by CINAHL as well as Medline by Tom Ferguson (Ferguson, 1995). Five years later, Gunther Eysenbach identified consumer informatics as a branch of medical informatics and provided one of the earliest definitions. "Consumer health informatics is the branch of medical informatics that analyses consumers' needs for information; studies and implements methods of making information accessible to consumers; and models and integrates consumers' preferences into medical information systems. Consumer informatics stands at the crossroads of other disciplines, such as nursing informatics, public health, health promotion, health education, library science, and communication science, and is perhaps the most challenging and rapidly expanding field in medical informatics; it is paving the way for health care in the information age" (Eysenbach, 2000, p. 1713). The impact of this definition can now be seen in the American Medical Informatics Association (AMIA) definition of consumer informatics located at http://www.amia.org/programs/working-groups/programs/consumer-health-informatics. Much of the same language is used in both definitions (American Medical Informatics Association, n.d.). In addition to the Society for Participatory Medicine, other examples of national groups and associations supporting consumer informatics include:

- Informatics for Consumer Health (ICH)—http://informaticsforconsumerhealth.org/
- AMIA Working Group for Consumer Health Informatics—http://www.amia.org/applications-informatics/consumer-health-informatics
- Partnership for Patients: A Common Commitment—http://www.healthcare.gov/compare/partnership-for-patients/about/index.html

Along with the emerging definition and support for consumer informatics was the movement from Web 1.0 to Web 2.0 and Health 2.0 that takes advantage of the developing technologies and interactive nature of the Internet.

Moving From Web 1.0 to Web 2.0 to Health 2.0

In 2004, Tim O'Reilly coined the term Web 2.0 to describe the changing nature of the Internet after the dotcom bust. Combining the symbol 2.0 with the word web suggested a new and updated version of the web. He defined Web 2.0 as a set of economic, social, and technology trends characterized by user participation, openness, and networking. In explaining the difference between Web 1.0 and Web 2.0, O'Reilly provided several examples. Britannica Online, representing Web 1.0, is a reference written by experts and depends on the knowledge of these experts to ensure its accuracy. Wikipedia (http://www.wikipedia.org/), representing Web 2.0, is written by the public and depends on end-user edits to ensure its accuracy.

Another example of the differences between Web 1.0 and Web 2.0 is the concept of indexing. With Web 1.0, one thinks in terms of a taxonomy represented by a standard language with a specific term and definition for each item or concept. With Web 2.0, one thinks in terms of tagging where each person selects the term they would use to label the item or concept (O'Reilly, 2005). In each of these examples the theme with Web 2.0 is collaboration to create user-generated content. The development of user-generated content through a process of collaboration synergistically opens up new doors to knowledge and questions about the accuracy of that knowledge.

The trend to Web 2.0 most likely began around the turn of the century, picking up momentum over the decade. In 2010, Facebook bypassed Google as the most visited site on the Internet. This was seen by many as the passing of the flag from Web 1.0, based on searching for information, to Web 2.0, based on creating and sharing information. Table 1.3 identifies the beginning date for several well-known social media applications.

Table 1.3 *Development of Social Media Applications and/or Device*

Year	Device and/or Application
1978	Computerized Bulletin Board
1998	Blogger
2000	Friendstar
2002	My Space
2003	Linkedin and Facebook
2005	YouTube
2007	iPhone
2009	Twitter
2010	iPad and Pinterest

Source: Adapted from Bennett, S. (2012).

Wisdom of Crowds

In 2004, Surowiecki published *The Wisdom of Crowds: Why the Many Are Smarter than the Few and How Collective Wisdom Shapes Business, Economies, Societies and Nations.* Surowiecki proposed that the aggregation of information in groups can produce decisions that are often better than that made by an individual. This would suggest that when examining group efforts at problem-solving, the problem solving ability or the intelligence of the group is greater than that of any individual in the group.

However, additional research has demonstrated that using the collective wisdom of groups is not a panacea for solving all types of problems. The "wisdom of a crowd" approach can be very effective for well-defined problems, where each member of the group provides his or her input independent of the other members. A well-defined problem is a problem that has one correct solution. For example, how many pieces of candy are in a jar? If each person in a group were to guess the answer, several people could be way off base, but the correct answer is very likely to be close to the average of the individual scores. However, if the group is permitted to discuss the problem and achieve a consensus, they are less likely to achieve the correct answer. In other words, the wisdom of the crowd is usually inaccurate when well-defined problems are solved by group consensus.

In health care, many if not most problems are ill-defined. Ill-defined problems are problems that can be managed via several different options, none of which are perfect. Research on how groups manage ill-defined problems is limited. Two studies conducted at Massachusetts Institute of Technology (MIT) and Carnegie Mellon University (CMU) found converging evidence that groups participating in problem-solving activities demonstrate a general collective intelligence factor that explained the group's performance on a wide variety of tasks. "This 'c factor' is not strongly correlated with the average or maximum individual intelligence of group members, but is correlated with the average social sensitivity of group members, the equality in distribution of conversational turn-taking, and the proportion of females in the group" (Woolley, Chabris, Pentland, Hashmi, & Malone, 2010, p. 686). "A group's interactions drive its intelligence more than the brain power of individual members" (Marshall, 2010). Certain characteristics of the individuals within the group and the group's ability to work together as a whole can influence the effectiveness of the group, whether they are online or face-to-face. These findings are important to nurses working with both online and in-person support groups.

The term Health 2.0 began to appear in the online and published literature around 2007. The term Health 2.0 extends the definition of Web 2.0 and concepts associated with Web 2.0 to health care, such as the power of collected wisdom. In 2008, the California Health Care Foundation published a report, titled *The Wisdom of Patients: Health Care Meets Online Social Media*. In this report, Health 2.0 is defined as "the use of social software and its ability to promote collaboration between patients, their caregivers, medical professionals, and other stakeholders in health" (Sarasohn-Kahn, 2008, P.2). Other related terms such as eHealth, Patient Empowerment 2.0, Health Care 2.0, Medicine 2.0, and Nursing 2.0 also begin to appear, along with a discussion concerning which of these is the more inclusive term (Van De Belt, Engelen, Berben, & Schoonhoven, 2010). Van De Belt et al determined, for their purposes, Medicine 2.0 was the more inclusive term and that Health 2.0 was included as part of Medicine 2.0. In 2010, Van De Belt et al searched both the peer-reviewed professional literature and the gray literature, finding 46 unique definitions. An analysis of these definitions identified 7 themes:

1. Patient and Consumer
2. Web 2.0
3. Professional
4. Social Networking
5. Change
6. Collaboration
7. Health Information of Content.

In this book we have selected Health 2.0 as the more inclusive term. The term Health 2.0 refers to the use of social media, via electronic devices, electronic health information exchange platforms, and mobile applications to promote collaboration among stakeholders and health care providers. This collaboration includes the empowered patient/consumers within the health care system, with the goal of improving the health and quality of life for individuals, families, and communities. Achieving this goal requires, at a minimum, stakeholders that have achieved digital literacy.

LIERACY IN THE WORLD OF SOCIAL MEDIA

There are a number of different types of literacies that have been identified in the literature. Some examples include emotional literacy, numeric literacy, scientific literacy, and health literacy. In this chapter the discussion is limited to basic literacy and those literacies that relate directly to the use of social media. Successful use of social media tools to achieve the goals of Health 2.0 is dependent on basic literacy, computer literacy, information literacy, digital literacy, and health literacy. These specific literacies are both overlapping and interrelated, as demonstrated in Figure 1.1.

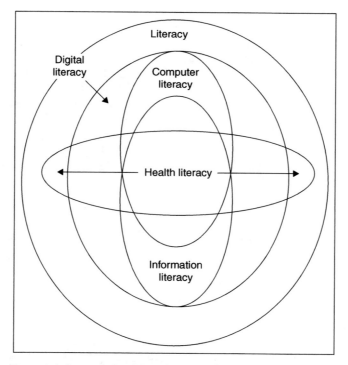

Figure 1.1 Interrelationships of literacies required for Health 2.0.

In each of these types of literacy, basic literacy is the foundational skill. Without a basic level of literacy the other types of literacy become impossible and irrelevant. The assessment of a consumer/patient's potential to benefit from social media tools begins with an assessment of basic literacy.

A Definition of Basic Literacy

An international effort to address the need for a literate population was initiated in 1946 with the formation of the United Nations Educational Scientific and Cultural Organization (UNESCO). As part of this effort, UNESCO offered one of the first definitions of literacy and one that is still quoted today. "A literate person is one who can, with understanding, both read and write a short simple statement on his or her everyday life" (UNESCO Educational Sector, 2004, p. 12). As the needs of society changed, the UNESCO definition evolved, and in 2003 UNESCO proposed an operational definition that attempted to encompass the several different dimensions of literacy. "Literacy is the ability to identify, understand, interpret, create, communicate and compute, using printed and written materials associated with varying contexts. Literacy involves a continuum of learning in enabling individuals to achieve their goals, to develop their knowledge and potential, and to participate fully in their community and wider society" (UNESCO Educational Sector, 2004, p. 13). UNESCO points out that this definition requires careful thought in order to incorporate it into the various circumstances in which individuals lead their lives. When considering Health 2.0, one of the primary aspects of how people lead their lives is how they live their online lives.

In the United States, the U.S. Department of Education, Institute of Education Sciences, National Center for Education Statistics conducts the National Assessment of Adult Literacy (NAAL), which is a nationally representative and continuing assessment of English language literary skills of American adults. The NAAL definition of literacy includes both knowledge and skills and assesses three types of literacy—prose, document, and quantitative. A description of each can be seen in Exhibit 1.1.

The focus of both the national and international definitions is the ability to take in and understand information that is presented in printed or written format. The assumption is that this includes the ability to understand both text and numeric information. If one can read information in printed format, it could be expected that this individual could read and understand the same information on a computer screen. However, computer literacy involves much more than the ability to read information from a computer screen. In fact, the term computer literacy, with its limited focus, is becoming outdated.

Exhibit 1.1 *National Assessment of Adult Literacy—Three Types of Literacy*

Prose literacy
The knowledge and skills needed to search, comprehend, and use continuous texts such as editorials, news stories, brochures, and instructional materials.

Document literacy
The document-related knowledge and skills needed to perform a search, comprehend, and use non-continuous texts in various formats, such as job applications, payroll forms, transportation schedules, maps, tables, and drug or food labels.

Quantitative literacy
The quantitative knowledge and skills required for identifying and performing computations, either alone or sequentially, using numbers embedded in printed materials such as balancing a checkbook, figuring out a tip, completing an order form, or determining the amount.

Source: National Assessment of Adult Literacy (NAAL; 2003).

Definition of Computer Literacy/Fluency

The National Academy of Science has coined the term FIT Persons to describe people who are fluent with information technology. These people go beyond proficiently in using a computer and are able to express creatively, reformulate knowledge, and synthesize new information using a wide range of information technology. FIT Persons possess three types of knowledge.

- Contemporary Skills—the ability to use current computer applications such as word-processors, spreadsheets, or an Internet search engine. This means using the correct tool for the right job. Spreadsheets when manipulating numbers; word processors for manipulating text, and so on.
- Foundational Concepts—underlie the how and why of information technology. This knowledge gives the person insight into the opportunities and limitations of social media and other information technologies.
- Intellectual Capabilities—the ability to apply information technology to actual problems and challenges of every life. An example of this knowledge is the ability to use critical thinking when evaluating health information on a social media site (Committee on Information Technology Literacy, National Research Council, 1999).

While these three types of knowledge might be easily conceptualized in a formal curriculum, it is more of a challenge to apply these types of knowledge and skills to the assessment and education of a patient/consumer. This is the challenge for health care providers as we work to educate and, in turn, empower patients/consumers.

Definition of Information Literacy

The American Library Association (ALA) has supported the development of information literacy standards since the 1980's. As part of this effort they have established standards of information literacy for higher education, high schools, and even for a personal digital assistant (PDA). The ALA defines information literacy as "a set of abilities requiring individuals to recognize when information is needed and have the ability to locate, evaluate, and use effectively the needed information" (Library Association, 2000, p. 2). This definition has gained wide acceptance. However, with the extensive growth of social media, there are increasing calls for revising the definition as well as the established standards from over a decade ago. "Social media environments and online communities are innovative collaborative technologies that challenge traditional definitions of information literacy ... information is not a static object that is simply accessed and retrieved. It is a dynamic entity that is produced and shared collaboratively with such innovative Web 2.0 technologies as Facebook, Twitter, Delicious, Second Life, and YouTube" (Mackey & Jacobson, 2011, p. 62).

For example, what are the different types of knowledge and skills needed to evaluate information posted on Facebook, versus Wikipedia, versus a peer-reviewed article posted online before publication, versus a peer-reviewed published article. Are different writing skills needed when participating in an online dialog as opposed to preparing a term paper? Are there standards that apply to text messaging, especially if the message is between health care colleagues or being sent to a patient? These questions are the challenges facing health care providers in the world of social media.

Definition of Digital Literacy

The term digital literacy first began appearing in the literature in the 1990s, however, to date there is no generally accepted definition. Interestingly, there are a number of Digital Literacy Centers supporting the development of digital literacy. Some examples include:

- Syracuse University's Center for Digital Literacy, located at http://digital-literacy.syr .edu/
- University of British Columbia, the Digital Literacy Centre, located at http://dlc.lled .educ.ubc.ca/
- Microsoft Digital Literacy Curriculum, located at http://www.microsoft.com/ About/CorporateCitizenship/Citizenship/giving/programs/UP/digitalliteracy/ eng/default.mspx
- National Telecommunications and Information Administration Literacy Center, located at http://www.digitalliteracy.gov/

There are also a number of books published on digital literacy. A search of Amazon for books with "Digital Literacy" in the title produced 53 results. The American Library Association Digital Literacy Task Force posted a working definition on their online community. This definition describes digital literacy as "a broad term to encompass information literacy abilities requiring individuals to recognize when information is needed and have the ability to locate, evaluate, and use effectively the needed information, as well as competencies in creating content, reflecting on one's own conduct and social responsibility, and taking action to share knowledge and solve problems. Digital literacy also is associated with the ability to use computers and other devices, social media and the Internet" (American Library Association Digital Literacy Task Force, 2011, para. 1). The work of the task group is not yet complete and the final definition has not been presented to the larger organization for approval.

In a white paper commissioned by the Aspen Institute Communications and Society Program and the John S. and James L. Knight Foundation, "Digital and media literacy are defined as life skills that are necessary for participation in our media-saturated, information-rich society. These include:

- Make responsible choices and access information by locating and sharing materials and comprehending information and ideas,
- Analyze messages in a variety of forms by identifying the author, purpose, and point of view, and evaluating the quality and credibility of the content,
- Create content in a variety of forms, making use of language, images, sound, and new digital tools and technologies,
- Reflect on one's own conduct and communication behavior by applying social responsibility and ethical principles, and
- Take social action by working individually and collaboratively to share knowledge and solve problems in the family, workplace, and community, and by participating as a member of a community (Hobbs, 2010, pp. vii–viii).

As both these definitions demonstrate, except for basic literacy, digital literacy is a more comprehensive concept than any of the other social media-related literacies discussed in this section of the chapter. The definition goes beyond the comfortable use of technology demonstrated by the digital native. Digital literacy is not just about knowing how to use the tools; it's about understanding the implications of digital technology and the impact it is having, and will have, on every aspect of our lives. "Though most people think kids these days *get* the digital world, we are actually breeding a generation of digital illiterates. How? We are not teaching them how to really understand and use the tools. *We are only teaching them how to click buttons.* We need to be teaching our students, at all levels, not just how to click and poke, but how to communicate, interact, and build relationships in a connected world" (Murphy, 2011).

For the purposes of this book, digital literacy is defined as including:

- Competency with digital devices of all types, including cameras, eReaders, smartphones, computers, tablets, video games, and so forth. This does not mean that one can pick up a new device and use that device without an orientation. Rather, one can, using trial and error as well as a manufacturer's manual, determine how to effectively use a device.
- The technical skills to operate these devices as well as the conceptual knowledge to understand their functionality.
- The ability to creatively and critically use these devices to access, manipulate, evaluate, and apply data, information, knowledge and wisdom in activities of daily living.
- The ability to apply basic emotional intelligence in collaborating and communicating with others.
- The ethical values and sense of community responsibility to use digital devices for the enjoyment and benefit of society.

Definition of Health Literacy

While health literacy is concerned with the ability to access, evaluate, and apply information to health-related decisions, there is not a generally accepted agreement of the definition of this term. A systematic review, in 2011, of the literature that had been published on Medline, PubMed, and Web of Science identified 17 definitions and 12 conceptual models of health literacy. Definitions of health literacy from the American Medical Association, the Institute of Medicine, and the World Health Organization (WHO) were found to be cited most frequently (Sorensen, et. al., 2012). Current definitions from these organizations are provided in Exhibit 1.2.

The focus in each of these definitions is on an individual's skills in obtaining, processing, and understanding the health information and services necessary to make appropriate health decisions. While these definitions are not incongruent with Web 1.0, they do not address a networked world. In recognition of this deficiency, Norman and Skinner introduced the concept of eHealth as "the ability to seek, find, understand, and appraise health information from electronic sources and apply the knowledge gained

---

Exhibit 1.2 *Definitions of Health Literacy*

- American Medical Association defines health literacy as "a patient's ability to obtain, process, and understand basic health information and services needed to make appropriate health decisions" (American Medical Association, 2004).
- The Institution of Medicine uses the definition of health literacy developed by Ratzan and Parker and cited in *Healthy People 2010*. Health Literacy is "the degree to which individuals have the capacity to obtain, process, and understand basic health information and services needed to make appropriate health decisions" (Committee on Health Literacy Institute of Medicine, 2004, p. 4).
- The World Health Organization (WHO) defined health as "the degree to which people are able to access, understand, appraise and communicate information to engage with the demands of different health contexts in order to promote and maintain good health across the life-course" (Nutbean, 1998, p. 351).

to addressing or solving a health problem" (2006, p. e9). This definition acknowledges the need for computer fluency and the use of information literacy skills to obtain an effective level of health literacy. However, this definition is not especially sensitive to the impact of social media. For example, it does not address the individual as a patient/consumer collaboratively creating health-related information that could be used by others in making health-related decisions. Yet, there is increasing evidence that patients bring to the dialog a unique knowledge base for addressing a number of health related problems (Hartzler & Pratt, 2011). Creating a comprehensive definition and model for assessment of health literacy levels that includes the social media literacy skills necessary for Health 2.0 is now a challenge for health professionals.

While each of the social media-related literacies focus on a different aspect of literacy and have a different definition, they all overlap and are interrelated. Figure 1.1 demonstrates that interrelationship. In this figure, basic literacy is depicted as foundational to all other literacies. Digital literacy includes computer and information literacy as well as other social media-related knowledge and skills not currently included in the definitions of computer and information literacy. For example, using a Wii to play online games is not usually considered part of information or computer literacy, but clearly requires digital literacy. Health 2.0 requires both digital literacy and a basic knowledge of health, unrelated to automation. In other words, it overlaps digital literacy and basic literacy. All of the literacies require the ability to evaluate information.

EVALUATION OF ONLINE INFORMATION

As more and more consumers and health care professionals use the Internet to find information, it becomes critical for them to effectively evaluate the quality of that information. Remember, anyone can and does publish to the Internet; it is NOT a refereed source of information. This is especially critical when that information relates to health care decisions that could alter the life of the consumer.

Types of Health Care Information Sites on the Internet

There are three main types of health informational sites on the Internet:

- Static web pages,
- Web pages that request some personal information and provide a report back to the consumer based on the data supplied, and
- Consumer-generated information found on social media sites.

Web 1.0 provided the first type of health care information retrievable from the Internet—passive or static information. A web page with information about a specific condition is an example of this type of information. While the user searches for this information and reads the information found, the user does not interact with the website or input any information. Anyone can publish to these types of sites; some are by reputable organizations like the American Heart Association, some are government-sponsored sites, and some are consumer-published sites.

Do not confuse accessing information OVER the Internet with information published ON the Internet. Medline is a database of professional biomedical literature; it is a web-based searchable database. This is similar to the literature databases that one may have access to through a library. Most colleges/universities have arrangements to access these databases OVER the Internet. Many of them require a user-id and pass-word. These databases point to peer-reviewed information. MedlinePlus, an example of information ON the Internet, includes a number of high quality health related resources written for patients, families, and other consumers. This database is published on the Internet and is free (http://www.nlm.nih.gov/medlineplus/). MedlinePlus contains carefully selected links to web resources as well as interactive health tutorials. Other Internet sites may not be peer reviewed or written by authoritative sources.

The second type of health informational site requires the patient to enter personal health information. Many of these sites are looking to market some type of health-related product to the consumer or organizations with a cause, like heart disease or cancer. Some of these sites offer an opportunity to enter personal information and receive feedback, such as a risk assessment. Examples of these sites include Harvard Pilgrim Health Care (https://www.harvardpilgrim.org/portal/page?_pageid=213,38394&_dad=portal&_schema=PORTAL), The National Cancer Institute (http://www.cancer.gov/bcrisktool/), and The American Heart Association (http://www.heart.org/HEARTORG/Conditions/Whats-Your-Risk-Find-out_UCM_306929_Article.jsp).

The third type of health informational site involves the use of Web 2.0 applications. Web 2.0 is an umbrella term referring to web-enabled applications that are built around user-generated or user-manipulated content. Some examples include wikis, blogs, pod-casts, and social networking sites (see chapter 2 for more information on these tools). When these applications are used with health-related issues, they are included in the Health 2.0 movement.

Criteria for Evaluating Health Information

Traditional methods of evaluating the credibility of information on the Internet includes criteria related to a peer reviewed journal, the credentials of the author, and writing style of the publication (Standler, 2004). The standard for credibility was peer reviews or scholarly journals and the reputation of the publishing company. This, however, provides no protection against fraud, as there are incidences of fraud in medical research published in peer review journals. This also provides little or no help in the social media world, as most posts are not peer reviewed—more on this later. Next, one would consider the credentials of the author. The credentials of the author are also not of much help in the social media world, as one needs to either know the field in order to recognize the "experts" or trust what the author published about his/her credentials is the truth. The last traditional method is the writing style. While this may have some validity in the social media world, many posts on social media sites tend to be more informal and not scholarly in writing style.

How does one protect him/herself from using poor information to make health care decisions? For Web 1.0, we traditionally looked at selecting sources more likely to be reliable, like NIH, Cleveland Clinic, WebMd, and so forth; evaluating that information based on a set of criteria, like authority/credibility, accuracy and currency, coverage and scope, objectivity, and reasonableness; and using evaluation checklists to make sure all criteria were considered (see Exhibit 1.3).

There are many evaluation checklists available. Most of them include the same points, but are expressed in different ways. In summary, these checklists consist of four to five main criteria one should use to critically evaluate the sources of the information. Here are two examples of such sets of criteria:

- Authority of author, Accuracy of content, Objectivity, Currency, and Coverage (Alexander & Tate, 2005).
- Credibility, Accuracy, Reasonableness, Support (Harris, 2010).

Exhibit 1.3 *Evaluation of Information From the Internet*

Authority/Credibility: Who wrote or is responsible for the content on the web page? What are the credentials of this person(s)? If it is an institution, what is the purpose of this institution? What is their reputation? Do they provide contact information?

Accuracy/Currency: How current and comprehensive is the information? Is there a publication date listed? Is currency relevant to the topic area? Is it presenting a complete picture of the topic (both sides of an issue)? Does it contain generalizations with no supporting evidence or links? Are there references or citations? Can you corroborate the information with other sites? Is the grammar correct? Are words spelled correctly?

Coverage/Scope: Is the content sufficient in extent and depth of coverage for the intended audience? Did it answer the obvious questions? Does it give enough detail on the topic? Did it make generalizations?

Objectivity/ Reasonableness: Does the site cover the content with fairness, objectivity (controlled bias), and consistency? Is there a hidden agenda, like trying to sell you a product? Is the writing slanted?

Note how authority can also refer to credibility; accuracy of content can refer to currency; and objectivity can refer to reasonableness.

Some of these same criteria, such as currency and accuracy, can also apply to social media sites. One must also consider websites from the perspective of the intent or purpose of the site. Some websites may be advocacy sites with a purpose of influencing the user toward a specific issue or cause. Two examples of these websites are ACLU (http://www.aclu.org) and the Democratic Party (http://www.democrats.org/). Social media sites can also fall into this category of websites. Other types of websites with their own aims or purposes include:

- Entertainment/gaming—The primary aim of these sites is to entertain, although sometimes they get caught up in enticing you to purchase a game or some other item. They have a variety of URL endings depending on the sponsoring organization. Three examples are http://games.yahoo.com, http://film.com, and http://kidshealth.org/kids/. The last site has games or word finds about health for kids to play.
- Informational—The purpose of these sites is to provide factual information. They tend to end in edu or gov. Three examples are http://usa.gov (formerly firstgov.gov), http://www.cdc.gov, and http://owl.english.purdue.edu/owl/.
- Marketing/Business—The purpose of these sites is to sell a product or service. Most of them end in com, but some of them now take on one of the new top-level domains (TLD), like pro. Some examples include http://www.amazon.com, http://www.microsoft.com, http://www.beltone.com, and http://smiles.pro.
- News—Most news sites end in com and serve to present current information or news about what is happening worldwide, regionally, and locally. Two examples in this group are http://www.cnn.com and http://www.nytimes.com.

Social Media and Health 2.0 Criteria

Another type of website that has populated the Internet over the past few years includes sharing and/or community sites. These websites have evolved from Web 2.0 tools. Each of these types of sites can provide quality information, misinformation, or biased information. Using traditional criteria for evaluating information on Web 1.0 sites may not be effective when applied to Web 2.0, Health 2.0, or social media sites. For example, is the patient who writes about their condition and treatment issues a credible source? They may have no health care provider credentials, but may be expert in how they are responding to treatment and what symptoms they present.

When using types of resources like Health 2.0, patients need guidelines on how to evaluate the information from these sites and how to apply the information to their health care decisions. Many of the sites that offer educational materials deal only with teenagers and issues of safety. An excellent resource for these types of materials can be seen at http://www.ftc.gov/bcp/edu/pubs/consumer/tech/tec14.shtm. However, there are several resources that have been developed to teach patients safe access to quality information. The data that can be applied to Health 2.0 sites is limited. The National Library of Medicine at NIH (Figure 1.2) provides access to examples of these types of resources at http://www.nlm.nih.gov/medlineplus/evaluatinghealthinformation.html, as does Evaluating Online Sources of Health Information from the National Cancer Institute (Figure 1.3) at http://www.cancer.gov/cancertopics/cancerlibrary/health-info-online/.

The best advice one can give consumers at this point is to use their own best judgment in deciding how far to explore these sites and what information to enter and share publically with others. With experience, individuals will develop "Internet street smarts" or a gut reaction to a site and how the site is designed. The following general questions will help guide that development:

- Who is maintaining this site and why? Who is paying for this project?
- Can a cookie or other technology be used to track this information back to me? Is this a concern to me? How might this affect me?
- What is included in the disclaimer posted on the site?
- What are the Terms and Conditions to use this site?
- What is included in the privacy statement for this site?
- Do I trust they will follow their privacy statement or Terms and Conditions?
- Can I trust that the patients/consumers posting to this site are who they say they are? Can that be verified in some way?

In addition, some traditional criteria, such as how current is the information, may also apply. However, the best advice may be to pay close attention to where the information comes from and back up what you find with authoritative sources, such as recognized health sites and your health care provider. Health 2.0 sites involve not only the evaluation of information that is on these sites, but how one can and/or should participate in the creation of information. The following section discusses that issue.

Guidelines for Participating in Online Groups

Information and guidelines for participating in online groups can be divided into six topic areas. The topics provide a framework for what should be included in patient education programs. These topics are:

- Deciding why one wants to participate,
- Setting realistic expectations about the activity and what one will gain by participating,
- Finding an appropriate group,
- Joining and participating in a group, and
- Discontinuing participation in a group.

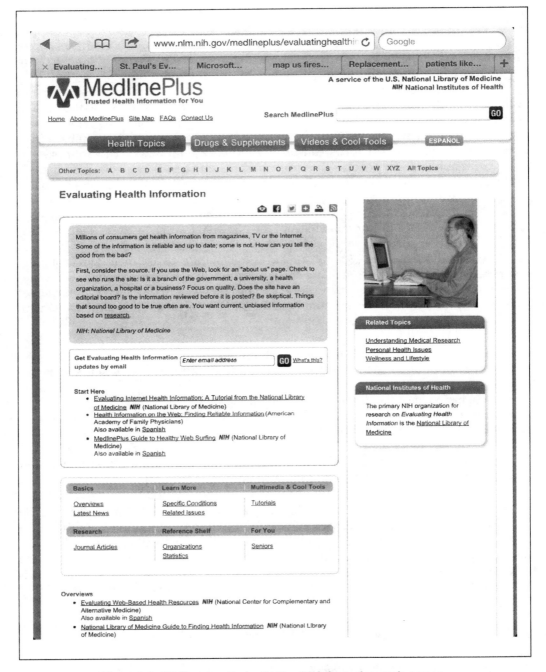

Figure 1.2 Medlineplus: Evaluating health information, main screen.

Table 1.4 lists common reasons why patients are interested in joining online groups and some of the cautions a nurse can share with patients in terms of these reasons.

When initially joining an online group, the new person is joining an ongoing discussion. It can be helpful to have realistic expectations. If the group has been interacting

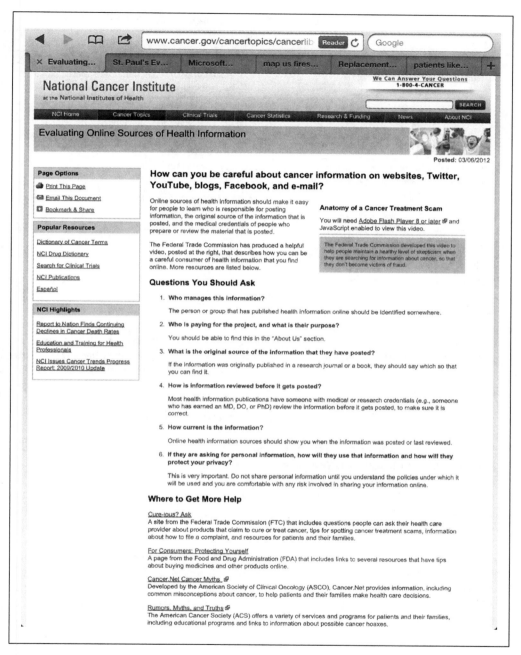

Figure 1.3 National Cancer Institute: Evaluating online sources of health information.

for some time, the amount and depth of the information discussed can be overwhelming. The flow of information can appear disorganized. Different online groups may also have different personalities. Some groups will take the initiative in helping a newcomer, while others will suggest the new person spend some time reading the archives.

Table 1.4 *Reasons to Participate in Online Groups and Related Cautions*

Reason	Caution
I would like to talk to someone else who has this same problem.	Each person is different. Your symptoms and your personal situation may be very different from someone else with the same diagnosis.
I want to know if anyone else is having this same symptom, side effect, or problem.	It may be just a coincidence that someone else is experiencing the same symptoms, side effect, or problem, or it can be an early alert for a previously unrecognized problem. More information will be needed.
I can find out about other potential treatments from other patients who are also researching this problem.	Some of the treatments discussed may be experimental or even outdated.
Someone is always online 24/7.	Be careful, since the first response may not be the last or best answer to your question.
I can find out if there are several other people with this issue.	A group consensus is not always a corrent answer.

Over time, the group can become inactive or drift off target, leaving some members to feel they are losing a friend or support network.

In selecting groups, patients should be encouraged to search for groups that are associated with known organizations, such as major medical centers. They should look for groups with easy to find information about who they are and why the group is being sponsored. They should use caution with groups that ask for personal health information in order to learn about the group; sites that have numerous advertisements, making it hard to read the content without reading the ads; and sites that stress how much they offer, with little or no information about who has established the site.

When participating in an online group, patients/consumers should:

- Use caution in establishing personal relationships since health problems, especially newly diagnosed health problems, can increase their vulnerability.
- Be careful not to isolate themselves from family and established friends.
- Avoid providing too much personal information, especially when tired and anxious.
- Think carefully about how much privacy they are willing to trade for information.

One of the things that can be difficult for patients who are active members of an online group is the loss of a member. If a patient decided to leave a group for any reason, they could indicate they are leaving the group. They are not obliged to give any explanation for their decision, but a brief good-bye as opposed to just disappearing can be reassuring to an ongoing group. Several other aspects of participating in online groups are discussed throughout this book.

SUMMARY

As consumers and health care professionals become more empowered with stronger levels of literacy, electronic devices, and web based platforms to access, share, and receive information a paradigm shift is occurring. This paradigm shift is moving patients/consumers and providers to a virtual world that requires new guidelines, standards, and health policies to ensure the safe and effective use of social media. This book is an introduction to the world of Health 2.0 and the wealth of opportunities offered by this new digitalized world.

DISCUSSION QUESTIONS

1. What specific literacy skills should be included as part of a baseline patient assessment for patients being seen for the first time in any health care establishment?
2. You are being assigned to a new unit in an acute care setting. The unit is designed for patients who have both a significant mental health and physical illness. To learn more about mental health from a patient perspective, you are interested in joining an online support group designed for patients with depression. Should you (a) contact the site before joining and explain your interest; (b) Sign in and then introduce yourself, including your professional background and reason for joining; (c) Sign in, lurk on the site, but never participate; or (d) Select another approach. Explain your selection and why you did not select the other options. Before you complete your answer, you may want to examine some of these sites to see if they provide any directions or check the additional resources located in the Appendix.
3. The hospital where you are employed is creating a new transparency policy, making more information about the institution available online. Currently, a number of quality measures including infection rates, patient satisfaction scores, employee turnover rates, and so on, are viewable via the Internet. Should unit-specific data and scores be posted on the hospital's website, open to the general public to see? Should hospital-wide data and scores be posted? Explain your answer. Share a list of data items you would and would not post. Discuss how you reached this conclusion about these items.
4. As a nurse educator, you have been asked to prepare a tutorial sheet as part of a patient education discharge packet on understanding and using health information on the Internet. List the key points you would include in this document. Share what format or manner you would use to create the document.
5. Please review the website located at http://www.cancer.gov/cancertopics/cancerlibrary/health-info-online and answer the following questions:
   - Is the website sensitive to the different types and levels of literacy?
   - Does the website prepare people to safely participate in online groups?
   - Does the criteria for evaluating information apply to both Web 1.0 and Web 2.0 type of sites?
   - What additional information would you include on this site?

EXERCISES

Exercise 1: A Rose by any Other Name—Is Maybe Not a Rose

Purpose: *The purpose of this exercise is to appreciate the implications of the terms used to describe the individuals, families, and groups utilizing health care services.*

Objectives
1. Analyze the different meanings for the terms used to identify individuals, families, and groups utilizing health care services.
2. Explore the implications of the terms used to identify individuals, families, and groups utilizing health care services.
3. Develop appropriate definitions for terms commonly used to describe individuals, families, and groups who use should be health care services.

Directions

Note: This activity can be done as a group exercise or as an individual assignment.

1. Use an Internet search engine to find three or more definitions for each of the following terms:
   Patient
   Client
   Consumer
   Community.
2. Using this information, create your own definition for each of these terms.
3. Use an Internet search engine to find three or more definitions for each of the following terms:
   Empowered
   Engaged.
4. Using this information, create your own definition for each of these terms
5. Use each of the terms in step 3 to modify the terms in step 1. This will create a list of phrases, starting with empowered patient and ending with engaged community.
6. Use your word processer to create a glossary that includes a definition for each of these phrases.

Exercise 2: Can You See Me Now?

Purpose: *To explore the difference in personal responses to virtual communication or voice communication versus an actual face-to-face (F-2-F).*

Objectives

1. Describe the difference in feelings or emotions that can be experienced in online versus F-2-F communication.
2. Analyze the difference in feedback loops associated with F-2-F communication versus online communication.

Directions

1. Select a former teacher who has had a major positive impact on your education
2. Create *but do not send an email* letting the person know the impact they have had on your education.
3. Create a script you would use to make a telephone call to this person.
4. Modify the script for you to use with an online video call (i.e., Skype) to this person.
5. Create a script of what you would say if you were able to invite this person to lunch
6. Modify the script, if needed, if the meeting was scheduled to take place in the person's office.
7. Set-up a role-play with a classmate where you can review your email and rehearse your scripts. Do *not have* the scripts in front of you during the role-play experience. Use your memory of what you wanted to say to talk in the F-2-F role-plays.
8. In a small group, discuss the overall experience. Explore how you felt during the actual events. For example, did you feel nervous, embarrassed, or pleased with the opportunity?

In which of the three situations did you have more control? How did the F-2-F conversation go when your classmate who was playing the role of the teacher began to respond to your comments? At any point did you get off topic? Did you cover all your points in your script?

9. As a group, create a list of key points to guide your online communication with both colleagues and patients.

Exercise 3: Patient Is Not a Third Person Word

Purpose: *The purpose of this exercise is to explore the role of the patient as perceived by the patient.*

Objectives

1. Analyze the level and type of communication a patient may expect when talking with their health care providers.
2. Contrast and compare the definition of an ePatient and the definition of a patient that you created in Exercise 1.

Directions

1. Watch the You Tube video located at http://www.youtube.com/watch?v=2vejkD0Rl3o.
2. It has been suggested that social media is a" game changer." As a small group online or in an F-2-F setting, discuss the implications of this video for your communication with patients/consumers.

Exercise 4: If Two Heads are Better Than One, are More Heads Even Better?

Purpose: *The purpose of this exercise it to consider the implications of research related to group process and the use of social media in health care.*

Objectives

1. Explain the concept of group intelligence as opposed to individual intelligence.
2. Discuss how access to group intelligence may impact the decisions individuals make about their health care.

Directions

1. It has been suggested that patients working together in social networks with access to the same information as health care providers are increasingly functioning as peers in the health care team. Watch the video located at http://www.nsf.gov/news/news_videos.jsp?cntn_id=117795&media_id=68461&org=NSF.
2. Now go to the website https://www.inspire.com/groups/lung-cancer-survivors/ and review some of the postings. Do not join this group unless you or a family member, close friend, or so forth, are dealing with lung cancer. Read the different comments.

3. Create a blog with your classmates. Discuss how individual patients and/or families are using this group as a resource in making decisions related to their health care. Is this an effective approach to making these decisions? Support your answer with your opinion and with data.
4. Should digital literacy be a job requirement for all professional nurses? Explain your answer.

Exercise 5: Did I Say that Clearly?

Purpose: *The purpose of this exercise is to explore the level of literacy required for understanding health-related information from different online resources.*

Objectives
1. Measure the level of basic literacy required to access different health-related information resources.
2. Analyze the relationship between basic literacy and an individual's decision to utilize different health care resources.

Directions
1. Go to http://www.nlm.nih.gov/medlineplus/ and search on the term lung cancer
2. Copy and paste a paragraph from each of the first five results.
3. Use Microsoft Word to measure the reading level required for each paragraph.
4. Calculate the average reading level of your sample.
5. Go to the website https://www.inspire.com/groups/lung-cancer-survivors/.
6. Copy and paste a paragraph from the first five postings.
7. Use Microsoft Word to measure the reading level required for each paragraph.
8. Calculate the average reading level of your sample.
9. Look over both sets of data for differences in style and tone.
10. Create a PowerPoint presentation outlining your findings and the implications of your findings for patient education concerning health related online resources.

Exercise 6: Is this Information Credible?

Purpose: *The purpose of this exercise is to explore a social media site and evaluate it using selected criteria.*

Objectives
1. Apply selected criteria to evaluating a social media site for content quality.

Directions
1. Find a social media site that addresses a health care issue and is not a .gov or .edu site. This should be a site from a health care consumer to other health care consumers—a site like http://laughingatmynightmare.1000notes.com/.

2. Select one of the traditional criteria for evaluating health care information from the Internet—credibility, accuracy, currency, authority, scope, or so on. In addition, answer the questions found in the section Social Media and Health 2.0 Criteria in this chapter.

3. Using the criteria from step 2 and those questions, evaluate the information on this site. Did the criteria work? Would you recommend a patient with this problem follow this site? Why or why not? What problems did you find in applying the criteria and answering these questions?

4. Create a PowerPoint with your findings and recommendation.

REFERENCES

Alexander, J., & Tate, M. (2005). *How to recognize an informational web page.* Retrieved from http://www.widener.edu/libraries/wolfgram/evaluate/informational.asp

American Library Association. (2000). *Information literacy competency standards for higher education.* Chicago, IL: American Library Association.

American Library Association Digital Literacy Task Force. (2011). *Office for information technology digital literacy task force charge.* Retrieved from http://connect.ala.org/files/94226/4_1_2011_working_dig_lit_tf_charge_pdf_12069.pdf

American Medical Informatics Association. (n.d.). *Informatics areas: Consumer health informatics.* Retrieved from http://www.amia.org/applications-informatics/consumer-health-informatics

Anonymous. (1999). Ready for the empowered consumer? Providers need retailer's attitude. *Healthcare Benchmarks, 6*(1), 1–4.

Austin American-Statesman. (2006). *April 14, 2006—Tom Ferguson, M.D.* Retrieved from http://doctom.com/

Bennett, S. (2012). The history of social media (1978–2012). Retrieved from http://www.mediabistro.com/alltwitter/social-media-history_b18776

Berkman, N., Sheridan, S., Donahue, K., Halpern, D., Viera, A., Crotty, K., ... Viswanathan, M. (2011). *Health literacy interventions and outcomes: An updated systematic review.* Retrieved from http://www.ahrq.gov/clinic/tp/lituptp.htm

Brennan, P., Moore, S., & Smyth, K. (1991). ComputerLink: Electronic support for the home caregiver. *Advances in Nursing Science, 13*(4), 14–27.

CDC. (n.d.). *Ten great public health achievements—United States, 2001–2010.* Retrieved from http://www.cdc.gov/washington/docs/greatachievements.pdf

Committee on Information Technology Literacy, National Research Council. (1999). *Being fluent with information technology.* Washington, DC: National Academy Press.

Consumers Union of U.S. (2012). Our history. Retrieved from http://www.consumerreports.org/cro/aboutus/history/printable/index.htm

Eysenbach, G. (2000). Consumer health informatics. *British Medical Journal, 320*(24), 1713–1716.

Ferguson, T. (1995). Consumer health informatics. *Healthcare Forum Journal, 38*(1), 28–33.

Ferguson, T. (2007). *e-patients: How they can help us heal healthcare.* Retrieved from http://e-patients.net/e-Patients_White_Paper.pdf

Guo, K. (2010). Consumer-directed health care understanding its value in health care reform. *The Health Care Manager, 29*(1), 29–33.

Harris, R. (2010). *Evaluating internet research sources.* Retrieved from http://www.virtualsalt.com/evalu8it.htm

Hartzler, V., & Pratt, W. (2011). Managing the personal side of health: How patient expertise differs from the expertise of clinicians. *Journal of Medical Internet Research, 13*(3), e62.

Hibbard, J., Greene, J., Sofaer, S., Firminger, K., & Hirsh, J. (2012). Consumers' and providers' responses to public cost reports, and how to raise the likelihood of achieving desired results. *Health Affairs, 31*(4), 843–851.

Hobbs, R. (2010). *Digital and media literacy: A plan of action.* Aspen Institute Communications and Society Program and the John S. and James L. Knight Foundation.

Mackey, T., & Jacobson, T. (2011). Reframing information literacy as a metaliteracy. *College & Research Libraries, 72*(1), 62–78.

Marshall, J. (2010). *How to measure the wisdom of a crowd.* Retrieved from http://news.discovery.com/human/group-intelligence-wisdom-crowd.html

Murphy, S. (2011). *Digital literacy is in crisis.* Retrieved from http://socialmediatoday.com/suzemuse/273828/digital-literacy-crisis

Norman, C., & Skinner, H. (2006). eHealth literacy: Essential skills for consumer health in a networked world. *Journal of Medical Internet Research, 8*(2), e9.

O'Reilly, T. (2005). *What is Web 2.0?* Retrieved from http://oreilly.com/web2/archive/what-is-web-20.html

PriceWaterhouseCoopers Health Research Institute. (2012). *Social media "likes" healthcare: From marketing to social business.* New York, NY: PriceWaterhouseCoopers Health Research Institute.

Sarasohn-Kahn, J. (2008). *The wisdom of patients: health care meets online social media.* Retrieved from http://www.chcf.org/publications/2008/04/the-wisdom-of-patients-health-care-meets-online-social-media

Simons, J. (1967). Consumer attitudes toward prepaid dentistry. *Journal of the American Dental Association, 75*(3), 673–677.

Standler, R. (2004). *Evaluating credibility of information on the internet.* Retrieved from http://www.rbs0 .com/credible.pdf

Surowiecki, J. (2004). *The wisdom of crowds: Why the many are smarter than the few and how collective wisdom shapes business, economies, societies and nations.* New York, NY: Doubleday.

Thompson, M., & Cutler, C. (2010, First Quarter). Health care consumerism movement takes a step forward. *Benefits Quarterly,* 24–28.

UNESCO Educational Sector. (2004). *The plurality of literacy and it's implications for policies and programmes: Position paper.* Paris: United Nations Educational Scientific and Cultural Organization.

Van De Belt, T., Engelen, L., Berben, S., & Schoonhoven, L. (2010). Definition of health 2.0 and medicine 2.0: A systematic review. *Journal of Medical Internet Research, 12*(2), e18.

Weber, D. (1997). The empowered consumer. New demands for access, information and services are changing the face of healthcare delivery. *Healthcare Forum Journal, 40*(3), 28–33.

Woolley, A., Chabris, C., Pentland, A., Hashmi, N., & Malone, T. (2010). Evidence for a collective intelligence factor in the performance of human groups. *Science, 330,* 686–689.

Zinman, S., Budd, S., & Bluebird, G. (2009). *The history of the mental health consumer/survivor movement.* Retrieved from http://promoteacceptance.samhsa.gov/archtelpdf/history_consumer_movement.pdf

CHAPTER 2

Software Applications Supporting Social Media

Irene Joos

LEARNING OBJECTIVES

At the completion of this chapter the reader will be able to:

1. Discuss the historical development of social media.
2. Identify potential uses for and issues with using social media.
3. Describe selected social media terms and concepts.
4. Use selected social media tools.

TERMS

Alexa rankings	Microblogging
Apps	Profile
Blog	Simple Markup Language
Blog archive	Social media
Blogger	Social networking
Blogosphere	Status update
Contacts	Tags
Cyberbullying	Timeline
Data mining	Virtual worlds
Friending	Wall
Friends	Wikis
Microblog	

Social media sites are an integral part of modern everyday life. Just look at students, family, and friends and how they spend their time. Notice how many businesses, including health care facilities, have Facebook, Twitter, and YouTube icons on their marketing materials or websites. Most colleges and universities have a social media presence for marketing to prospective students or keeping in touch with alumni.

You can find social sites for just about everything, from global sites like the "friending" site Facebook and the "following" site Twitter, to niche sites with special interests. We share text, photos, images, audio, and video and interaction on social networking sites. Exhibit 2.1 contains some interesting facts about social media usage from number of users, to number of *tweets* per day, to Alexa rankings.

We all use the term social media in everyday conversations but what does the term social media mean? Meriam-Webster's online dictionary defines social media as "forms of electronic communication (as websites for social networking and microblogging) through which users create online communities to share information, ideas, personal messages, and other content (as videos)" (Social Media, n.d.). Cohen (2011) goes further

---

Exhibit 2.1 *Some Social Media Statistics and Interesting Facts*

Social Media Site	Interesting Statistics
Facebook[1]	▪ More than 800 million users (would make it the 3rd largest country in pure numbers if it were a country)
	▪ More than 50% of active users log on any given day
	▪ Average user has 130 friends
	▪ More than 340 million users access Facebook from mobile devices
	▪ 200 million – the number of users added in 2011
Twitter[2]	▪ 200 million tweets per day
	▪ Alexa Traffic Rank is 9 globally and 8 in the United States
YouTube[3]	▪ Alexa Traffic Rank 3 globally and in the United States
Flickr[4]	▪ Alexa Traffic Rank 44 globally and 36 in the United States
	▪ More popular with 18–34 year olds with college education
	▪ More than 51 million members who upload about 4.5 million photos daily
	▪ Smartphones are more likely to be used to take pictures than the iPad
General[5]	▪ 43% of adults use an online social networking site on a typical day (5-1-2011)
	▪ 28% of adults watch a video on a video sharing site on a typical day (5-1-2011)
	▪ Social media commerce is on the rise along with mobile social media via smart phones and tablets
	▪ In 2007 the iPhone took social media mobile
	▪ 34% of Internet users read someone else's experience about health or medical issues on news groups, websites, or blogs
	▪ 25% of Internet users watched an online video about health or medical issues

Data sources for this page include the following:

[1] Facebook http://www.facebook.com/press/info.php?statistics and Bennett, S. (2012). Retrieved from (http://mediabistro.com/alltwitter/social-media-internet-2011_b17881

[2] Alexa at http://www.alexa.com/siteinfo/twitter.com

[3] Alexa at http://www.alexa.com/siteinfo/youtube.com#

[4] Alexa at http://www.alexa.com/siteinfo/flickr.com and http://advertising.yahoo.com/article/fickr.html

[5] The Pew Internet Organization. http://www.pewinternet.org/Static-Pages/Trend-Data-(Adults)/Online-Activities-Daily.aspx and Fox (2011). From http://www.pewinternet.org/~/media//Files/Reports/2011/PIP_Social_Life_of_Health_Info.pdf

on her website to include 30 definitions of social media. The common threads running through these 30 definitions include:

- Online web-based technologies making it platform independent,
- Interactive dialog for sharing information, opinions, experiences, links, and media such as pictures, text, and video,
- Communication any time,
- Enhanced speed of interacting, and
- User-driven or -generated content.

Social media is reliant on Web 2.0 tools such as blogs, podcasts, wikis, and so on that one uses in the process of communicating and interacting with others over the Internet; media refers to the tools. Do not confuse it with social networking, which refers to the act or process of using these social media tools to build online communities through groups, friends, and followers.

The purpose of this chapter is to present basic social media concepts and to introduce selected social media tools. This chapter covers text, image, audio, video, wikis, virtual worlds, and social network tools and selected examples. It does not cover social bookmarking (http://delicious.com/), news aggregators (http://digg.com/), or online gaming (http://www.warcraft.com/) concepts.

While every attempt was made to be accurate with examples and links, this is a rapidly changing field with a lot of jockeying for position—it is ever changing, and by the time this book is published, some of the URLs and sites may no longer exist. For example, Yahoo! 360 and Microsoft LiveSpaces blogging sites were recently closed, in 2009 and 2011, respectively.

HISTORICAL DEVELOPMENT

The purpose of this section of the chapter is to provide the reader with an appreciation for the development of social media as we know it today. This section presents selected forerunners to our current social media climate.

The Beginning of Social Networking

While many believe social networking using social media tools is a new phenomenon, initial social networking opportunities were in existence in the late 1970s with Usenet and BBS (Bulletin Board Systems) systems. Usenet and BBS sites permitted users to post information to newsgroups or bulletin boards. Technical and research staff in universities, the military, and research institutions were the primary users of these early tools. There was no access for the general public. At that time, these were all text-based systems that users accessed over slow Internet connections, usually through a university and a home dial-up 300 baud modem. System equipment for access included TTY (TeleTYpewriter) terminals and acoustic couplers to cradle the phone once the user connected to the mainframe system. These early systems provided online platforms or web-based technologies to interact with others; they were the forerunners of today's chat rooms, RSS feeds, blogs, and Groups that Yahoo and Google employ (Chapman, n.d.).

Next were online services like CompuServe (1979), Prodigy (1980), and AOL (1985) that offered the first PC-based connection to the Internet and service to individuals and businesses (Chapman, n.d.). These early services were originally text-based services that provided mainly email access, but quickly added functions like chat (IRC or Internet Relay Chat and ICQ, meaning I seek you and CQ for Morse code calling any station), *instant messaging for* PCs, shopping, forums, news, weather, and games (ICQ, n.d.). These functions followed the early development of PCs, the installation of PCs in individual homes, and the commercialization of the Internet, opening it up to the masses.

The Initial Browser-Based Social Networking Sites

The introduction of browsers in the early 1990s provided a more user-friendly interface than the earlier browser-based sites (BBS) and made them easier for nontechnical users (Chapman, n.d.). In the mid to late 1990s TheGlobe (http://www.theglobe.com/), GeoCities (now closed, http://geocities.yahoo.com/index.php), Six Degrees (open to members only, http://www.sixdegrees.com/), and LiveJournal (http://www.livejournal.com/) were launched. TheGlobe and GeoCities permitted each user to create a customized website, chat rooms, and messaging. GeoCities required you to join one of six "cities" like Hollywood, SiliconValley, and WallStreet. These cities represented categories for content of the webpages. Six Degrees was the first modern social network. It permitted users to create a profile and friend other users through a series of contact lists. Users had access to bulletin boards, messaging, and email. It had a short life span from 1997 to 2001, but it has reopened to previous members only (Edwards, 2011). It may at some point open to the public. In 1999, LiveJournal became the first social networking site with a blogging focus. In December 2007, a Russian Internet company, SUP, purchased LiveJournal, and established LiveJournal Inc. to run it (LiveJournal n.d.). Most of its operation was moved to Russia in 2009 (Edwards, 2011).

The early 2000s brought many changes in social networking sites. Friendster (http://www.friendster.com/) permitted the expansions of "friends" through the friends of friends concept. In 2009, MOL Global, an Asian Internet company, bought it and in 2011 redesigned the site as a social gaming site with 115 million users (MOL Global, n.d.; Rao, 2009). Another early social networking site was Hi5 (http://hi5.com/). It boasts of over 25 million monthly visitors, is the 10th top youth website, the 6th largest gaming site, and has 5 million friend requests per day in over 200 countries and 50 languages, (Raice, 2011; Quick Facts, n.d.). In 2011, Hi5 was purchased by Tagged (Raice, 2011). Tagged also focuses on games and entertainments.

There are also many niche (Nations, n.d.) and company-sponsored social networking sites:

- 43 Things for goal setting (http://www.43things.com/)
- BlackPlanet for African Americans (http://www.blackplanet.com/)
- LinkedIn for business networking and resume posting (http://www.linkedin.com/)
- Care2 for green and health living (http://www.care2.com/)
- Digg for sharing news (http://digg.com/).

As more of these companies came into being, more and more people were learning to connect on a human level over the Internet.

The more current social networking sites include MySpace (http://www.myspace.com/), Facebook (http://facebook.com), and Twitter (http://twitter.com/). On the international scene there are other popular social media sites like Bebo which is popular in Canada, the United Kingdom, and Ireland (http://www.bebo.com/) and Google's Orkut that is popular in India and Brazil (http://www.orkut.com/). New on the scene is Google+ (http://www.google.com/+); how popular it might become is yet to be seen. The point here is that this is a constantly changing arena as these sites grow, develop, and merge. What is popular in one country may not be as popular in another country. However, the concept of online social networking is an international phenomenon.

Media Sharing Sites

In addition to social networking sites, there are also media sharing sites that developed in early 2000. Media sharing sites provide storage and sharing of multimedia files with other users. These developed in line with the introduction of digital cameras and the ability to take pictures with smartphones. Photobucket (http://photobucket.com/) is one of the more popular photo sharing sites; Flickr (http://www.flickr.com/) is a major photo and video sharing site. They permit creation of albums for storing the photos and videos. YouTube (http://www.youtube.com/) followed those sites in 2005 to permit hosting and sharing of videos up to 15 minutes long; longer uploads are permitted if:

- Your account is in good standing,
- You verify your account with a mobile phone, and
- Your account has no worldwide Content ID blocks on any content (Uploading Longer Videos, 2012).

Mobile and Streaming Media Sites

In 2007, Apple rolled out the iPhone and soon afterward rolled out the iPad. While there were other devices that permitted real-time updates to social media sites, the iPhone is credited with making this easier to do. With the added apps for most social networking sites, it became possible to update them anytime and anywhere. With the movement to broadband connectivity and 4G speeds, real-time updates increased the number of people lifecasting, that is, broadcasting virtually everything they do. Two of the earlier sites were Ustream.tv (http://www.ustream.tv/) and Justin.tv (http://www.justin.tv/). Tumblr (https://www.tumblr.com/) is a cross between blogging and lifestreaming. At these sites, viewers can watch the birth of eagles and bears, and so forth. Most of these sites can be integrated into a website or blog for easy access.

People are social beings who have always been interested in interacting. Technology and more specifically the Internet makes it easier to expand one's ability to interact with many more individuals without the physical boundaries of distance. The development of social media follows the technical innovations that give people access to the broader world, from the movement from dial up modems to high speed connectivity to the movement from mainframes to mobile devices. From the movement of text based systems to real-time video, social media has become a large part of our lives, whether doing something as simple as looking up movie reviews as ordinary movie goers, using social media sites to obtain support when going through a tough time, or keeping in contact with family and friends.

With technology easier to use and more robust, the general public became more computer literate. Technology is now an integral part of everyday activities, from planning a party to making travel arrangements. As socialization moves online, it is impacting and redefining the concept of privacy. These changes impact health care providers and consumers alike, and, in turn, change the expectations of providers and patients, blurring professional and personal boundaries. To understand this impact, one must first develop a basic level of social media understanding and literacy.

USES

Communications and interaction with family and friends is the key primary use of social media sites. Increasing numbers of grandparents are using social media sites to stay in touch with children and grandchildren when distances or time are issues, while children are using them to monitor aging parents. With our mobile society and need to move where jobs take us, social media sites allow us to maintain friendships.

People are also turning to the social media sites for entertainment. There are many opportunities at these sites to watch entertaining videos or play simulation games and traditional board games. For example, your mother loves to play Scrabble, but her Scrabble buddies have moved away or are no longer able to play. You know that Facebook has a Scrabble opportunity, so you and she now play Scrabble online a couple of times a week. In an article by Mulvihill titled "Facebook: From Social Media Site to Entertainment Portal," she suggests that Facebook and Google+ are attempting to become the portal to entertainment (Mulvihill, 2011). You can now rent movies from your Facebook interface.

Corporations, government agencies, and educational institutions are using social media sites for brand monitoring and marketing. This is a less expensive way to advertise your products, obtain public opinions, receive feedback, communicate issues, send alerts, review proposals, and let the public know what key political events are occurring. In the educational arena, creative use of social media is the new trend, as is the integration of media into the classroom (Brennan, Monroy-Hernandez, & Resnick, 2010). The question is no longer if, but rather when and how to integrate social media into the educational process.

In the health field, patients are using social media sites to connect with other patients for support purposes and to share helpful hints in dealing with their conditions. It enables physicians to stay up-to-date on new procedures, treatments, and medical research. Sermo is one example of an online physician-only network for discussion about clinical issues, health care reform, practice management and more (http://www.sermo.com). For others, it is a way to network with other professionals as well as to job search. Many hospitals are now using social media sites as teaching tools.

The use of social media sites will only grow. What role will nurses play in this growth? That is up to nurses, employers, and nursing and health care professional organizations. Multiple examples of uses in health care are provided in Chapter 4.

ISSUES

While there is a magnitude of benefits to be gained from using social media, there are also issues, challenges, and problems that must be addressed. There are a number of current research studies examining the effects of this environment on users who are immersed in social media (Park, Kee, & Valenzuela, 2009; Tokunaga, 2011; Yang, 2011). The CQ Researcher (http://www.cqresearcher.com) devoted two issues to looking at social networking as it related to privacy and the impact of the Internet on thinking (Clemmitt, 2010; Greenblatt, 2010). The main concerns that have been reported to date relate to (1) personal safety and privacy, (2) liability, (3) employment fallout, and (4) changes in our body and mental processes.

Personal Safety and Privacy

Personal safety issues run the gamut from stalkers, to child predators, to criminals looking to steal your identity. Most social media sites now include options for making personal profiles private and available only to selected users. It is the responsibility of users to make sure that they use these options and read the privacy statement on these sites. Users also need to understand that what is posted, private or not, is material that others can discover during the legal discovery process and then use in litigation. This includes a user's social network account user name and password, as was demonstrated in *McMillen v. Hummingbird Speedway, Inc.*, Case No. 113-2010 CD (*McMillen v. Hummingbird Speedway, Inc.*, September 9, 2010). During discovery, the defendant asked the plaintiff if he belonged to any social network sites and, if so, requested that he provide his user name, login name(s), and password(s) in an attempt "to determine whether or not plaintiff has made any other comments which impeach and contradict his disability and damage claims" (p. 2). The judge ordered the plaintiff to provide his user names and passwords to his two social networking sites and to not delete or alter those accounts. It does not matter what your privacy settings are; there is *no* guarantee of confidentiality when posting online.

Over the past several years there have been several news stories regarding cyberbullying and what can or cannot be done about it. These stories are especially disturbing when a young person commits suicide because of an attack by a cyberbully. Cyberbullying is defined as the online posting of mean-spirited, hostile messages about a person with malicious intent to harm that person emotionally or physically. It is an attempt to systematically harass a single person. Trolling, on the other hand, is the misuse of social media sites to annoy everyone on that site by posting inflammatory or off the topic responses. For example, if you purposely post a comment, "all obese people are lazy and obese by choice," on an obesity support social media site, you are inciting responses from members of that community. The intent is to provoke an emotional response or disrupt the site rather than single out one person for attack.

Data mining, of both your public and private data, including deleted data, by a social media site is an additional privacy concern. Data-mined information is shared with third-party partners who then use that data to target and tailor their ads directly to individuals. In an article titled "Third-Party Advertisers Tracking Users in Google Ad Network," Grant Gross states that "Google has now sanctioned behavioral targeting on its network ..." (Gross, 2008). For a more complete understanding of Google practices regarding third parties, check out its ever-changing privacy policy at http://www.google.com/intl/en/policies/privacy/.

Another issue here is the trivial nature of certain discourse and detailed personal facts on many social media sites. Do any of your contacts really care if you ate pancakes for breakfast or that you are grocery shopping? But these trivial postings can put you at risk, for example, when dealing with a potential stalker. In addition, an inappropriate or just uncomplimentary picture of yourself can result in a lost opportunity for a job or new friend without you ever knowing what really happened. What about your statement "I won't be posting for the next week since I will be in Las Vegas?" This is an announcement to the public that you won't be at home in the next week and has the potential to invite criminals into your home. If you want to let others know you went on vacation to Las Vegas, do so AFTER you return home.

Liability

The second area of concern relates to liability or defamation. When does freedom of speech cross over to be defamation? Do users have the right to say what they want on these social media sites? While the Constitution guarantees freedom of speech, if you post information that is false and that information causes harm to someone, you have defamed that person. That person can then sue for the damages you have caused.

Rumors abound on social media sites and spread rapidly. The old saying "think before you speak" has new meaning in the world of social media, and especially blogging. A rumor is an unverified statement that one might make on a blog site that can easily and quickly spread or disseminate. In some cases these are intentional and in other cases they are accidental when blogging before thinking.

In the health field, HIPAA regulations come into play as to what can and cannot be said about patients on social media sites. Chapter 9 covers this topic and provides some good examples of inadvertent HIPAA violations.

Employment Fallout

The third area of concern deals with employment fallout. Most individuals are aware that future and present employers are monitoring these social media sites as to how current and prospective employees represent themselves and ultimately their employer. Employers have not hired people because of their online persona that reflects an image that the employer distains. Colleges and universities are also monitoring social media sites as part of the admission process.

An increasing number of employers are utilizing social media policies to define appropriate social networking behaviors. In some situations, employers, as a part of their employment policies, require that their employees not have blogs or other social media accounts in order to protect the company from liability as well as deal with safety concerns for the employee because of the nature of the job. This is especially true in the criminal justice field.

Some employees, including nurses, have lost their jobs or have been subject to disciplinary actions by licensing boards because of information or comments they posted on social media sites. What do you need to know about responsible online behavior? The NCSBN (National Council of State Board of Nurses) and the ANA have both worked on guidelines for nurses when using social media sites. Chapter 9 covers this issue and provides links to those documents.

Our Bodies and Minds

Nicholas Carr, in his book *The Shallows*, paints an interesting picture of some of the issues whenever new media emerges (Carr, 2010). He argues that "when people start debating whether the medium's effects are good or bad, it's the content they wrestle over" (p. 2). He argues that "our focus on content can blind us to these deep effects" of the medium on our bodies and minds (p. 3). Some of the chapter titles are intriguing: "Tools of the Mind," "The Image of a Book," "The Church of Google," "The Juggler's Brain", and "Human Elements." While at this point we don't know what impact social media will have on our bodies and minds, he cites some interesting research in Chapter 7, "The Juggler's Brain." This early research indicates that daily use of digital media accessible through tablets, smartphones, and laptops is altering our brain's pathways by creating new ones and weakening old ones and promoting cursory reading, distracted thinking, and superficial learning.

CQ Researcher (http://www.cqresearcher.com) devoted the September 24, 2010 issue to "The Impact of the Internet on Thinking" (Greenblatt, 2010). What impact is spending so much time using digital devices to access social media sites having on our bodies and minds? We know some of this as repetitive strain injuries, eye strain, back strain, and so on. But what effect does the increasing use of digital media have physiologically and psychologically on our brains? The verdict is out on this until more research occurs. Early results are causing a stir on some social media sites.

Some people are starting to write about the addictive nature of social media (Gaudin, 2010; Khalid, 2011). A few social media sites now discuss "digital detox" vacations (Sharpsteen, 2012; Yang, 2011). At these technology-free vacations, people leave their digital devices at the door! In the Yang article, he has an interesting series of assessment questions for determining if you are addicted and makes some "detox" suggestions. While many of these are first-person accounts, some research results are starting to emerge from places like the University of Chicago, Booth School of Business.

This section discussed uses and issues with social media; what follows will discuss a few social media tools.

SOCIAL MEDIA GENRE

Blogs

Blogs or web logs are nothing more than online journals, posts, or entries in chronological order that one updates frequently. Blogs can take the form of personal diaries, group causes like political or social issues, or corporate marketing, and they usually focus around a particular topic or subject. They may include reflections, commentaries, comments, images, videos, and, many times, hyperlinks to other articles, videos, and podcasts of interest to the blogger. See Figure 2.1 for what a blog might look like and Exhibit 2.2 for URLs of a few common blog sites.

Terms used in discussing blogging include:

Blog sites are online sites that provide the application or tool for creating blogs.

Blogger is the person who creates and maintains the blog site. This is also the name of one of the most common blogging sites.

Blogosphere is a term used to describe the collective community of all bloggers and their blogs.

Blog comment refers to comments left on a blog post by readers of the post. The ability to leave comments on a blog post depends on the settings that the blog administrator uses.

Blog archive is an area of the blog page where the site places old posts. The visitor can access these generally by date.

Tags are keywords added to the blog in the tag field for easier searches and aggregation.

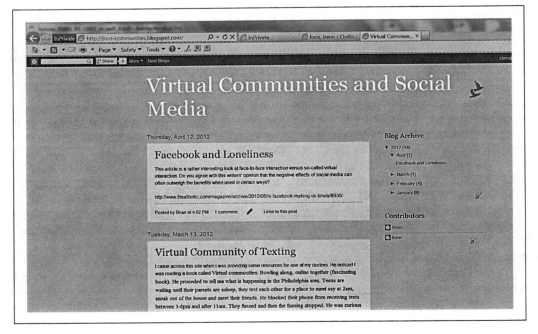

Figure 2.1 *Simple homepage and post using Blogger.com.*

Exhibit 2.2 *A Few Common Blog Sites*	
Blog Site URL	**Blog Site Name**
http://blogger.com/	Blogger
http://wordpress.com/	WordPress.Com
http://livejournal.com/	LiveJournal
http://twitter.com/	Twitter
https://www.tumblr.com/	Tumblr
http://friendfeed.com/	FriendFeed
http://www.qaiku.com/	Qaiku

Blogs are interesting and valuable for several reasons. They go beyond a news story with facts to a personalized discussion of a topic. Blogs provide an opportunity for interactive online dialog with politicians (http://www.Whitehouse.gov/blog/), an opportunity to manage student and teacher blogs (http://edublogs.org/), an ability to read selected news articles and blogs at Huffington Post (http://www .huffingtonpost.com/), an opportunity to share personal lives and experiences (http://hudds53.wordpress.com/), and an ability to dialog about health issues at http://technorati.com/blogs/directory/living/health/. Some institutions are using them to update employees on workplace issues and policy changes, provide support to patients, provide for interactive focus groups, report on new trends in nursing practice, and the list can go on and on.

With the growth in popularity of blogging, specific blog search engine sites like BlogScope (http://www.blogscope.net/) and Technorati (http://www.Technorati.com) have emerged. These sites provide a searchable database of blogs. In addition, Yahoo and Google have searchable databases for blogs, just as as they do for images. Dedicated blog search sites can update as quickly as every few minutes. Exhibit 2.2 provides the URL and name of selected blog sites. One may also happen upon a blog of interest at a website by clicking on its blog icon or accessing them under the What's New item on the navigational bar for the site.

Earlier blogs were in the form of HTML updates and required knowledge of HTML tagging. The late 1990s saw an explosion of blogging with the advent of Web 2.0 tools that made it easier to post to one's blog. One can use a hosted blog service like blogger.com or host the blog on your own server with WordPress or LiveJournal. These sites provide directions for using their specific blog application through their help section.

Tips for starting a blog include:

- Determine the purpose of the blog.
- Decide the focus or topic for the blog and the intended audience.
- Check to see if your school and/or employer has any policies related to blogging or resources supporting blogging.
- Select a blog application by comparing several different blog applications to criteria important to you. Consider such things as ease of use, cost, hosting service, functions, privacy controls, and so on.
- Create an account on the blog.
- Design the blog. Most blog applications have templates one can select.
- Configure the blog's settings. Most blog applications have some settings that deal with marketing the blog. There are also formatting and layout settings that you can select.
- Be sure to check the privacy settings. Start with a more restrictive setting until one knows how to use the various features of the blog.
- Use a conversational tone and post the first blog. Add additional posts on a regular basis. People will come back if one posts regularly, has interesting topics or opinions, and writes in a clear manner.
- Once comfortable with the design, experiment with enhancements to the blog like pictures, videos, and adding gadgets to the blog. Gadgets are objects like a search box, poll, and so on.
- Monitor the blog and related comments setting the stage for acceptable code of conduct. Check Tim O'Reilly's "Call for a Blogger's Code of Conduct" (posted at http://radar.oreilly.com/archives/2007/03/call-for-a-blog-1.html) and related discussion on this.
- Before posting, consider how parents, spouse or partner, children, employer, and colleagues might interpret the blog or tweet.

Microblog is a term to describe a subset of blogging that limits posts to brief updates. *Tweets* in Twitter are microblogs. Think of it like sending a text message to a group of friends. This limitation of 140 characters forces the poster to convey an idea or message in a succinct manner. Most microblogs also permit one to enhance the post with images, videos, sound, and links, but the idea is to keep the posts short, to the point, and to pay attention to file size for images, videos, and sound.

Microblogs are relatively newer phenomena with the advent of Twitter in 2006. Twitter delivers tweets to "followers" or people who have signed up to follow the blog. To restrict followers, most sites have a setting one can use that requires acceptance of all new followers. To gain an understanding of microblogs consider how they have moved into the mainstream of communications with politicians, sports figures, movie stars, most businesses and educational institutions, and news organizations (both print and television). Microbloggers communicate with others through tweets ranging on wide topics including what you are currently doing. Why? It takes much less effort to tweet than to update other social media. In 2012, the biggest movement now seems to be using microblogging for marketing and public relations. Microblogs have become a source of real-time updates during times of unrest and natural disasters that provide information about the events and the needs of the victims.

A few popular microblogging sites are Twitter (http://twitter.com/), Tumblr (http://www.tumblr.com/), FriendFeed (http://friendfeed.com/), which Facebook recently acquired, and Qaiku (http://www.qaiku.com/). As with many social media applications, there is considerable activity in terms of acquisitions and closings. For example, Google acquired Jaiku in 2007 and shut it down on January 15, 2012 (Perez, 2011).

Social Network Sites

Social network sites are probably the most popular of the social medium sites, with Facebook leading the way. Many people have integrated them into their daily lives and can't imagine life without social network sites. These sites are sometimes called virtual communities since they host a community of users and facilitate both public and private communication with members of the community. Social network sites permit people to:

- Construct a public or private profile,
- Identify a list of others with whom they share a connection, and
- View and interact with their list of connections generally around some concept like friends or interests (Boyd & Ellison, 2007).

Additional concepts used in discussing social media sites include:

Profile is what the user tells others about himself or herself in accordance with a completed form. The profile is now being replaced by the Timeline.

SNS is an abbreviation that refers to social network sites.

Social networking is the practice of enlarging ones circle of friends or business acquaintances by making connections through others. While this is possible on these sites, it isn't their prime purpose. For most users, being in contact with family and friends is their primary purpose.

Friends and *Contacts* are the terms that most often describe relationships.

Friending is the act of adding someone to your list of friends.

Wall is the term that describes a place where others can leave a message on the profile of someone else. The wall is now being replaced by the Timeline.

Status update is the term for updates in the member's life at this time.

While people always found a way to network with others, the Internet has opened unparalleled potential for such interaction. With the growth of mobile devices and wireless connections, users are only beginning to exploit this potential.

There are several reasons why social network sites have become so popular with a number of *people.* These sites make it possible for people to connect when they share common interests and activities. There are no geographical distance restrictions. With the click of a mouse, one can easily maintain relationships with people all over the world. There are no time restrictions. You may write status updates any time or post comments to a friend's wall any time of the day or night. For some it is a place to hang out with friends and contacts, review pictures, listen to posted music or watch posted videos from friends. Virtual communities create a world where people can share in discussions, exchange information, and stay current with happenings within their circle of friends.

There are several reasons why social network sites have become so influential with a number of *organizations* and *groups.* Businesses are now using social media sites for marketing and feedback purposes. Politicians use them to get their message out on their accomplishments and to gauge how citizens are responding to a number of political issues. The entertainment industry uses them to connect with their fans. Educational institutions are using them to keep in touch with donors, alumni, and parents. Students are using them for study partners and homework help, while parents check up on homework deadlines and requirements. Business colleagues use these sites for networking. Health care organizations use them to communicate with patients and provide information. Health care professionals use them to interact with each other and with patients.

For an example of how one community is using Foursquare, look at what Minneapolis is doing. While the city has had thousands of followers, the city did not feel it connected on a deeper level with its citizens. They switched to Foursquare and now engage their citizens by having them check in "… via a smartphone app or SMS to Foursquare, … share their location with friends while collecting points and virtual badges. Foursquare guides real-world experiences by allowing users to bookmark information about venues that they want to visit and surfacing relevant suggestions about nearby venues" (Basu, 2012, para 4).

Getting started with a social network site begins with deciding the focus of the social network site. Will it be for personal, professional, or informational use? Next, select the social network site or sites to use, for example, Facebook, MySpace, Foursquare, or LinkedIn. Different sites have a different focus and are used for different reasons. It is often wise to maintain one site for personal networking and a different site for professional networking.

Facebook (http://www.facebook.com/) is the most popular personal networking site today. MySpace (http://www.myspace.com/) has been around for a while, but seems to have reached a plateau. Foursquare, according to its website, "makes the world easier to use" and focuses on location-based mobile device users (https://foursquare.com/about/), LinkedIn (http://www.linkedin.com/) is a professional networking site gaining in popularity with professionals and professional groups, while Google+ (https://plus.google.com/) and Stumbleupon (http://www.stumbleupon.com/) are the newest additions. There are also many others for targeted groups like academia.edu (http://academia.edu/) for academic researchers, CafeMom for mothers

---

Exhibit 2.3 *Selected General Social Network Site URL and Site Name*

URL	Social Network Site Name
http://www.facebook.com/	Facebook
http://www.myspace.com/	Myspace
http://www.linkedin.com/	LinkedIn
https://plus.google.com/	Google+
https://foursquare.com/	Foursquare
http://www.stumbleupon.com/	StumbleUpon
http://badoo.com/	Badoo
http://www.cloob.com/	Cloob.com

(http://www.cafemom.com/), Flixster for movies (http://www.flixster.com/), and the list goes on and on. If you have friends overseas, there are sites that are very popular in certain countries, like Badoo (http://badoo.com/) in Europe and Latin America and Cloob (http://cloob.us/) in Iran. See Exhibit 2.3 for the URLs and site names of some selected social network sites.

Once one decides the purpose or focus of the site, selects a site, and creates an account on that site, consider these tips for getting started:

DOs

- Post an update status often but not too often. To be part of this virtual community one must participate, but don't go overboard. Have something to say first.
- Be cautious. Set much of the information on your personal network site for private viewing by family and closer friends only. There are people out there that may subvert personal information.
- Be careful about discussing one's private life; this is essentially a public forum. Post only things that you don't mind your parents or employers seeing.
- Be to the point. People don't want to read pages and pages for one status update.
- Use proper spelling. Phrases and incomplete sentences are acceptable if others can understand them. Use some common shortcuts like LOL (laughing out loud, not lots of love) but only if those that read them understand them.
- Link to other sites instead of trying to write long explanations of what is already at another location.

DON'Ts

- Post photos or say things that are incriminating. There are lots of examples of people who posted photos that landed them in jail or court.
- Post photos that include the location where the photo was taken.
- Indiscriminately post photos of others.
- Accept every friending request.
- Post just to post.
- Post where you are all the time.
- Be careless about what you post.

See Figure 2.2 for a sample user profile using Facebook's new Timeline.

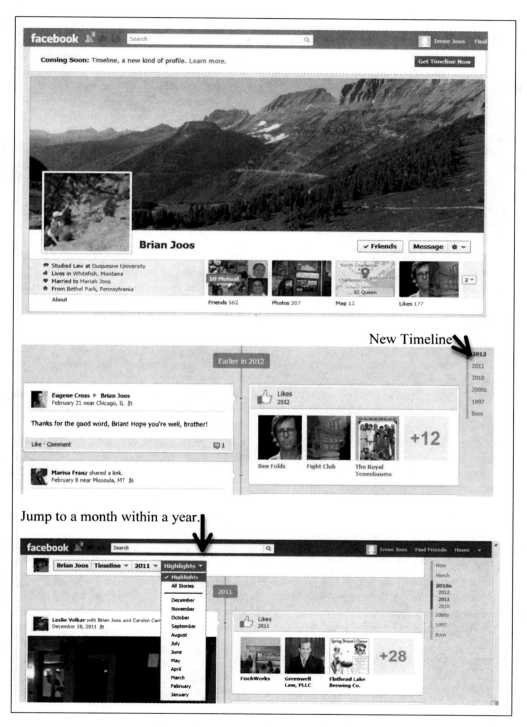

Figure 2.2 *Sample facebook profile page.*
Source: Used with permission of Brian Joos.

Wikis

Wikis are applications or websites that permit people to quickly comment on, edit for the purpose of improving, and collaborate in sharing their expertise for the benefit of the web pages contained on the wiki website. A wiki is a quick collaboration tool that uses the web. Ward Cunningham developed the first known wiki (http://c2.com/cgi/wiki?WikiWikiWeb) in 1994. Early wikis were the purview of software developers and programmers but unknown to the general public.

In 2001, things changed with the development of Wikipedia, the most notable free-content encyclopedia. In 2003, Jimmy Wales and Larry Sanger founded the Wikimedia Foundation, Inc., to host and manage Wikipedia. However, many in the academic world do not consider this a reputable source for information because it adds and deletes information solely via user generated content. This peer review process, which is based on everyone being able to contribute, is a paradigm shift from the expert-based traditional peer review process used in academia. There is still much useful information on Wikipedia. Research studies are demonstrating this resource is an increasingly important source of health-related information. Many of the webpages contain extensive resources at the bottom and others have notes that ask for contributions to enhance newly developed pages. Figure 2.3 depicts the main screen of Wikipedia. Note the translation into many different languages.

While Wikipedia raised questions about the reliability of the information on a wiki site, Wikileaks raised questions about what information should be shared by whom. Wikileaks (founded 2006) is dedicated to publishing submissions of private, secret, and classified information from anonymous sources. The goal of Wikileaks "is to bring important news and information to the public. We provide an innovative, secure and anonymous way for sources to leak information to our journalists (our electronic drop box). One of our most important activities is to publish original source material alongside our news stories so readers and historians alike can see evidence of the truth" (Wikileaks, n.d., para 1). They intend to reveal to the public what might otherwise remain secret by virtue of government policy. They seek a more transparent government when governments seek less transparency. Their publication of secret government documents has raised many questions about the appropriateness of posting this type of information for everyone and anyone to read.

As Wikipedia demonstrates, wikis have become an extremely valuable, easy to use tool for cooperatively developing ideas and publishing documents with a simple write, edit, and save approach. Wikis allow users to edit any page or to add new pages through their web browser. A user does not need any new software to collaboratively participate. One can link keywords from one page to any other page. The goal of the wiki is to involve users in the creation and collaboration of the wiki pages for true user-generated content.

Some common terms:

Wiki is the software or site hosting the wiki pages.

Wiki page is a single page on the website.

Simple Markup Language is the code that permits the writing and publishing of a wiki page through a web browser. One does not need to know the code as the wiki uses a WYSIWYG (what you see is what you get) interface.

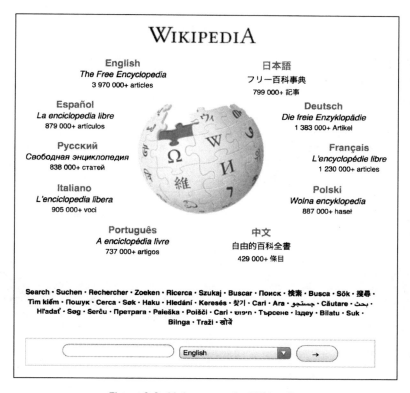

Figure 2.3 *Main screen for Wikipedia.*

There are many uses for wikis. In the academic world users exploit wikis for working on group projects, taking notes, and making lists; in the professional world, users employ wikis for creating knowledge bases around certain topics like scientific and medical research, for working together to develop policies and procedures, for stimulating creative problem solving—the list can go on and on.

Getting started with a wiki begins by first deciding what one intends to do with this wiki. Second, decide if it is for internal or external use. These answers can help one decide which wiki application to use. Note that some colleges and universities as well as course management applications have built-in wiki software. Some free wiki sites are wikispaces (http://www.wikispaces.com/), pbworks (http://pbworks.com/), and wikia (http://www.wikia.com/Wikia). See Exhibit 2.4 for URLs and Site names.

The third step is to create an account and set up the first page. See Figure 2.4 for a sample wiki page for a course where the students are going to select their group members and work on their group project using wikispaces. If this is a private wiki for a class or group of patients, adjust the privacy settings accordingly and invite members to join. Lastly, visit the wiki frequently to make updates and see what others are adding and revising.

Podcasts

A podcast is an audio or video file that the podcaster generally delivers in a series or in episodes. For example, your professor's lectures would be a series of podcasts covering the content for the course. A group of podcasts around diabetes might contain directions on how to monitor blood sugar, watch for signs and symptoms of complications,

Exhibit 2.4 *A Few Sample Wiki URLs and Their Site Names*

http://www.wikipedia.org/	Wikipedia
http://www.wikispaces.com/	Wikispaces
http://pbworks.com/	PBworks

http://wikimediafoundation.org/wiki/Home
    Note this site hosts many different wiki projects
    to "**Imagine a world** in which every single human
    being can freely share in the sum of all knowledge.
    That's our commitment."
	Wikimedia

http://www.wikia.com/Wikia	Wikia
http://www.medpedia.com/	Medpedia

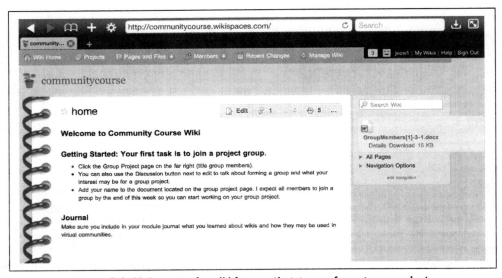

Figure 2.4 *Main page of a wiki for creating groups for a group project.*

administer medication, and so on. Accessing podcasts is as simple as subscribing to a podcast through web syndication or downloading it from a variety of social media sites to a computer or media player. Many blog and social networking sites permit the insertion or links to podcasts combining both the advantages of instant information with audio or video files. Do not confuse this with streaming media, which is real-time listening to or viewing of movies or television programs over the Internet.

Some common terms:

Podcaster is the host or person making the podcast.

Vidcast, vcast, and *vodcast* are terms that describe a video clip to be viewed on a portable device. These can be as simple as adding voice to a PowerPoint presentation and converting it to an MPEG4 file.

Web feed is a format for data to provide users with frequently updated content. The most commonly known one is RSS (really simple syndication).

Podcasts are an excellent way to provide information or to entertain. Podcasts are used to provide professional education, employee orientations, continuing education, and review of policies and procedures, and so on. They are an inexpensive way to reach many people and provide information to people who have irregular work hours, travel regularly for their jobs, need to review material repeatedly, or need updates on changing information. Use them to deliver audio or video content on a regular basis, reach a wide audience, or provide something of note.

To find podcasts, check portals like Lifehacker (http://lifehacker.com/183411/ technophilia-find-great-podcasts) or sites like Pandia Powersearch (http://www.pandia .com/powersearch/index.html#radio), which lists all the search engines by categories, one of which is podcasting.

To start creating a podcast, determine what the podcast is to accomplish. What is the purpose of the podcast? Is this the best medium for that? Second, determine the need for either a voice or video podcast. Is it important for listeners to see the podcast content? Is hearing voice enough? Third, select the correct equipment and software to produce the podcast. Podcasts require a computer with Internet access, a sound card, a microphone, headphones, a web cam if making video podcasts, and software. There are a variety of software sound recorders like Sound Recorder that comes with Windows, Audacity (http://audacity.sourceforge.net/), Windows Live Movie Maker (comes with Windows), or CamStudio (http://camstudio.org/) for capturing screen movement. A more expensive program like Camtasia (http://www.camtasiasoftware .com/) has more features for editing and capturing screen shots. One's first attempt need not be perfect and sometimes simple is best. Next, write the script (unless this is to be impromptu), keeping in mind the length of the podcast, and then practice with it. Next, make adjustments and then record the podcast. Last, upload the podcast to a social media site. It can be one already discussed like a blog or social network site or a specific site like Podbean.com (http://www.podbean.com/), which specializes in podcasts.

A few resources that one can use to learn how to make a podcast are:

- http://how-to-podcast-tutorial.com/ for general information,
- http://www.how-to-podcast-tutorial.com/17-audacity-tutorial.htm for using Audacity,
- http://www.howstuffworks.com/internet/basics/podcasting.htm for an overview and then http://www.howstuffworks.com/internet/basics/podcasting3.htm for actually podcasting,
- http://www.labnol.org/software/tutorials/convert-powerpoint-video-upload-you-tube-ppt-dvd/2978/ for converting PowerPoints to MPEG files.

Photo and Video Sharing

Photo and video sharing is the sharing of pictures or video with others. People have always shared their pictures with family and friends. Initially, this was in print form and then on CDs. The first time that people shared pictures through the Internet was in the early 1990s. Picture sharing through the Internet increased in convenience and popularity with the advent of digital cameras and smart-phones that had camera and video capabilities. Earlier means of sharing photos over the Internet included email attachments. Two of the earliest Internet sites that permitted the sharing of photos were Shutterfly (http://www.shutterfly .com/) and SnapFish (http://www.snapfish.com/). These two sites developed photos and sold an assortment of other photo type products like calendars and cards. In the early 2000s, Photobucket (http://photobucket.com/) and Flickr (http://www.flickr.com/) emerged. These two companies not only permit photo sharing but also video and other image sharing. Most social network and blog sites permit the uploading of photos or videos. And of course the most popular video sharing site is YouTube (http://youtube.com/).

Some photo and video sharing terms include:

All rights reserved means the copyright holder (the person who created the photo or video), reserves the right to determine how others may use this creative work. No one can use it without the creator's permission.

Creative Commons by Attribution is release of photos for use by another entity as long as that entity gives credit to the creator. It gives "others the permission to distribute, remix, tweak and build upon your work" (Creative Commons, n.d.).

Creative Commons by Attribution-NoDerive "allows for redistribution, commercial and noncommercial, as long as it is passed along unchanged and in whole, with credit to you" (Creative Commons, n.d.).

Folksonomy is a less structured way of classifying content; in this case, tagging or assigning keywords to photos and videos to permit easier retrieval.

People use photo- and video-sharing sites as an easier means of sharing their life with family, friends, and others. Others use them as a place to easily store and organize photos and videos as well as to backup photos and videos stored on their computers. If one has space limitations on another site like a blog or social network site, the owner can link to the photo(s) or video(s) on the photo or video sharing site. Businesses use them to market their products and to provide a portfolio of past projects for perspective clients to view. Some patient groups, like the AIDS.gov blog use them to share experiences with each other and with family as well as capture fund raising and educational events. See Figure 2.5 for the New Media page on this website. Note the photo and video sharing link on the New Media tools list.

And lastly, use photo- and video-sharing sites for educational purposes as well as entertainment. One of the most popular sites for video sharing is YouTube. Search on YouTube for dialysis and look at all the results ranging from instructional (what it is), to patients' experiences with living with kidney disease resulting in routine dialysis, to the marketing of dialysis products.

Three concerns that arise with photo and video sharing deal with privacy, piracy, and censorship.

Privacy

Privacy is a major concern with photos and videos. As health care professionals, you know about HIPAA and sharing patient information. But what about patients who take a video during their hospital visit that includes other patients and then posts it on a video-sharing site? What about taking pictures of your colleagues during a social at a conference and sharing them online without their consent? Some people believe the best policy here is to obtain permission to post pictures of others online. Others believe

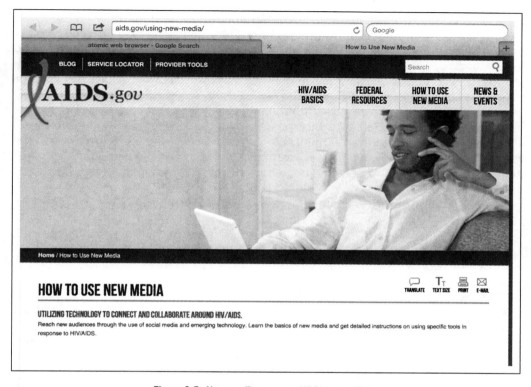

Figure 2.5 *New media page on AIDS.gov website.*

you should just not post pictures that you would not want your mother, grandmother, or employer to view. The law is not clear on this issue so it will be interesting to see how it develops.

The other privacy issue relates to the tags on these photos that many people don't know are there, but that can provide information (metadata) about where the picture was taken, with what camera, when, and so forth. The best practice here is to disable that feature on your cameras and smartphones or remove the data when editing a picture in photo editing software.

Piracy

Piracy is another issue, especially with photos. While one might not think that someone might want to use personal photos or videos, this has become a major issue. There are people blogging about finding themselves on marketing materials when a friend notices it. Some as far away as Australia! When posting photos and videos, it is important to identify the restrictions on using them. Some of the online sites set the default to free to use or Creative Commons by Attribution. Make sure the setting for materials posted is appropriate. If one posts a lot of images, consider investing in a service such as Tineye (http://www.tineye.com/), which produces a plug-in to a browser that can search for images that are posted on other sites.

Censorship

Censorship is in some people's minds more important when dealing with photos and videos because of the graphic nature of this medium. What is obscene and pornographic to one person may not be to another. For example, would pictures of male body builders during competition be obscene or not, or pictures of two nude bodies entwined? Different cultures have different beliefs and values about showing nude or almost nude bodies. Different professions view images of the nude body differently. There are also value and ethical implications for some of these images. Is watching a teenager getting drunk at a party an acceptable image to convey to others? Again, the key here is responsible use of this medium and caution when uploading photos and videos to websites.

Here are a few tips for starting to use photo and video sharing sites:

- Decide the purpose of the photo or video. Is it for personal sharing of activities with family and friends or is it for professional or instructional purposes?
- Take a picture or create a video (actually take lots of pictures and select the best to share).
- Transfer the picture or video to a computer.
- Edit the pictures or video if desired. Enhance the photos and videos with subtitles and sound.
- Upload the altered images or videos to your favorite sharing site. Learn how to do this in the help sections on these sites or through help guides and tutorials on the Internet.
- Place appropriate meta tags (keywords) and descriptions with photos and videos. This makes them easier to find and organize.
- Create galleries for displaying photos and videos in organized groups.

Virtual Worlds

Virtual worlds are Internet simulated environments where inhabitants interact with other inhabitants. Surprisingly, they have been around since 1968 when Ivan Sutherland developed the first computer-based virtual reality (Safko, 2010). Virtual worlds began with early simulators like the one at the Smithsonian where you tried to land an aircraft on a carrier. Many students use simulators as part of their nursing education. Today one speaks of 2D and 3D virtual worlds as in Second Life (http://secondlife.com/). These are shared "worlds" that provide interaction in real time, provide some rules for changing the "world" or interacting with it, and use avatars to represent users.

Some virtual world terms include:

Avatar is a graphical representation of a user or player. Users generally design their own avatars.

MUVE is a multiuser virtual environment that both the designers and the users create. They include multiple users, rich immersion environment, access through the Internet, and interaction between users acting through avatars.

By far the largest use of virtual worlds is for entertainment such as gaming as in *World of Warcraft* (http://us.battle.net/wow/en/) and *Everquest* (http://www.everquest2.com/).

Community building, education, and military training increasingly are turning to virtual worlds to provide necessary experiences. They provide people with the ability to participate in imaginary communities in a safe environment. Olsen asks the question, "Are virtual worlds the future of the classroom?" (Olson, 2006). Since that publication, there have been many writings about some of the educational virtual worlds. For example, *River City*, developed by Harvard but now with a licensing agreement with Activeworlds (http://rivercity.activeworlds.com/), *Whyville* http://www.whyville.net/smmk/nice), *SecondLife* (http://secondlife.com/), and simulated virtual clinics (http://www.license.umn.edu/Products/Minnesota-Virtual-Clinic-Medical-Education-Software__Z05174.aspx) are a few of these "worlds."

To start using virtual worlds, first decide its purpose. Is a virtual world an option for achieving the goals? Second, conduct a search to see what is available in the area of interest. This includes searching on YouTube for what others in your area of interest are doing. View some of these videos to "see" them in action. Open an account on a site that has potential for achieving the goals. Next, evaluate the costs in both time and money of this endeavor. Lastly, make a decision.

SUMMARY

Social media allow interaction between people regardless of time or distance. This chapter presented a brief historical look at the development of social media sites, a look at uses and issues, and then covered selected social media genre.

DISCUSSION QUESTIONS (PLEASE SUPPORT YOUR RESPONSES)

1. Take a look at Exhibit 2.1. What other fun facts can you share with your classmates about social media statistics? Select 2, share them, and then present why you believe they are fun facts.
2. What impact do you believe online social media sites are having on our privacy and security? Provide some examples.
3. How are online social media sites changing our interactions with others, for better or for worse? What might this mean to you in your practice?
4. What impact does always being connected have on our health? On our social behaviors? On our ways of learning? On the delivery of health care?
5. What are the issues when adding music to a podcast? Provide two resources that address these issues and summarize what they said.
6. Should you obtain permission to use pictures you took of your friends before you post them to the Internet? What does the law say? What is ethically and morally right? Explain the rationale for your response.

EXERCISES

Exercise 1: Social Media—What Is It? Why Is It Growing?

Purpose: *The purpose of this exercise is to explore the world of social media regarding definitions and statistics and to relate that to personal experiences and the practice of nursing.*

Objectives

1. Develop a workable definition of social media.
2. Relate usage statistics to personal experience and implications for the practice of nursing.

Directions

1. View this video from YouTube for a short review of social media: http://www .youtube.com/watch?v=jQ8J3IHhn8A&feature=related.
2. Find one other article or site defining social media. Share this with your classmates.
3. Discuss with classmates the critical components in defining social media. (This could be done in class or in the discussion forum in a course management application.)
4. Write a definition of social media for use in this course and when working with patients.
5. Using sites like Pew Foundation, Alexa, and Marketinggum.com, obtain some statistics about social media usage. Discuss:
   - What social media do you use and why? How do you "fit" with the statistics?
   - What implications do these statistics have for the practice of nursing? You don't have to use all of them but a few that are relative to your life and practice.
   - What one concern do you have about use of social media? Support your answer with at least one reputable resource.

Exercise 2: Social Media Effects on Our Lives

Purpose: *Some research results about the effects of social media on our lives and bodies are just surfacing. The purpose of this exercise is to examine the possible effects social media are having on our lives personally and professionally.*

Objectives

1. Examine the literature on social media's impact on people's lives.
2. Discuss implications of this information on your nursing practice and your personal life.

Directions

1. Listen to this podcast: http://www.npr.org/player/v2/mediaPlayer.html?action=1&t=1 &islist=false&id=88552617&m=88552581 Morning Our Electronically Tethered Lives.
2. Read the article "A Social-Media Addict Tries to Disconnect" by Kiran Khalid at CNN (located at http://www.cnn.com/2011/12/14/tech/social-media/khalid-social-media-unplug/index.html?iref=allsearch). Do you believe people can be addicted to social media? Support your stand with resources or examples.
3. Go to http://www.cqresearcher.com and see what they might be writing about regarding social media's impact on our thinking (Sept 10, 2010). What one thing stood out for you on this issue? Why?.
4. Research social media's impact on users. Use both the Internet and online literature databases (available through your library). Focus on an issue like liability, bullying, privacy, safety, and piracy. Prepare a short synopsis of the major points you found
5. Provide your classmates with a copy of your synopsis.

Exercise 3: Blog Comparison

Purpose: *Both professionally and personally, one needs to be able to compare current and emerging technologies in order to make good decisions. The purpose of this exercise is to compare two blog software applications using appropriate criteria and logic.*

Objectives
1. Select two similar blog software applications.
2. Compare the two applications using selected criteria.
3. Select the best one for the purpose of your blog.

Directions
1. Decide on the purpose of your blog. Alternatively you could decide to keep a blog for this course or book that would include timely links to resources and what you are learning.
2. Find two blog software applications to compare (Blogger, WordPress, Typepad, LiveJournal, etc.). Alternatively you may also use the blog that may be part of your course management software like Blackboard and compare it with one of the free ones.
3. Develop criteria on which to evaluate them. What is critical to you when selecting a blogging site? What features are essential to you? You must identify at least five. Why did you pick those criteria?
4. Compare the two sites on those criteria. Make sure you end with your selection and rationale for that choice.
5. Submit your comparison in a Word document table style following the directions of the professor.

Exercise 4: Blogging and YOU

Purpose: *When one first starts to blog, it can be an intimidating experience. The more you do it, the easier it becomes; you might also find out that you enjoy communicating ideas this way. The purpose of this exercise is to create a blog account and make several entries and enhancements to the blog over the course of the semester.*

Objectives
1. Create a blog account.
2. Post entries on appropriate topics.
3. Create enhancements to your blog.
4. Comment on others blogs.

Directions
1. Create your blog account. NOTE: If you have a student gmail account you will need to check if blogging has been enabled. If not, you will need to create your own gmail account if using blogger.com. You might want to consider using the blog site you recommended in Exercise 3.

2. Review any of the following for directions on how to use the blog you selected
   - http://www.ehow.com/blogging/ for Blogger, WordPress, and LiveJournal
   - http://www.ehow.com/video_4774531_create-blog.html
   - http://websitesetupguide.com/basic/blog-wordpress.htm?gclid=CL_n_ LWI9q0CFYPc4AodDX3Ssw
   - Also note, you may find other How To's to help with learning how to use the blog application you selected.
3. Make sure you set your blog to private and invite classmates and the professor to access and comment on your blog.
4. Make your initial post on what you learned about selecting and creating your blog
5. Comment on at least two other classmates' blogs.
6. Add five more posts to your blog dealing with wikis, social networking, virtual worlds, issues with health care blogs, and one topic of your choice. Make sure you use resources to support your statements or include links to appropriate sites and articles you found helpful.
7. Add one enhancement to your blog such as a picture or gadget like a poll or newsreel from Google.

Exercise 5: Finding Blogs and Blog Directions

Purpose: *Since many consumers turn to blogs, the purpose of this exercise is to have you investigate the world of blogs in areas of your professional interests.*

Objectives
1. Use one of the blog search sites discussed in this chapter.
2. Locate two blogs of interest to you that relate to health care or nursing.
3. Follow these two blogs for 4 weeks.
4. Summarize the nature and type of posts on these two blogs.

Directions
1. Go to BlogScope (http://www.blogscope.net/) and Technorati (http://www.Technorati.com).
2. Type in your search string for the type of blog you would like to find. Alternatively you can also check out places like 10 Health care Bloggers We're Thankful For (http://www.fiercehealthcare.com/special-reports/10-healthcare-bloggers-were-thankful) geared toward health care executives and Blogging e-Nursing (http://bestmastersin-nursing.com/2011/top-25-social-sites-for-nurses/#more-12).
3. Select two blogs to follow and follow them for 4 weeks.
4. Answer these questions: What was the nature of these two blogs? What kinds of posts were made? Who is the person running the blog? How reputable is the information on these two blogs?

Exercise 6: Social Networks—Comparison

Purpose: *The purpose of this exercise is for you to compare two different social networking sites in terms of ease of use, help guides for learning how to use them, and privacy settings and statements.*

Objectives

1. Develop appropriate criteria for comparing social networking sites.
2. Use developed criteria to compare social media sites.
3. Recommend a social media site.

Directions

1. Select two different social networking sites – Facebook, LinkedIn, Foursquare, and so on. The two you select is your choice.
2. Develop criteria on which to evaluate the two sites. What is critical to you when selecting a social networking site? What features are essential to you? You must identify at least five.
3. Why did you pick those criteria?
4. Compare the two sites on those criteria and recommend one of them.
5. Submit your comparison in a Word document table style.

Exercise 7: Wikipedia and Quality

Purpose: *The purpose of this exercise is to understand what types of information are available about health on a common wiki site.*

Objectives

1. Explain the accuracy of information found on Wikipedia related to health information.
2. Evaluate resources provided at the end of a wiki page.
3. Examine the role health care providers should play on these sites.

Directions

1. Go to Wikipedia (http://en.wikipedia.org/wiki/Main_Page).
2. Search on two health related topics of interest to you.
3. Answer these questions:
   - Was the information accurate?
   - Where there resources listed at the end where you can validate the facts provided?
   - Where those resources reputable? Explain your answer.
   - What role do you see nurses and other health care providers playing in adding and editing this information on Wikipedia? Why?

Exercise 8: Wikis—Using a Wiki to Work on a Project

Purpose: *Some organizations are turning to wiki servers to assist in working on group projects or documents like policies and procedures. This exercise was designed to provide you with experience using a wiki service to collaborate on a group project.*

Objectives

1. Collaborate on a project using a wiki site.
2. Produce a document or project using a wiki site.

Directions

1. Read M. Brain's work *How Wikis Work*. Retrieve it from http://computer.howstuffworks. com/internet/basics/wiki.htm. This is a tutorial on getting started with Wikispaces, one of the most commonly used wikis for education and communities. Now view this video on creating project websites, http://www.youtube.com/watch?v=df2rC2QfvFc.
2. Create an account on http://www.wikispaces.com/ or http://pbworks.com/. One person will create the wiki site. As an alternative, the professor may create a class wiki and have the class form groups on the wiki for their project.
3. Adjust the settings on the wiki to private and invite your group to participate.
4. Create a document on some aspect of social media or create a virtual community around some topic of interest using the wiki to work on the project. Alternatively the project could be a guide for patients viewing health information on social media sites.
5. Edit and refine the document with input from all members.
6. Submit the final document to the professor.

Exercise 9: Podcasting—Creating and Distributing

Purpose: *There are many uses and variations of podcasting. They are used increasingly to educate on what something is, how it works, and why you would do something. The purpose of this exercise is to experience creating and uploading a podcast.*

Objectives

1. Create a podcast following the guidelines provided.
2. Upload the podcast to your blog.
3. Evaluate one podcast of classmates.

Directions

1. Select a topic for your podcast. It should be something related to the topics covered to date in this book or something health related.
2. Decide on whether you will create a voice or video podcast. A video podcast can be as simple as a PowerPoint with voice added and saved in the correct format.
3. Decide on the length. Try to keep it under 4 minutes.
4. Select the appropriate software. Here are just a few examples but there are many others out there:
   - If doing a simple voice podcast, try using Audacity (download and install a free version for your operating system from http://audacity.sourceforge.net/download).
   - If using some visuals, use the voice feature of PowerPoint and save in Windows Media format, Windows Live Movie Maker, or Mac iMovie.
5. Create your podcast. Review it and rerecord if necessary.
6. Upload it to your blog.
7. View one of your classmates' podcasts. Was it clear and easy to follow? What was the message? How was the quality of the audio and/or video? What was one thing that was great about it? What would you do to improve it?

Exercise 10: Photo and Video Sharing

Purpose: *The purpose of this activity is to learn what is involved in uploading and using photo sharing and video sites and to acquaint you with two issues with sharing photos and videos.*

Objectives

1. Discuss issues surrounding photo and video sharing practices.
2. Upload photos to a photo sharing sight.
3. Adjust the appropriate settings.

Directions

1. Review this video (http://www.youtube.com/watch?v=-lSkY4X3yNA), http://www
.youtube.com/watch?v=Zil-e5Bh82E) and read this article (http://www.ehow.com/
print/how_7662952_remove-camera-information-photos.html).
2. Review either Photobucket or Flickr sharing sites for their statements about who can
do what with your photos.
3. On your blog, discuss the issues surrounding photo sharing and safe practices
4. Comment on two other student's blogs.
5. Create an account on either Photobucket or Flickr. You can use the Help system at
each of these sites or any How To-type documents available on the Internet. Make
sure when you create your account that you select the appropriate option for how you
want your photos shared.
6. Check the information settings on your camera for the metadata file.
7. Upload a few photos (making sure you remove tags on them).
8. Invite your professors to view your images.
9. Add to your blog what you learned from doing this.

Exercise 11: Virtual Worlds

Purpose: *Since virtual worlds are an increasingly discussed area and students and patients
will be coming to us with these experiences, the purpose of this exercise is to learn about virtual
worlds and their potential in the health care arena.*

Objectives

1. Investigate the potential of using virtual worlds in nursing and patient education.
2. Experience a virtual world.

Directions

1. Go to this link http://secondlife.com/whatis/?sourceid=0410-sergoog-slSecondLife-
wisl&gclid=CKeXspKrlKUCFQ915Qod71i_QA#Intro. View the introduction and
welcome videos. See if you can find anything related to your area of interest. NOTE:
YouTube has some demos of what some schools of nursing are doing.
2. Create an account on *Second Life*.
3. Spend some time looking around and learning how to navigate.
4. Discuss these questions:
  - How do you think this could be used in nursing and patient education?
  - What do you perceive as the advantages/disadvantages of learning/training this
  way?
  - How difficult do you think it is for learners to learn how to work in this virtual
  world?
  - Would you consider taking the time and resources to develop a virtual environment? Explain your response.

REFERENCES

Basu, I. (2012). Getting the Most Out of Foursquare. *Digital Communities*. Retrieved from http://www.digitalcommunities.com/articles/Getting-the-Most-Out-of-Foursquare.html?elq=8a43ff0f435a46a4a33398378d3de175)

Bennet, S. (2012). *The Numbers Just Keep On Getting Bigger: Social Media And The Internet 2011 [STATISTICS]*. Retrieved from http://www.mediabistro.com/alltwitter/social-media-internet-2011_b17881

Boyd, D., & Ellison, N. (2007). Social network sites: Definition, history, and scholarship. *Journal of Computer-Mediated Communication, 13*(1), Article 11. Retrieved from http://jcms.indiana.edu/vol13/issue1/boyd.ellison.html

Brennan, K., Monroy-Hernandez, A., & Resnick, M. (2010). Making projects, making friends: Online community as catalyst for interactive media creation. *New Directions for Youth Development, 128*, 75–83.

Carr, N. (2010). *The shallows.* New York, NY: W.W. Norton & Company.

Chapman, C. (n.d.). *History and evolution of social media.* Retrieved from http://www.webdesignerdepot.com/2009/10/the-history-and-evolution-of-social-media/

Clemitt, M. (2010). Social Networks: Are online social networks eroding privacy? CQResearcher. Retrieved from http://library.cqpress.com/cqresearcher/document.php?id=cqresrre2010091700&type=hitlist&num=0

Cohen. H. (2011). *30 Social media definitions.* Retrieved from http://heidicohen.com/social-media-definition/

Creative Commons. (n.d.). About the licenses. Retrieved from http://creativecommons.org/licenses/

Curtis, A. (2011). *The brief history of social media.* Retrieved from http://www.uncp.edu/home/acurtis/NewMedia/SocialMedia/SocialMediaHistory.html

Edwards, J. (2011). *10 Key turning points in the history of social media.* Retrieved from http://www.cbsnews.com/8301-505123_162-42750171/the-10-key-turning-points-in-the-history-of-social-media/

Facebook (2012). News. Retrieved from http://www.facebook.com/press/info.php?statistics.

Flickr (n.d.). Retrieved from http://advertising.yahoo.com/article/flickr.html

Fox, S. (2011). The social life of health information, 2011. Retrieved from http://www.pewinternet.org/~/media/Files/Reports/2011/PIP_Social_Life_of_Health_Info.pd

Gaudin, S. (2010). *Social networking addicts updating from bed, bathroom.* Retrieved from http://www.computerworld.com/s/article/9172378/Social_networking_addicts_updating_from_bed_bathroom/

Greenblatt, A. (2010). Impact of the Internet on thinking: Is the web changing the way we think? *CQResearcher*. Retrieve from http://library.cqpress.com/cqresearcher/document.php?id=cqresrre2010092400&type=hitlist&num=0

Gross, G. (2008) Third-party advertisers tracking users in Google ad network. Retrieved from http://abcnews.go.com/Technology/PCWorld/story?id=4959131

ICQ (n.d.). *Webopedia.* Retrieved from http://www.webopedia.com/TERM/I/ICQ.html

Khalid, K. (2011). *A social-media addict tries to disconnect.* Retrieved from http://www.cnn.com/2011/12/14/tech/social-media/khalid-social-media-unplug/index.html

LiveJournal. (n.d.). About us: Our company. Retrieved from http://www.livejournalinc.com/aboutus.php#ourcompany/)

McMillan versus Hummingbird Speedway. (2010). Retrieved from http://www.ediscoverylaw.com/uploads/file/McMillen%20v%20Hummingbird%20Speedway.pdf

MOL Global. (n.d.). About us. Retrieved from http://www.molglobal.net/about-us/

Mulvihill, A. (2011). *Facebook: From social media site to entertainment portal.* Retrieved from http://www.econtentmag.com/Articles/ArticleReader.aspx?ArticleID=78027

Nations, D. (n.d). *Top niche social networking sites.* Retrieved from http://webtrends.about.com/od/socialnetworking/tp/top_social_networking_sites_s.htm

Olson, S. (2006). *Are virtual worlds the future of the classroom?* Retrieved from http://news.cnet.com/Are-virtual-worlds-the-future-of-the-classroom/2009-1041_3-6081870.html

Park, N., Kee, K., & Valenzuela, S. (2009). Being immersed in social networking environment: Facebook groups, uses and gratifications, and social outcomes. *CyberPsychology & Behavior 12*(6), 729–733. doi: 10.1089.

Perez, S. (2011). *Google axes more services: Jaiku, buzz, code search, & more.* Retrieved from http://techcrunch.com/2011/10/14/google-axes-more-services-jaiku-code-search-more/

Pew Internet Organization (n.d.). Retrieved from http://www.pewinternet.org/Static-Pages/Trend-Data-(Adults)/Online-Activities-Daily.aspx

Quick Facts. (n.d.). Retrieved from http://about.tagged.com/blogs/

Raice, S. (2011). Tagged acquires facebook competitor Hi5. *The Wall Street Journal.* Retrieved from http://blogs.wsj.com/digits/2011/12/14/tagged-acquires-facebook-competitor-hi5/

Rao, L. (2009). *Malaysian payments company mol global snaps up friendster.* Retrieved from http://techcrunch.com/2009/12/09/malaysias-mol-global-to-buy-friendster/

Safko, L. (2010). *The social media bible: Tactics, tools & strategies for business success.* Hoboken, NJ: John Wiley & Sons.

Sharpsteen, A. (2012). *Time for a digital detox?* Retrieved from http://www.standard.net/stories/2012/01/16/time-digital-detox

Social Media. (n.d). *Merriam-webster: An encyclopedia britannica company online.* Retrieved from http://www.merriam-webster.com/dictionary/social%20media

Tokunaga, R. (2011). *Friend Me or You'll Strain Us: Understanding Negative Events That Occur over Social Networking Sites.* Cyberpsychology, Behavior, and Social Networking. July/August 2011, 14(7–8): 425–432. doi:10.1089/cyber.2010.0140

Uploading Longer Videos. (2012). *YouTube.* Retrieved from http://support.google.com/youtube/bin/answer.py?hl=en&answer=71673

Wikileaks. (n.d.). Retrieved from http://wikileaks.org/About.html

Yang, T. (2011). *There is such a thing as being too connected.* Retrieved from http://lifestyle.inquirer.net/18255/there-is-such-a-thing-as-being-too-connected

CHAPTER 3

Selecting Devices and Related Hardware to Support Social Media

Debra M. Wolf

LEARNING OBJECTIVES

At the completion of this chapter the reader will be able to:

1. Discuss mobile devices and related hardware used to access social media.
2. Identify leading manufacturers of computer technology and mobile devices.
3. Explore accrediting agencies approving devices and related hardware.
4. Outline criteria to assist in purchasing mobile devices and related hardware.
5. Explore how health care providers can use mobile devices to support consumer's health needs using social media.

TERMS

Camcorder	Notebook computer
Cellular phone	PC video camera
Desktop computer	Portable media players
eReaders	Smartphone
Laptop computer	Short message service (SMS)
Malware	Software programs
Mobile applications (apps)	Tablet computer
Multimedia message service (MMS)	Tablet
NetBook computer	Webcam

Social media requires the appropriate electronic device(s), software, and/or mobile applications (referred to as apps). More specifically, to fully participate in a virtual networked world using social media, one must have the appropriate electronic device(s), software, and apps that support their interests. This chapter presents the most common type of devices currently being used to view, hear, and share information on the Internet. Emphasis is also placed on devices that enhance health care delivery and enable the consumer to address their personal health needs. Using these devices, individuals are migrating to a new era of health called Mobile Digital Health or mHealth.

A FRAMEWORK FOR UNDERSTANDING DEVICES THAT SUPPORT SOCIAL MEDIA

Every day, newspapers, magazines, television, and radio programs are advertising the latest and greatest devices, promoting sales of the most recently released devices, related software, and mobile applications. To evaluate the pertinent information within this barrage of advertisements, consumers must determine what benefits a device and related software or application has to offer. In addition, consumers need to understand how these products can support their current need to participate in social media activities. The purpose of this chapter is not to review all possible electronic devices that can be used for social media. The focus is on the most commonly used items, including computers, tablets, cell phones, smartphones, portable media players, video/camera devices, and eReaders.

COMPUTERS AND SOCIAL MEDIA

Computer Configurations

Computers come in many different configurations (see Figure 3.1). A desktop computer refers to a combination of individual interconnected wired or wireless devices such as a monitor, keyboard, tower, speakers, camcorder, and mouse that is usually stationary for daily use atop a desk or office table. A laptop computer is similar to a desktop computer but includes all the items in one device and is smaller and more convenient to move and transport. Ultrabooks™, introduced by Intel, are the latest style of laptop computers and are thinner and lighter than older laptop models (Consumer Reports, 2012). A notebook computer is comparable to a laptop but is typically lighter in weight, smaller in size, and less powerful. Depending on the manufacturer, a notebook's display screen uses flat-panel technology to reduce bulkiness. For those who want an even smaller computer for accessing the Internet, manufacturers are now producing "netbook" computers, which are even smaller than notebook computers. These computers are typically used for accessing Internet-based applications.

The terms desktop, laptop, notebook, and netbook used to describe the different types of basic computer configurations are not mutually exclusive but rather overlap. Each manufacturer has its own configurations for these types of computers. Think of them on a continuum where one manufacturer's 12-inch screen will be a laptop, while another manufacturer will classify their 12-inch screen as a notebook. Figure 3.2 demonstrates this overall pattern.

Adding to the confusion, similar terminology is frequently used to describe similar devices. For example, a "tablet computer" (see Figure 3.1) is a mobile computer that combines the functionality of a notebook computer but with the feeling and effect of a tablet surface (TopTenREVIEWS, 2012a). This means the screen part of the laptop can be swiveled and collapsed to take the form of a paper tablet, hence the name tablet computer. This type of computer has larger-built in storage and

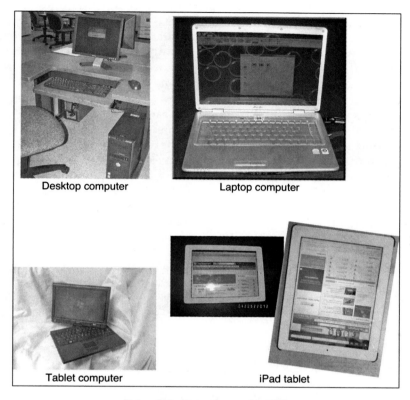

Figure 3.1 *Computer and tablet.*
Source: Courtesy of Irene Joos. Used with permission.

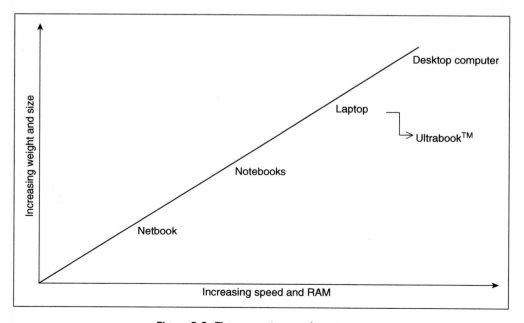

Figure 3.2 *The computer continuum.*

uses a keyboard and pen as the primary input device. This configuration is not to be confused with a "tablet" (see Figure 3.1). A tablet is an electronic device that is thin, flat, lightweight, but smaller than a laptop computer screen, in which one touches the screen to interact with the device. A tablet generally relies on the touch screen's virtual keyboard, with no physical keyboard attached, and has less built in storage. This device supports the use of mobile applications and has the capability of connecting to the Internet.

While laptops, notebooks, and netbooks are more compact and mobile, desktop computers are still very common among most consumers. Since 1979, the U.S. Census Bureau has collected information regarding the population's use of the Internet (U. S. Census Bureau, 2009). The latest survey revealed that 68.7% of the population had Internet service in their home, up from 61.7% in 2007. These statistics compare to the Pew Internet and American Life Project (2010), which revealed that 62% of adults own desktop computers (slightly down from 68% in 2006). Interestingly, the report also revealed that 55% of Americans now own laptops, which could explain the decrease in desktop ownership. This increase in computer and Internet usage supports the belief that many adults now have the tools in their possession to actively participate in social media. Often, these adults are connecting outside the home. Fifty-four percent of individuals who own a laptop use wireless Internet to surf the net from a location other than home (Pew Internet & American Life Project, 2010).

Selecting a Computer

Depending on what computer list or resource one reviews, the top ten computers in today's market vary by sales, preference, and performance. Common brands that appear on most lists include Apple, Hewlett Packard (HP), IBM, Dell, Acer, and Toshiba. Squidoo (http://www.squidoo.com), a web-based platform whose mission is to share common interests and information from individuals who are passionate about certain topics, posted the top 10 laptop computers for 2012. Their list of manufacturers includes Apple, Lenovo, Toshiba, HP, and Dell (Squidoo, n.d.), which is very similar to the list found on Amazon or other sales marketing websites. Depending on the brand, software, and services, prices for computers can vary greatly. Usually, when one searches the market, desktop computers are found to be lower in cost than the more popular laptop brands.

Although there are numerous websites that offer reviews on electronic devices, each website ranks products for different reasons. For example, some may rank on features such as processors (speed); RAM (memory); hard drive (storage); and input & output devices (such as optical drives, webcams, screens), while others rank on help and support (via telephone, chat, or email) and warranty. The actual rankings may be of limited value, for what is listed as the top brand will vary based on the ranking criteria used.

What is more important here is what one should look for when buying the device. When buying a computer, one needs to obtain as much RAM as they can afford because, as software programs are updated, they usually require more memory to use with any speed. Next, obtaining the latest processor will also support software upgrades as they become available. Finally, the size of the hard drive is important for storing program and data files. The most important question to ask is what one intends to do with the computer or electronic device. That dictates what value or ranking one places on storage, speed, memory, or input/output devices.

When selecting computers or electronic devices, there is a series of questions one needs to ask.

- What do I need the device for – work, leisure, fun, or travel?
- What design or configuration is best for me – desktop, laptop, or tablet?
- What screen type is preferred – mouse or touch screen?
- What size, height, or weight is important – net book vs. notebook vs. laptop?
- What performance is expected – processor (speed), RAM (memory)?
- What additional functionality is needed – audio, video, camcorder, speakers, Wi-Fi?
- Will battery life be important?
- Will technical help and/or support be needed, if so, in what format (telephone, chat, email)?
- What are the known issues with the device?
- What is compromised when smaller devices are selected? Are the compromised items critical to one's needs?

A list of websites that offer reviews on electronic devices include:

- Consumer Reports (http://www.consumerreports.org/cro/index.htm)—requires a membership fee
- TopTenREVIEWS (http://www.toptenreviews.com/)—free
- PC Magazine (http://www.pcmag.com/)—free
- PC World (http://www.pcworld.com)—free
- C|NET (http://reviews.cnet.com)—free

TABLETS AND SOCIAL MEDIA

As stated above, a tablet is an electronic device that is thin, flat, lightweight, but smaller than a laptop computer, in which one touches the screen to interact with the device. This device supports the use of mobile applications and has the capability of connecting to the Internet. In 2010, Apple released the first iPad tablet, which used this type of touch screen technology. A benefit of touch screens is the freedom of an individual to be more mobile, removing the need for individuals to use keyboards, styluses, or pens. Currently, tablets, like the iPad, have no inner ability to print documents. Nor do they have USB ports to connect removable storage devices, that allow for storage or transporting of data. However, if one is technologically savvy, there are ways of transferring information to another device that does have printing capabilities. For example, one could email a file to an inbox of a device that does have printing capability or store it in the "cloud."

Selecting a Tablet

Today, the iPad (third generation) is believed to be the leader of all tablets with "faster graphics, 4G wireless options (meaning fourth generation), a better camera, and a 1080 HD screen" (CNET, 2012, para. 3). Other brands that are showing close competition include Samsung Galaxy Tab 10.1, Motorola Xoom, and T-Mobile G-Slate. The same type of questions used to choose a computer can be used to select a tablet. Key features that need to be explored when purchasing a tablet include:

- Webcam—includes a front- and/or back-facing camera (meaning one can take pictures or videos of self or others using the tablet in any direction).
- Battery life—including time to recharge battery.
- Warranty—such as parts, service, or technical support.
- GPS—options available.
- Ports—are USB ports included or needed.
- Hardware—processor, memory, speakers, microphones.
- Screen—size and shape.
- Display—resolution, color, image.
- Size—weight, height.
- Operating system—are upgrades available or optional?
- Connectivity—is the tablet Wi-Fi and/or Bluetooth enabled. Do you need a monthly contract for Internet access?
- Ease of use.

Government Health IT (2012) shared that "Forrester Research reported earlier this year that sales of tablets in the United States in 2010 totaled roughly 10.3 million units, and the firm expects that number to more than double in 2011 to 24.1 million units" (p. 8).

Use of Tablets in Health Care

Tablets are quickly being adopted into clinical settings because of their mobility factor, greater integration with electronic health records (EHRs), and ease of use (Government Health IT, 2011). With features like high-resolution screens, radiologists are using tablets to view scans and make diagnoses. The U.S. Food and Drug Administration, in 2011, approved the first diagnostic radiology application for mobile devices, including the Apple iPad and iPhone.

Cardiologists at Swedish Medical Center are using tablets and mobile apps to access patients' personal health information via the institution's EHR when outside of the organization's facility (Carr, 2011). This type of remote access allows physicians to respond to patients and other professional needs in a timelier manner. In addition, these physicians are using medical imagery to display vivid animations of heart conditions on a tablet to educate patients about their current condition. The imagery displayed on the tablets is helping patients to better understand the severity of their conditions. This new form of educating patients is removing the "hand-drawn sketches" typically used to reflect a leaking heart valve compared to a normal heart valve (Carr, 2011, para. 6).

With the advanced interconnections between health care providers, mobile computers and tablets are excellent devices to begin reaching out to patients or individuals within the community through social media networks. University of Michigan Health System is currently offering tablets to their residents, patients, and families. For example, patients and family waiting in the surgical areas are offered tablets to listen to music or play Sudoku (University of Michigan Health System, 2012). Radiology residents are using tablets to access references, monitor patients, or complete tasks such as surgical scheduling (University of Michigan Health System, 2012).

Tablets and Mobile Applications

A significant difference between a computer and a tablet device is the 3rd party software called mobile applications, which tablets support. Mobile applications, also known as "apps," are software developed for small handheld devices such as mobile phones, tablets, or PDAs (Viswanathan, n.d.). Apps are typically distributed through online stores and downloaded to a device, whereas software programs were historically purchased as a CD-ROM, but more recently are being downloaded directly from a software site. An example of a common app used today is Skype. Skype enables video/audio chatting between two or more users through Internet connections.

Today there are approximately one million different apps available to consumers, which translates to one app for everything you do (BGR, 2011; Freierman, 2011). Apps can provide users with weather information, translate speech to text, identify constellations from a picture of the sky, provide GPS navigation, or even help women to plan or prevent pregnancy. Apps vary in price, ranging from being free to costing more than a thousand dollars. In addition, apps are device-specific, meaning an iPhone app may or may not work on other brands of mobile phones, and an app for a tablet may not work on an iPhone. Within the health care arena, apps are popping up everywhere, allowing users to schedule online appointments, find doctors by city/specialty/insurance, or to keep track of weight loss goals. A new app aimed specifically for physician use is called Drchrono and can be accessed at http://itunes.apple.com/us/app/drchrono-ehr/id369191782?mt=8. Drchrono is a cloud-based platform for the iPad that includes an electronic medical record, e-prescribing, and paperless billing app. Additional information on apps can be found in Chapter 4. Exhibit 4.1 describes the different types of cloud-based platforms.

Several medical applications are also emerging for tablets, such as the three-dimensional human anatomy application (Government Health IT, 2012). Doctors and nurses are using iPads in the exam room to review information with patients, write prescriptions, and order labs (Government Health IT, 2012). These encounters are excellent opportunities to introduce the patient to their EMR or their personal health record (PHR), if one exists; share quality websites that may be used for additional reading; share information about their diagnosis; or to share virtual websites the provider has initiated to support the patient's needs. Tablets, with wireless functionality, make an ideal tool to easily access patients' charts regardless of location. With tablets, health care providers have the ability to connect to patients from multiple locations.

With increased mobility, however, comes increased security risks. The occurrence of a hacker or misplaced tablet could pose a serious threat to both health care professionals and patients if security and cautionary measures are not taken. Malware refers to software that is purposely designed to damage, disable, or obtain sensitive information and can impact tablets. Caution needs to be taken to protect tablets by using anti-malware programs. There is no universal definition of malware. One blog that explores the true definition is located on C|NET and accessed at http://forums.cnet.com/7723-6132_102-530771/how-do-you-define-malware/.

Individual preferences and the intended use should dictate what type of computer or tablet one buys. Exhibit 3.1 offers a general list of factors one can consider when buying a computer or tablet. A video of how to select a laptop is provided by PC World (http://www.pcworld.com/). The video discusses and demonstrates various laptop components and characteristics that should be considered (PCWorld, 2010). The video can be accessed at http://www.pcworld.com/article/187748/laptop_buying_guide_selecting_the_right_laptop_for_you.html.ConsumerReports.org

---

Exhibit 3.1 *Factors to Consider When Selecting a Computer or Tablet*

Computer type	Desktop, laptop, notebook, netbook, or tablet
Manufacturer	Reputation and history with product
Size and weight	Light, heavy, bulky, meets traveling needs
Ergonomics	Size (screen display, button size), shape
Power	Electrical cord or battery life
Where to buy	Online or retail store. Caution for a specific model can be configured differently for a retail store vs. buying online from manufacturer (ex. graphics cards can differ but the model number and name of computer could be the same)
Service, Help, or Support	Free or charge, time period, reputation
Warranties	Time period and coverage
Device components	CPU (processor), graphics, RAM (memory), monitor display, hard drive (storage), and optical drives (CD-DVD-DVR) options
Method of interaction	Keyboard—is it a separate piece of equipment that also uses a mouse, or is it accessible through a touch screen using finger prompts or a stylus
Hidden cost	Unknown accessories (ex. is webcam included, wireless software, USB ports), Internet service provider fee
Educational support	Training opportunities
Internet connectivity	Wireless (Wi-Fi) networking capability as well as wired connections

---

(http://www.consumerreports.org/cro/index.htm) also offers consumers a buyer's guide for computers and tablets, but an online subscription is required to access the content.

CELLULAR PHONES AND SOCIAL MEDIA

In 1973, the first cellular phone was introduced by Dr. Martin Cooper (working for Motorola), weighing 4.4 pounds (Heeks, 2008; Teixeira, 2010). Merriam-Webster defines a cell phone as a portable, usually cordless, telephone for use in a cellular system (Cell phone, n.d.). Cellular phones, also referred to as cell phones or mobile phones (see Figure 3.3), are perhaps the most common and easily accessible mobile electronic device that supports wireless communication via radio waves or satellite transmissions available to consumers today. Not only are they small enough to be carried conveniently in a pocket or purse, but their large spectrum of functionality makes them a top pick for consumers to share information and communicate with other individuals.

Today, the handheld cellular phone has undergone a rapid technological and engineering evolution and has advanced to what is being called the smartphone. A smartphone is a cell phone that includes additional software functions, such as email and Internet browsers (Smartphone, n.d.). Within the health care arena, the use of smartphones has quickly been adopted. A survey conducted in 2011 revealed 74.6% ($n = 1101$) of nurses owned a smartphone or tablet, with 43.7% ($n = 342$) owning an Apple iPhone/iPod touch screen and 22% ($n = 172$) having an Apple iPad (Springer, 2011). The following section presents the differences between cell phones and smartphones, demonstrating how both are being used in health care settings and in social media activities.

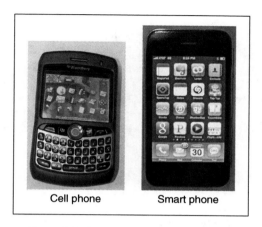

Figure 3.3 *Cell phones and smartphones.*
Source: Courtesy of Irene Joos. Used with permission.

Cell Phones

Originally, cell phones were created to allow individuals to communicate using voice in a synchronized process. Today, the basic cell phone offers the consumer the ability to communicate using voice and short message service (SMS), also known as "text messaging" and multimedia message service (MMS), meaning the ability to send and receive different forms of media such as pictures, videos, or graphics. Depending on the cell phone model one selects, its functionality, and the provider, the service plan will vary. For example, a basic cell phone with a minimal service plan may only offer voice communication. A higher level cell phone and service plan may offer voice communication along with SMS and MMS functionality. For some people, a basic cell phone for synchronized voice communication is the best option; for those who are seeking to use social media via a cellular phone, a smartphone is the better choice.

Smartphones

In 1992, the first smartphone was introduced by IBM as a prototype (Fendelman, n.d.). Since then, smartphone functionality has extended its capabilities from not only offering voice communication, but to offering Internet access, media players, cameras, and more (Teixeira, 2010). From a technical perspective, today's top smartphones have faster processors, Internet browsers, longer battery life, tight security features, quality audio and video displays, cameras, touch screen technology, and large internal memory. In short, a smartphone is a combination of a cell phone, camera, personal digital assistant, and a highly mobile technical operating system. Individuals who have smartphones can call others, send secure text messages, browse the Internet, play games, take photos, and download software; just to name a few activities. In other words, today's most advanced cellular phones are capable of doing most things we need from a computer and a phone, dubbing them as "smartphones."

When choosing between a mobile device such as a cell phone or smartphone to access the Internet or social media sites, the operating system is a critical factor to consider. Operating system (OS) refers to the software mobile devices used to manage the functionality the service provider offers within their products. Some of the current OSs include:

- iOS—offered with Apple's iPhone, allows multitasking by running more than one app at a time.
- Blackberry OS—offered with Blackberry smartphones.
- Google's Android OS—an open-source platform that is customizable.
- Windows Phone—the OS developed by Microsoft to support consumers using a new user interface that is more user friendly.

Choosing an operating system is as important as choosing the mobile device. Depending on where one is employed or what educational institution one attends, there may be resources that would support individuals in buying a cellular phone. A company employing sales agents may offer or require their employees to have a mobile device for ease of communication. The company may offer the employee access to an existing service provider through a business plan or may offer an expense allowance. In addition, businesses may have policies or guidelines one must follow if using mobile devices to exchange information with the consumer or other businesses partners. For example, Yale University (n.d.) shares guidelines that all smartphones, whether personally owned or University-provided, must be password protected, use encryption to protect data, and have a limitation on number of messages stored.

Service Providers

One of the first steps in selecting a cell phone or smartphone is to decide on a service provider to support your cellular needs. As noted above, various websites will provide a review of the various service providers one can choose. Some of the current providers include, Verizon Wireless, AT&T, Sprint, T-Mobile, and Boost Mobile. Key factors that need to be considered when selecting a provider include:

- Type of provider—do they offer services that require a one- to two-year contract (including a discounted phone) or are their services prepaid (phone may not be included).
- Plans offered—this can be very confusing for consumers. Types of plans include:
  - Individual plans—designed for one individual, with one phone line/service.
  - Family plans—designed for multiple people, using several phone lines/service, but all under one primary plan.
  - Data plans—designed to receive data in addition to voice communication using the Internet, Wi-Fi, or satellite. For example, email.
  - Business plans—designed for businesses to meet all employee's needs, including information sharing.
  - Prepaid plans—designed to allow consumers to pay in advance for services. Usually no extended contracts are needed.
  - Unlimited voice, voice and text, or unlimited everything – depending on the plan, these options allow unlimited use of the phone and data services. For example, there may be no limits on the number of minutes one uses to send and receive voice communication, no limit on the number of SMS/text messages one sends or receives, or no limit on the number of MMS files sent.

▪ Phones offered.
▪ Features or functionality.
▪ Additional benefits to consider include:
   — Voicemail—allows messages to be received and stored for future use.
   — Caller ID—allows the name and number of person calling to be displayed.
   — Call waiting or forwarding—allows the notification of an incoming call while actively having a phone conversation, or allows calls to be forwarded to your cell phone number. (e.g., calls received at work or home can be forwarded to your cell phone if you are away).
   — 3-way calling—allows 3 individuals to participate in one conversation.
   — Conference calling—allows multiple individuals to participate in one conversation.
   — Roadside assistance—offers vehicular roadside assistance via phone call.
▪ Fees one needs to consider include:
   — Roaming fees—charges applied if calls are outside of one's calling plan.
   — Activation fee—one-time charge to initiate services.
   — Cancellation fees—or early termination charges, occur if services are terminated prior to agreed contract length.
▪ Help & support.

Short Message Service

Today, individuals use cell phones and smartphones to send text messages and communicate with others in a non-synchronized fashion. In order to send a text message using SMS functionality, the phone number of the individual is needed. Once the phone number is entered, the selection of the "SMS function" versus the "Call function" is made, opening a small window screen. The sender types their short message on the cellular device using the phone keys, keyboard, or touch-screen virtual keyboard. The typed message is sent directly to the other person's cellular phone. Once received, the individual is alerted depending on what sounds the individual selected. If the receiver of the message has their sound off, no sound notification occurs, only a visual light or icon on the phone alerting them that a message is waiting. The text message is stored on the phone until the individual removes the note. This process is referred to as "texting." Due to its ease of use, freedom to communicate without speaking, and accessibility at all times, text messaging has grown tremendously.

In 2011, over eight trillion text messages were sent (MobiThinking, 2012). This functionality opens the door for communicating (texting) messages to patients regarding flu vaccines, health updates, or news releases one should to be aware of. In addition, one could send text messages reminding patients of their next office visit or lab testing that needs to be completed. As a wound skin nurse, a diabetic nurse, or a heart failure nurse, the opportunities are endless for extending nursing services to patients upon discharge. With a well-defined policy and list of guidelines, patients can be educated on how to use social media to connect with health care personnel to ask questions, attend educational workshops, or to follow up on their status after discharge. Again, the opportunities are endless.

Although SMS/text messaging is very popular, there are certain environments where SMS/text messaging should not be used based on the type of cell phone one has and the level of functionality it contains. AMCON Software (2011), a manufacturer of telecommunication products used in health care settings for advanced communication, released a white paper that introduced hospitals to using SMS and email communication to send critical messages of high priority to staff. The purpose of the white paper was to illustrate that health care organizations need to purchase smartphones that contain "smartphone application messaging," which includes encryption functionality. AMCON highlighted eight reasons why hospitals should not use SMS and email for critical communication unless a smartphone with encryption functionality was used. The following reasons were highlighted:

- Messages sent via SMS lack security and encryption—patient personal health information must be protected as noted through the HIPAA and HITECH Acts,
- SMS cannot integrate with your hospital's staff directory or on-call electronic schedules,
- SMS cannot show full traceability or escalations—meaning one cannot confirm if the message was received, acknowledged, or ignored,
- SMS cannot ensure priority delivery of messages—regardless of content or critical value, all messages are sent and received with other messages, which could be delayed,
- SMS inboxes cannot separate critical hospital notifications from those sent by friends and family,
- SMS only works over cellular networks—without the security of Wi-Fi delivery in your facility,
- SMS cannot be set to use priority ring tones or repeat notifications for important messages, and
- SMS incurs unnecessary cost—requiring one to purchase an additional plan to allow for this functionality, or applying a cost per SMS sent or received depending on the service plan one has purchased (AMCON Software, 2011).

Smartphones in Health Care

With the increased acceptance of cellular phone use and the recent release of smartphones, individuals now have access to the Internet 24/7. This means individuals can access various social networking sites, blogs, or wikis on demand or when prompted via text alert or email communication. Through the use of a mobile app, one can receive tweets from several twitter sites to stay abreast of the latest and greatest news. This high level of acceptance is a golden opportunity for health care professionals to be creative and initiate communication with patients using social media. Creating a blog, a wiki, or twitter site and enrolling patients to receive weekly health-related updates is an excellent way of promoting a healthier lifestyle. Alerts can be customized based on one's diagnosis or illness. The opportunities are endless to initiate one- or two-way communications using modern technology and social media tools.

The Centers for Disease Control and Prevention (CDC; 2012) shared an example of this creativity by presenting a study conducted in Kenya that found using a smartphone to collect disease information was faster and cheaper than traditional paper survey methods. In addition, the study found data collected via smartphone had fewer errors and was more available for data analysis. Another type of opportunity in using smartphones is in academia. Phillippi and Wyatt (2011) discuss the use of smartphones in nursing education. The mobile device supports quick access to educational materials such as clinical guidelines or instructional videos prior to performing certain skills needed to care for a patient. Although Phillippi and Wyatt share common concerns in using smartphones, such as cost and disease transmission, they believe there are ways of overcoming the adverse possibilities.

The future of cell phones is unpredictable, considering how far we have come since 1973. One thing that is certain is the level of functionality and the ability to support individual consumers' needs will continue to grow exponentially. Teixeira (2010) quoted Dr. Martin Cooper, the first person to test and use cellular phones as saying:

- "The future of cellular telephony is to make people's lives better–the most important way, in my view, will be the opportunity to revolutionize health care,"
- "Technology makes your life better, more convenient, safer, educates you, entertains you and mostly makes you more productive,"
- "We could not have predicted the annoyance that people have when the phone rings at the opera, but it doesn't take a cellular phone to make people be rude," and
- "The cell phone in the long range is going to be embedded under your skin, behind your ear along with a very powerful computer who is in effect your slave" (Teixeira, 2010).

The functionality of cell phones is now being integrated to other forms of technology. For example, the "USB Skype mouse" is a combination cell phone and computer mouse, allowing an individual to make a Skype connection through their computer mouse (PCMag.com, n.d.).

In 2011, The World Health Organization completed a global observatory report and stated there were roughly five billion cell phone subscriptions, which reflects over 85% of the population as having commercial wireless service (World Health Organization, 2011). The study also reflected that roughly 85% of business travelers use smartphones. With the improved subscription plans using 3G and 4G software, the number of smartphone users is continuously increasing (Egencia, 2010). With the increased use of smartphones, there is an excellent opportunity for health care providers to promote healthier lifestyles through social media. Just imagine the opportunities!

Protecting Mobile Devices

With the increased usage of mobile wireless devices, there is also a rise across the country in device theft (Federal Communications Commission, n.d.). The Federal Communications Commission (FCC, n.d.) offers consumers information on how to protect one's device and data from being lost or stolen. The FCC offers suggestions on:

- How to safeguard yourself against wireless device theft by:
    - Using the device discreetly in public locations.
    - Never leaving the device unattended.
    - Recording the device's model number, serial number, and unique device identification number and storing it in a convenient location.

— Reviewing the service provider's agreement or warranties; additional insurance may be needed.
- How to protect the data on your phone by:
  — Utilizing a password for access at all times.
  — Using anti-theft software or apps—these programs allow you to locate the phone from any computer, lock the device, remove sensitive data such as contact information, or to release a loud sound drawing attention.
  — Caution on storing information on a mobile device, especially if used to access social networking sites using apps.
- What to do if your wireless device is stolen, such as:
  — Using anti-theft software to track the device using the GPS indicator and locking the phone.
  — Reporting the loss to your service provider and to the police.
  — Changing usernames and passwords for email, banking, or social networking accounts if accessed using the mobile device (if anti-theft software was not used).

With the advancement of cellular phone technology and its integration within the health care setting, mobile devices like smartphones and iPads are key devices supporting social media. The ability to send and receive information (health-related or not) to various individuals in multiple locations is simple using cellular networks or secure wireless Internet systems. Having the correct cellular phone, computer, or tablet with the functionality needed to protect information being shared is a critical factor that must be considered when purchasing mobile devices. See Exhibit 3.2 for a listing of factors one needs to consider when purchasing mobile cellular phones.

Exhibit 3.2 *Factors to Consider When Selecting Cellular Phones*

Security and encryption	PIN required to retrieve messages, lock feature to prevent use, remote access to phone if lost or stolen
Integration functionality	Ability to access other database systems and devices
Manufacturer	Reputation and history with product
Assigning message priority	SMS messages sent as critical, private, or confidential
Ergonomics	Size (screen display, button size), shape
Power	Electrical cord (house/car) and battery life
Where to buy	Online or retail store
Cellular coverage	Geographical area
Warranties	Time period and coverage
Hidden cost	Unknown accessories, separate costs for SMS communication, service plan, etc,
Tracking messages	Records message delivery and read status
Connection	Cellular or Wi-Fi connection
Notification options	Separate ringtones or sounds for priority SMS communication
Service and support	Retail store, phone, or web-based
Educational support	Training to use device

OTHER ELECTRONIC DEVICES SUPPORTING SOCIAL MEDIA

Portable Media Players: MP3 or MP4

A portable media player (PMP) refers to a mobile device that plays music, videos, and movies; stores images; and has hardware supporting Internet connectivity (depending on selected PMP models). Examples include MP3 or MP4 players. An example of an MP3 is the iPod by Apple, which is mainly used for music downloads and listening pleasure. MP3 players come in a variety of models, such as hard drive models, flash models, or ultra compact models (the smallest of all MP3 players).

The MP4 device allows a user to view text from electronic books, listen to music, watch movies, and access the Internet (based on model selection). Some of these devices have built-in speakers and voice recording capabilities. Battery life can extend up to 12 hours depending on usage, making the device a perfect match for the frequent traveler. The size of an MP4 ranges from 3.8 inches in height to 4.9 inches, allowing for easy storage in pockets or briefcases. In 2010, more than 46% of adults owned a PMP, and 16% of these individuals used them to access the Internet (Pew Internet & American Life Project, 2010).

Regardless of whether one uses an MP3 or an MP4, these devices provide excellent opportunities for health care professionals to design programs or podcasts that can be downloaded to the PMP, allowing individuals the ability to listen to or watch educational material while exercising or traveling. More importantly, MP4s are granting individuals access to the Internet. This access provides multiple opportunities to use the PMP to download information from a social media site. The information obtained could support healthier lifestyles through downloaded video programs, text message alerts, tweets, or by participating in virtual health communities such as WebMD (http://www.webmd.com/).

Camcorders, PC Video Camera, and Webcams

When surfing the Internet, individuals can find an abundance of sites that permit one to click and watch a video. In order to upload and make videos available via the Internet, one needs to have the right equipment. A camcorder is a free-standing electronic device capable of recording video and audio as its primary function. Historically, camcorder devices were referred to as movie cameras one would use to take home movies. Today, camcorders are relatively small mobile devices that fit in the palm of your hand. The devices record videos to a variety of memory tools such as cassette tapes, memory cards, DVDs, or CDs. These memory cards allow the uploading of videos to a computer to be relatively easy. This ease of transferring videos from a camcorder to a computer allows individuals to upload videos to social media sites without difficulty. Although this is one way of uploading a video to the web, other devices exist within computers and mobile devices that also support video sharing. For example, a PC video camera is "an input device that the operator uses to capture video. It may be used to send video images and email attachments, to make video telephone calls (Video conferencing), and to post live, real-time images to a web server" (Joos, Nelson, & Smith, 2010, p. 593). PC video cameras are usually built into the more portable computers such as laptops, notebooks, netbooks, or tablets.

Another type of device for producing videos is the webcam. Webcams are basically a video camera that attaches to a desktop computer (via a USB cable) and feeds real-time images to a computer or network using a Wi-Fi, USB, or cable connection. Today, video cameras are found in most computers, tablets, and smartphones. The use of video cameras by individuals is increasing in popularity in an attempt to share information and communicate via social media sites. For example, Youtube.com (http://www.youtube .com/) offers a variety of videos uploaded by individuals who want to share information or communicate a certain message. A search of Youtube.com for videos on diabetes produced, within seconds, over 72,000 videos that focus on diabetes and are available for free. However, caution is needed when viewing the videos. Not all videos come from a reliable source. The use of PC video cameras, camcorders, or webcams is popular for individuals to socialize on various social media sites. The opportunity exists for health care professionals to take advantage of these devices to further support their patients or extend their services through social media.

Personal Digital Assistant (PDA)

When personal digital assistants (PDAs) were first introduced in 1986, they served individuals as personal information managers by organizing calendars, contacts, notes, and tasks (Wikipedia, n.d.). Today, the role of PDAs has been absorbed by most smartphones. Since 1986, functionality within PDAs has advanced to connect to the Internet through Wi-Fi or wireless area networks, include a web browser, enable telephone communication, have touch-screen technology, and be Microsoft Office compatible (Wikipedia, n.d.).

While weight and screen sizes are nearly the same, PDAs (see Figure 3.4) are often cheaper than smartphones over their lifetime. Although the initial purchase prices are similar, PDAs do not require a wireless carrier contract like smartphones, which can become costly over time. Another highlighted difference between PDAs and smartphones lies in Internet connectivity. Smartphones can connect to the Internet anywhere a cellular signal is available. PDAs can only connect to the Internet through a wireless network or Wi_Fi hotspot.

A key opportunity in having a PDA is the ability to use the device to store and manage personal health information. Having the ability to connect with a computer, a PDA can become one's personal health record (PHR), if so desired. PHRs are discussed further in Chapter 6.

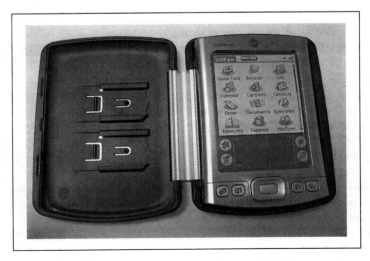

Figure 3.4 *Personal digital assistant (PDA).*
Source: Courtesy of Irene Joos. Used with permission.

eReaders

eReaders (see Figure 3.5) are portable devices used for reading books and other written materials that are in digital format (e-Reader, n.d.). These devices are designed primarily for reading documents created in electronic format that can be downloaded onto a mobile device. eReaders are the modern way of reading books, magazines, newspapers, journals, and so on. With an eReader, individuals can download a traditional paper or hardback book from Amazon or Barnes & Noble, enhancing readability for hours at a time. The electronic readers are equipped with a unique screen that ranges from 6″ to 9.5″ in size (TopTenREVIEWS, 2012b). While one can't print directly from an eReader itself, users can easily connect a USB cable to most eReaders to move a text or PDF file from the eReader to a computer for printing.

In 2011, a survey revealed that 41.5% ($n = 453$) of nurses owned an eReader, of which 61.4% of them were the Amazon Kindle (Springer, 2011). This usage by health care workers is an opportunity for nursing professionals to explore health-related apps or medical resources to share with patients to further expand one's health literacy. In 2010, one study revealed that only 4% of Americans owned some form of an eReader, and 46% of these individuals used their eReaders, to access the Internet (Pew Internet & American Life Project, 2010). A more recent study revealed that 28% of adults are using eReaders, with an additional 12% most likely to get one within the next 6 months (Biba, 2012).

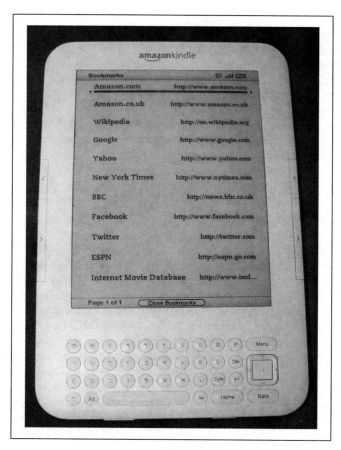

Figure 3.5 *eReader.*
Source: Courtesy of Irene Joos. Used with permission.

These data reveal an increased percentage of the population is using eReaders and will have accessed materials via the Internet. eReader mobile devices have the potential to support the social media needs of patients and consumers that could include using the Internet to seek health information. Health-related information can be created and marketed for the general population in a format that eReaders can download. Health care providers could promote the use of eReaders, allowing clients, patients, or other individuals access to a website they created that contains health-related information.

Selecting an eReader

One disadvantage of eReaders is the accessibility of "eReader Apps" for other mobile devices such as laptops, iPads, and iPhones. This accessibility allows one to read eBooks without an eReader device. The use of eReaders by health care professionals was explored in a study that consisted of twenty "2nd-year" medical students who were using the Kindle eReaders in clinics in place of medical textbooks (Shurtz & Isenburg, 2011). Results showed that major advantages in clinical settings were portability and searchability. The limitations centered on connection speed, navigation, and display views (Shurtz & Isenburg, 2011). When purchasing eReaders, factors one needs to consider include:

- Design (touch screen, screen size resolution, weight, etc.).
- Content (services, newspapers, magazines, blogs, eBook stores, etc).
- Memory.
- Battery life—including recharge time.
- Additional features—text to speech, grayscale levels, image formats.

Health care professionals should accept and use mobile devices to promote healthier lifestyles through their use. Engineers, analysts, and technical designers are advancing quickly in producing state-of-the art devices that will assist individuals to improve their level of health and information literacy. Health professionals can advance the advantages of Health 2.0, by encouraging consumers to utilize the various mobile devices. Nurses should encourage consumers to engage in using the devices to engage in quality websites and virtual health communities, to take charge of their health, and to be more participatory in their care. With a foundation in understanding what mobile devices have to offer, health care professionals can assist others in determining which device is better for one's health needs.

Using mobile devices to promote Health 2.0 through the use of social media is already actively pursued by some, but this is a minority. Individuals need to be cautioned when considering which tools and applications they will purchase to fully participate in virtual Health 2.0 communities. Some scholars believe health information technology (HIT) needs to focus on what is needed or requested by the consumer/patient, and not what works best for health standards or policy makers (Kibbe & McLaughlin, 2008). Research is needed to better understand what mobile device or related hardware will have the most impact in meeting patients' virtual needs, ultimately promoting healthier outcomes. With the overwhelming advancements in mobile devices and technology, the eReader is slower in being adopted than the smartphone and the tablet. There are two possibilities to consider; will consumers use their smartphone to replace the eReader, or will individuals with poor vision prefer the eReaders due to larger screens and formatting capabilities related to font size? The possibility of eReaders promoting a healthier lifestyle needs to be further explored.

FEDERAL SUPPORT FOR MOBILE HEALTH CARE (mHEALTH)

The U.S. Department of Health & Human Services (DHHS) supports the work of several agencies that are strongly influencing the use of mobile devices to obtain, store, and share personal information. For example, the Office of the National Coordinator for Health Information Technology (ONC) and the Office for Civil Rights (OCR) are two existing agencies that guide, approve, or certify various technologies or applications associated with health care or overall health. With the increased use of smartphones for personal and work-related needs, nurses and other health care professionals need to be knowledgeable of the implications and federal support that is available to assist them. Chapter 9 includes additional information concerning regulations and laws that impact the use of mHealth devices and apps.

Federal Agencies Regulating Technology

The ONC, in conjunction with the OCR, launched a privacy and security mobile device project designed to identify good practices for mobile devices (The Office of the National Coordinator for Health Information Technology, 2012a). The project's aim was to gather input from various groups, including subject experts, on how to protect and secure health information when using mobile devices, and more importantly, how to alert health care providers and make them aware of this type of needed protection when using mobile devices. Three panels were formed that explored:

- Setting the Federal Stage: Current Regulatory Framework, Guidance, Standards, & Toolkits for Providers and Other Health Care Delivery Professionals Using Mobile Devices,
- Real World Usages of Mobile Devices by Providers and Other Health Care Delivery Professionals, and
- Real World Mobile Devices Privacy & Security Practices, Strategies and Technologies (The Office of the National Coordinator for Health Information Technology, 2012a, para. 6).

Panel one provided an overview of the current Federal role in mobile health, listing five agencies. The Office of the National Coordinator for Health Information Technology (2012b) provides a full description of each agency as follows:

- Federal Communications Commission (FCC)—responsible for regulating interstate and international radiofrequency communications. Authorizes providers whose networks are used by various mobile devices such as smartphones or tablets to share or communicate health information. The agency develops technical rules for Wi-Fi networks.
- Food and Drug Administration (FDA)—responsible for the safety and effectiveness of a small subgroup of mobile medical applications, mobile apps that could be a potential risk to patients if they do not work as designed. In July 2011, the FDA released a draft of guidelines, for open comment, that would require vendors or manufactures of certain mobile medical applications or mobile medical apps to meet regulatory requirements (U.S. Food and Drug Administration, 2011). The FDA stated "a growing number of software applications are being developed for use on mobile platforms, which include smartphones, tablet, and personal digital assistants. As these mobile platforms become more user friendly, computationally powerful, and readily

available, innovators have begun to develop mobile apps of increasing complexity to leverage the portability mobile platforms can offer. Some of these new mobile apps are specifically targeted to assist individuals in their own health and wellness management. Other mobile apps are targeted at health care providers, as tools to improve and facilitate the delivery of patient care" (p 5). Some of the regulatory requirements being proposed by the FDA include:

- Establishment of registration and medical device listings—manufacturers of medical devices will need to register their products annually.
- Premarket submission for approval or clearance—manufacturers need to seek approval prior to placing their product on the market.
- All medical mobile apps must comply with quality system regulations—the mobile medical app and mobile platform must be safe and effective, with controls to ensure safe use and operation.
- Manufacturer must report any adverse event that is related to their device.
- Takes responsibility to correct all problems (U.S. Food and Drug Administration, 2011).
- Federal Trade Commission (FTC)—responsible for preventing fraudulent, deceptive, and unfair business practices protecting consumers' information. The FTC requires that consumers be notified if there was an electronic breach regarding one's personal health information.
- National Institute of Standards and Technology (NIST), U.S. Department of Commerce—a non-regulatory agency responsible for the advancement of innovation to improve quality of life. One division within the NIST is the Computer Security Division, responsible for creating standards, guidelines, tests, and metrics to protect information systems, and a leading resource for private businesses regarding information security.
- U.S. Department of Health and Human Services, Office for Civil Rights—responsible for implementing and enforcing the:
  - HIPAA Privacy Rule regarding protected health information (PHI) maintained by a health plan or provider that engages in electronic transactions.
  - HIPAA Security Rule, ensuring privacy, integrity, and availability of electronic PHI through standards. Violators face penalties of up to $50,000 per occurrence, with a yearly cap of $1.5 million for multiple violations.

SUMMARY

Today, both consumers and health care professionals are transitioning into a new era called mobile digital health or mHealth. Through the use of digital devices such as computers, tablets, smartphones, iPads, and eReaders, individuals will be able to manage their health and share their health information with the touch of a screen or the sound of one's voice. Digital engineering advancements have created a tremendous platform to promote healthier lifestyles. By 2013, tablets and smartphones are predicted to outsell personal computers (Government Health IT, 2012). With such technological advancement in wireless connections, Internet speeds, and intuitive processes, sharing health information between friends, family, health care providers, and virtual communities will be as easy as turning a paper page. Unfortunately, with this ease comes the increased opportunity for loss of privacy, lack of security, and misuse of personal health information. Currently there is a call to action for the government to initiate standards and develop policies to define guidelines that vendors must be held responsible for meeting.

DISCUSSION QUESTIONS

1. Select two cell phone providers available in your area. Explore the advantages and disadvantages of each, noting differences in service plans, warranties, costs, roaming charges, support, and so on. Look for online reviews of both companies. Discuss what plan you would choose if purchasing a cell phone for the first time, and why.
2. Compose a list of five computer manufacturers. Research each manufacturer to understand how long they have been in business and how long they have been selling computers. Search various blogs, tweets, and virtual communities to see how consumers are rating their products. Discuss your findings, highlighting five positive and five negative findings for each manufacturer. Share what social media sites you visited.
3. Review the U.S. Food and Drug Administration's posted draft of requirements guiding a manufacturer's role and responsibility in developing mobile medical applications at http://www.fda.gov/MedicalDevices/DeviceRegulationandGuidance/GuidanceDocuments/ucm263280.htm. Compose a comment reflecting your support for a section in the document or recommend a change in the document, including your reason for the suggested change.
4. In this chapter you were introduced to Marty Cooper, the inventor of the first cell phone. Several quotes were listed that shared his vision regarding the future of cellular phones. Read the article by Teixeira (2010) that can be found at http://news.bbc.co.uk/2/hi/programmes/click_online/8639590.stm. Reflect on Marty Cooper's vision. Discuss what visions you see in the next 20 to 30 years regarding cellular phones. Do you agree that, in the future, a cell phone will be embedded under the skin or behind the ear?
5. Portable media players are used frequently by travelers to watch movies, listen to music, and to access the Internet. Explore the various manufacturers of MP4 players. Discuss the advantages of having an MP4 player over a smartphone, highlighting other functions of the mobile device.

EXERCISES

Exercise 1: Choosing a Tablet

Purpose: *The purpose of this exercise is to evaluate the characteristics and functionality of tablets (e.g., iPad, Kindle Fire) and understand how they can be used to support the social media needs of practitioners and patients.*

Objectives
1. Explore the various characteristics and functionality of tablets.
2. Identify how tablets can be used to access social networking sites.
3. Discus how tablets can be used to support a healthier lifestyle.

Directions

1. Select five tablets for review
2. Using Exhibit 3.1, develop a list of specifications for comparing the tablets, including RAM, CPU, battery life, Internet connection, audio/video, price) and so on. Add additional features if these are important to you.
3. Use the list you have developed to eliminate three of the five tablets. For example, is the tablet too expensive to consider; is it missing a required feature? Select two tablets you would consider buying.
4. Find an online retail store that sells both products and compare the tablets again using your list.
5. Review and revise the list of specifications based on your analysis to this point
6. Compare the advantages and disadvantages of both tablets.
7. Utilize your list of specifications to select one of the two tablets for personal use
8. Identify how you would use the tablet to access a social networking site and support a healthier lifestyle.
9. Present your final selection in a two-page paper listing your rationale for choosing one tablet over the other; how the tablet will support your social networking needs; and support a healthier lifestyle. Include in your paper the reasons why you did not choose the other tablet.

Exercise 2: Transferring Knowledge

Purpose: *The purpose of this exercise is to assist an individual (who is not cell phone literate) in making a decision on which cellular phone to purchase (cell phone or smartphone) by translating information found on a marketing advertisement.*

Objectives

1. Assess the needs of an individual wanting to buy a cellular device.
2. Discuss the differences between a cell phone and a smartphone.
3. Translate terms used in an advertisement describing cellular devices.
4. Explore how cellular devices differ in supporting online activity involving social media.

Directions

1. Search the Internet for the top ten cellular devices. You can begin by reviewing the TopTenReviews @ http://cell-phones.toptenreviews.com/smartphones/ or any other reviews.
2. Identify the differences between a cell phone and smartphone, especially how they connect to the Internet and the specific features they offer.
3. Identify an individual who is interested in buying a cellular phone.
4. Assess their knowledge level regarding cellular phones; how they use the Internet; and their activity in using social networking sites.
5. Educate the individual on the advantages or disadvantages of cell phones versus smartphones. Explain which devices can be used to manage personal health information, access health-related websites, download mobile apps (that support a healthier lifestyle), and review what is included in the total cost of purchasing a cellular device (e.g., Cost of phone, service plan, accessories).

6. Review an advertisement marketing cell phones and smartphones with the individual
7. Translate the various features and terminology used on the advertisement for the individual (such as that CPU processor refers to the speed of the computer). Assist the individual in making a final decision
8. Share your experience in a blog or podcast describing the final outcome. Share your findings from the needs assessment and how the individual will or will not use the mobile device to promote a healthy lifestyle using social media solutions

Exercise 3: Removing the Confusion

Purpose: *The purpose of this exercise is to understand the difference between computers (desktop, laptop, ultrabook, notebook, netbook, tablet computer, and tablet device) and explore how each device enhances one's ability to surf the Internet and engage in social media activity.*

Objectives
1. Understand the differences between various computer models.
2. Identify the components of a computer that enhances communication within a virtual health community.

Directions
1. Define each of the following types of computers: desktop, laptop, ultrabook, notebook, netbook, tablet computers, and the tablet device.
2. Research the components of each computer (RAM, CPU, battery, etc), noting the advantages and disadvantages of each type.
3. Identify the computers that have video capabilities, a microphone, speakers, and wireless capabilities.
4. Explore the web to identify the most popular or most highly rated computer model for each type listed in step 1 above.
5. Visit a local retail store and compare your findings with what is being displayed. See how accurate your list is to the store's display.
6. Create an Excel spreadsheet comparing the computers, by listing the components, most popular model, the current retail price, and how your findings compared to the store's display.

Exercise 4: Developing a Health-Related Video

Purpose: *The purpose of this exercise is to understand how videos are being produced and uploaded onto a social media site.*

Objectives
1. Use a webcam, PC video camera, or camcorder to record a health-related message.
2. Explore the policy, terms, and conditions of a social networking site that supports the sharing (uploading) of video communications between members.

Directions

1. Identify a topic of interest involving a health-related need.
2. Find a mobile application that supports the health topic identified in step 1. Select a mobile app that can be downloaded to a cellular device, computer, or tablet.
3. Create a 2-minute script that introduces and promotes the mobile app usage, highlighting the benefits of the mobile app and encouraging individuals to maintain a healthier lifestyle.
4. Using a webcam, PC video camera, or camcorder, record a 2-minute video (using the script created above), encouraging others to try the mobile app.
5. Identify two social media sites to which you would consider uploading the video.
6. Explore the policy, terms, and conditions of the two sites.
7. Develop a PowerPoint (PPT) presentation of your 2-minute commercial and explain why you chose one social media site over the other to post your video. Include in your PPT presentation your institution's policy on posting videos the web. You are not to actually post the video, but to offer a strong rationale on why you should.

Exercise 5: Hypothetical Vision: Nurses Using Mobile Devices to Reach Patients

Purpose: *The purpose of this exercise is to envision how nurses can use mobile devices and related hardware to extend their services to individuals within the community.*

Objectives

1. Explore how nurses can use mobile devices to promote a healthier lifestyle.
2. Develop a proposal that presents the advantages and disadvantages of using social media to support individuals in the community.

Directions

1. Select a mobile device (computer, tablet, or smartphone) you would like to use to extend your services to individuals in the community through social media sites
2. Identify a topic of interest that involves your practice area
3. Outline an activity or service you would like to offer (using social media) that addresses the topic of interest. For example, a diabetic nurse may want to host a live, synchronized support group with patients she has educated on diabetes, which would require a computer, Internet access, and a video camera. Another example is the development of a blog for patients to share thoughts and ask questions; a blog that is monitored by a health care professional
4. Develop a PPT presentation (you will present to your CNO and CIO) that shares your vision. Introduce the topic, the type of interaction you are proposing, the social media tool (blog, wiki, live audio/video chats, etc) you anticipate using, and the audience you want to reach

REFERENCES

AMCOM Software. (2011). *Eight reasons SMS is unacceptable for Critical Hospital Communications: Is SMS good 4 hospitals? R U Sure?* Retrieved from http://www.ihealthtran.com/pdf/WP-US-8-Reasons-SMS-Unacceptable-Hospitals.pdf

Biba, P. (2012). *Ereader usage continues to grow, says Harris Poll; Almost 30% of US adults using them.* Retrieved from http://www.teleread.com/paul-biba/ereader-usage-continues-to-grow-says-harris-poll-almost-30-of-us-adults-using-them/

BGR. (2011). *Available apps across major mobile platforms approaching million-app milestone.* Retrieved from http://www.bgr.com/2011/12/05/available-apps-across-major-mobile-platforms-approach-million-app-milestone/

Carr, D. (2011). Healthcare puts tablets to the test. *InformationWeek Healthcare.* Retrieved from http://www.informationweek.com/news/healthcare/mobile-wireless/229503387

Cell phone. (n.d.). *Merriam-Webster Dictionary.* Retrieved from http://www.merriam-webster.com/dictionary/cell%20phone

Centers for Disease Control and Prevention. (2012). *Smartphones more accurate, faster, cheaper for disease surveillance.* Retrieved from http://www.cdc.gov/media/releases/2012/p0312_smartphone.html

Consumer Reports. (2012). *Computer buying guide.* Retrieved from http://www.consumerreports.org/cro/computers/buying-guide.htm

CNET. (2012). *Apple iPad.* Retrieved from http://reviews.cnet.com/ipad-3/ ?tag=rb_content; contentBody

Egencia. (2010). *Mobile Devices Integral to Effective Traveler Safety Strategies.* Retrieved from https://www.egencia.co.uk/public/uk/en/egencia-resources/egencia-white-papers/

e-Reader. (n.d.). *Dictionary.com.* Retrieved from http://dictionary.reference.com/browse/e-reader

Federal Communications Commission. (n.d.). *Stolen and lost wireless devices: FCC consumer facts.* Retrieved from http://transition.fcc.gov/Daily_Releases/Daily_Business/2012/db0410/DOC-313511A1.pdf

Fendelman, A. (n.d.). *How are cell phones different from smartphones?* Retrieved from http://cellphones.about.com/od/coveringthebasics/qt/cellphonesvssmartphones.htm

Freierman, S. (2011). One million mobile apps, and counting at a fast pace. New York Times, December 11, 2011. Retrieved from http://www.nytimes.com/2011/12/12/technology/one-million-apps-and-counting.html

Government Health IT. (2012). *Invited or not tablets are coming to your workplace.* Retrieved from http://www.govhealthit.com/news/invited-or-not-tablets-are-coming-your-workplace-julyaugust-2011

Heeks, R. (2008). Meet Marty Cooper-the inventor of the mobile phone. *BBC, 41*(6), 23–33. doi:10.1109/MC.2008.192

Joos, I., Nelson, R., & Smith, M. (2010). *Introduction to computers for healthcare professionals.* Sudbury, MA: Jones and Bartlett Publishers.

Kibbe, D., & McLaughlin, P. (2008). The alternative route: Hanging out the unmentionables for better decision making in health information technology. *Health Affairs, 27*(5), w396–w398. doi: 10.1377/hlthaff.27.5.w396.

MobiThinking. (2012). *Global mobile statistics 2012: All quality mobile marketing research, mobile Web stats, subscribers, ad revenue, usage, trends.* Retrieved from http://mobithinking.com/mobile-marketing-tools/latest-mobile-stats

The Office of the National Coordinator for Health Information Technology. (2012a). *Mobile devices roundtable: Safeguarding health information.* Retrieved from http://healthit.hhs.gov/portal/server.pt/community/healthit_hhs_gov__mobile_devices_roundtable/3815

The Office of the National Coordinator for Health Information Technology. (2012b). *Mobile devices roundtable: Panel 1 biographies & federal agency information.* Retrieved from http://healthit.hhs.gov/portal/server.pt?open=512&mode=2&objID=3847#federal

PCMag.com. (n.d.). *Top ten coolest combo devices.* Retrieved from http://www.pcmag.com/slideshow_viewer/0,3253,l%253D211933%2526a%253D211934%2526po%253D4,00.asp?p=n

PCWorld. (2010). *Laptop buying guide: Selecting the right laptop for you.* Retrieved from http://www.pcworld.com/article/187748/laptop_buying_guide_selecting_the_right_laptop_for_you.html

Pew Internet & American Life Project. (2010). *Mobile access 2010.* Retrieved from http://www.pewinternet.org/Reports/2010/Mobile-Access-2010/Part-3.aspx?view=all

Phillippi, J., & Wyatt, T. (2011). Smartphones in nursing education. *Computers, Informatics, Nursing. 29*(8), 449–454. doi:10.1097/NCN.obo13e3181fc411f.

Shurtz, S., & Isenburg, M. (2011). *Exploring e-readers to support clinical medical education: Two case studies.* doi: 10.3163/1536-5050.99.2.002. Retrieved from http://www.ncbi.nlm.nih.gov/pmc/articles/PMC3066586/

Smartphone. (n.d.). *Merriam-Webster Dictionary*. Retrieved from http://www.merriam-webster .com/dictionary/smartphone

Springer Publishing. (2011). *The Springer Publishing 2011 nursing ebook & smartphone survey.* Retrieved from http://springerpub.com/content/downloads/Springer-Publishing_2011_ Nursing_eBook-Smartphone_Survey.pdf

Squidoo. (n.d.). *Top rated laptop computers for 2012*. Retrieved from http://www.squidoo.com/ top-rated-laptop-computers-2009–2010

Teixeira, T. (2010). *Meet Marty Cooper—the inventor of the mobile*. Retrieved from http://news.bbc .co.uk/2/hi/programmes/click_online/8639590.stm

TopTenREVIEWS. (2012a). *2012 Best tablet PC comparison and reviews*. Retrieved from http:// tablet-pc-review.toptenreviews.com/

TopTenREVIEWS. (2012b). *2012 Best eBook reader reviews and comparisons*. Retrieved from http:// ebook-reader-review.toptenreviews.com/

University of Michigan Health System. (2012). *iPads help hospital rethink the textbook—and the magazine*. Retrieved from http://www.uofmhealth.org/news/hospital-ipad-use-0307

U. S. Census Bureau. (2009). *Computer and Internet use*. Retrieved from http://www.census.gov/ hhes/computer/

U.S. Food and Drug Administration. (2011). *Draft guidance for industry and food and drug administration staff mobile medical applications*. Retrieved from http://www.fda.gov/ MedicalDevices/DeviceRegulationandGuidance/GuidanceDocuments/ucm263280.htm

Viswanathan, P. (n.d.). *What is a mobile application?* Retrieved from http://mobiledevices.about .com/od/glossary/g/What-Is-A-Mobile-Application.htm

Wikipedia. (n.d.). *Personal digital assistant*. Retrieved from http://en.wikipedia.org/wiki/ Personal_digital_assistant

World Health Organization. (2011). mHealth: New horizons for health through mobile technologies. In *Global Observatory for eHealth series* (Vol. 3). ISBN 978 92 4 1564250. Retrieved from http://www.who.int/goe/publications/goe_mhealth_web.pdf

Yale University. (n.d.). *Smartphones: HIPAA Security Policy & Guidelines*. Retrieved from http:// www.yale.edu/hipaa/solutions/smartphones.html

CHAPTER 4

Applications and Tools Promoting Health 2.0 via Social Media

Debra M. Wolf

LEARNING OBJECTIVES

At the completion of this chapter the reader will be able to:

1. Demonstrate how health care institutions are utilizing social media to promote Health 2.0.
2. Explore driving forces supporting the development of Health 2.0 in the delivery of health care.
3. Examine the use of social media as a vehicle for delivering health care.

TERMS

Cloud

Digital games

EMRs (electronic medical records)

Exergame

Health 2.0

Health information exchange (HIE)

Mobile applications

Regional health information organizations (RHIO)

The empowered consumer, along with the high cost of health care, is now forcing a sea of change within the health care industry. Social media is both a tool and a force within this change. This chapter focuses on the use of social media to promote a healthier lifestyle, prevent illness, and manage chronic conditions among health care institutions, health professionals, and individual consumers, as well as analyzing how health care institutions are utilizing social media. Marketing strategies combined with individual consumer needs and preferences will ultimately decide how one accesses social media tools. As we know, there are two options: using the Internet via a web-based browser on one's computer, or using mobile applications installed on one's personal mobile digital device or smartphone.

WEB 2.0 TOOLS AND HEALTH CARE ORGANIZATIONS

Scientific discoveries, innovative technologies, and evolving patterns of health care delivery are driving and being driven by a culture of health care reform. Within this environment of continuous change, new mandates are established and laws are passed to meet the growing societal expectation for better health and better health care delivery for all. The move to Health 2.0 is one part of this larger picture. Examples of driving forces include:

- The passing of Executive Order 13335 in 2004, which requires all health care organizations to have some form of electronic medical record (EMR) by 2014 (U. S. Department of Health and Human Services [DHHS], 2007).
- The passing of the Health Information Technology for Economic and Clinical Health (HITECH) Act of 2009, offering financial incentives for health care organizations to implement EMRs by 2015 (DHHS, 2010). Part of the Meaningful Use requirements is that EMRs have the ability to communicate among other EMR systems. In response, health care organizations partner with vendors to select and implement new technology supporting Health Information Exchanges (HIE) administered through Regional Health Information Organizations (RHIOs). An HIE provides for the electronic movement of health-related information among organizations utilizing nationally recognized standards and policies (http://www.himss.org/content/files/HIETopicSeries_Fact%20Sheet%20071709.pdf).
- The increased emphasis on prevention of illness and other health problems as demonstrated by the release of the Institute of Medicine (IOM) report mandating the development of preventive care health reform guidelines to improve the health of populations worldwide (IOM, 2009).
- The increasing numbers of patients who are treated in same-day or outpatient settings, while patients who are treated in tertiary health care institutions are experiencing increased acuity. As a result, family and friends have an increasing hands-on responsibility as caregivers.
- The aging population has increased the demand for in-home support, assisted living facilities, and skilled long-term care providers.

With the increased availability of electronic health data, more practitioners are discovering that electronic mobile devices and social media can be important tools for promoting a higher level of quality patient care. In response, a number of organizations established initiatives combining the increasing availability of electronic patient information with the higher level of functionality offered within newer technology. Below are some examples of how the integration of technology is assisting with the delivery of patient care and ultimately improving the overall level of quality outcomes.

Mobile Access for Health Care Providers—University of Pittsburgh Medical Center (UPMC)

Health care organizations can design software interfaces that allow physicians, nurses, pharmacists, and other health care practitioners to access multiple applications or databases using electronic devices outside of a hospital setting and through the use of social media. With this technology, physicians can receive alerts of critical lab results or request consultations or other forms of critical information via smartphones or electronic tablets. The University of Pittsburgh Medical Center (UPMC), which is in the forefront of this trend to promote user access to multiple systems, facilitates—with one click of the mouse—clinician's access to multiple applications within the health care system via screen icons (UPMC Extra, 2007). This access provides practitioners who are not physically at the point of care the flexibility to view and utilize information needed for critical decisions about individualized patient care.

Hospital Mobile App Use for Consumers—Baptist Health Hospital, South Florida

Health care organizations are also turning to social media to create social networks through mobile apps by sharing:

- Educational opportunities for current patients or consumers within the surrounding community.
- Communication marketing strategies emphasizing new practices or services.
- Information to employees promoting healthier lifestyles.

One example of a health care organization that is marketing their services through mobile applications is Baptist Health Hospital. Located in South Florida, Baptist Health offers a free mobile application to consumers, which provides real-time information on the closest urgent care center and actual wait times (Page, 2011).

Marketing Health Care Information via a Website—Cleveland Clinic

Developing a website that markets a health care organization's services is part of the marketing strategies used by health care organizations today. These websites usually offer a variety of topics such as driving and parking directions, search engines to find a doctor, online services, and consumer health information by disease or department.

Within their websites, health care organizations usually display a section titled "Find Health Information" and provide a search engine which assists individuals to quickly navigate their website. Information such as specific diseases, contact information for clinicians, or specific departments treating patients with certain diagnoses can be searched. This approach is demonstrated on Cleveland Clinic's website http://my.clevelandclinic.org/default.aspx. Within seconds of using their online search engine (to search for a condition such as hypertension), a webpage displays results that includes the basic definition, treatments, research innovations, and any online health chats that may be available.

Using Web 2.0 technology, such as WebEx, Cleveland Clinic allows consumers to participate in live discussions with specialized clinicians. These "live health chats" offer clinicians a platform to promote healthier lifestyles and information on certain diseases or conditions to a select group of individuals who have a common interest. Basically, live chats are webinars that consumers can participate in to obtain additional information regarding certain diseases or medical conditions. Some institutions such as the Cleveland Clinic (n.d.) have moved beyond general information and are providing patients the option to view their medical record (through the website's homepage) including consults with their practitioners and images of tests completed within their facility.

Social Media Presence of Health Care Organizations

In an attempt to reach a wider range of consumers, many health care organizations have established a presence on social media sites such as Facebook, Twitter, or YouTube. These organizations display the related icons on their homepages, informing viewers of their virtual presence on these social media sites. By clicking on the icons, the viewer can open the related social media website for that organization.

In August 2011, the Department of Health and Human Services (DHHS) through the office of the Assistant Secretary for Preparedness and Response, announced a challenge to all multidisciplinary teams to develop an application leveraging Facebook to promote personal preparedness and strengthen public health promotion through social networks (Government Printing Office [GPO], 2011). The key activity within this challenge is for members of Facebook to identify three key persons they refer to as *Lifelines* who will be resources during any disaster. The goal of the challenge is ultimately to strengthen national health security by creating preplanned linkage of support (GPO, 2011).

Some physicians are using mobile applications that function through Facebook to connect to their community of patients. By integrating an EMR into Facebook, patients can receive alerts or reminders of medications they need to take, allowing them to manage their daily medication adherence. For example, teenage patients are signing up for "Iowa MedMinder," a Facebook application to see a full listing of all their medications needed for the day. With this application these young patients can click on drugs and doses taken at specific times creating not only a reminder of when medication should be taken, but a record of what medications were taken. These data are then transmitted to servers accessible by their physicians (Lewis, 2011a).

Although health care organizations such as hospitals are leading the virtual world in meeting consumers' and patients' needs via Web 2.0 and social media tools, other organizations are joining the movement. Long-term care (LTC) facilities, rehabilitation centers, personal care homes, and ambulatory centers that offer outpatient services for personal care, testing, or treatments are turning to Web 2.0 to market their services. For example, when searching for a nursing home facility to assist in caring for a family member, consumers can search the Internet and find an abundance of facilities. Another alternative to finding health facilities is Medicare. gov (http://www.medicare.gov/quality-care-finder/). This is an example of a social media site that assists individuals in finding and comparing health care resources such as:

- Hospitals
- Nursing homes
- Home health agencies
- Dialysis facilities
- Physicians.

With the increased use of Web 2.0 and various forms of social media, health care organizations and health professionals must understand the factors that impact how consumers will use their websites or services. The following section will present various factors to be incorporated into a strategic plan when designing and implementing virtual environments. In an attempt to attract consumers or offer extended services to patients and employees, health care organizations must have a presence using social media.

FACTORS IMPACTING HOW CONSUMERS, PATIENTS, AND HEALTH PROFESSIONALS USE SOCIAL MEDIA TO PROMOTE HEALTH 2.0

As technology and software development continues to rapidly advance, numerous driving factors are promoting the personal and professional use of social media. Individuals attempting to manage their personal health needs and health care organizations promoting their health services are turning to Web 2.0. Studies conducted through the Pew Internet and American Life Project (2011a) offer a variety of statistics on who is using the Internet (see Table 4.1) and who is using online communication for health information (Pew Internet and American Life Project, 2011b; see Table 4.2). Their research estimates that 78% of adults (18–65 years of age) who responded are using the Internet. Further

Table 4.1 *Percentage of Americans Using the Internet*

Adult population	
Total adults	78%
Men	78%
Women	78%
Race/ethnicity	
White, Non-Hispanic	79%
Black, Non-Hispanic	67%
Hispanic (English- and Spanish-speaking)	78%
Age	
18–29	95%
30–49	87%
50–64	74%
65+	42%
Household income	
Less than $30,000/yr	63%
$30,000–$49,999	85%
$50,000–$74,999	89%
$75,000 +	96%
Educational attainment	
Less than High School	42%
High School	69%
Some College	89%
College+	94%
Community type	
Urban	79%
Suburban	80%
Rural	72%

Source: The Pew Internet & American Life Project (2011a).

Table 4.2 *Peer-to-Peer Health Care Advice*

Who is more helpful when you need...	Professional sources like doctors and nurses	Fellow patients, friends, and family	Both equally
Times when professionals matter most			
An accurate medical diagnosis	91%	5%	2%
Information about prescription drugs	85%	9%	3%
Information about alternative treatments	63%	24%	5%
A recommendation for a doctor or specialist	62%	27%	6%
A recommendation for a hospital or other medical facility	62%	27%	6%
Times when non-professionals matter most			
Emotional support in dealing with a health issue	30%	59%	5%
A quick remedy for an everyday health issue	41%	51%	4%
Times when the two groups are equally helpful			
Practical advice for coping with day-to-day health situations	43%	46%	6%

N=3001 adults and the margin of error is +/– 3 percentage points for the full sample.
Source: The Pew Internet & American Life Project (2011b).

studies reflect that 59% of adults who use the Internet are looking for health information, 19% of adults have watched videos online regarding medical concerns, 18% of adults review drugs online, and 12% of adults have explored rankings of clinicians online (Pew Internet and American Life Project, 2011c). These findings demonstrate that an increased number of individuals are turning to the Internet to search for health information or communicate with clinicians regarding certain medical conditions. As might be expected these statistics have continued to change. Please see http://www.pewinternet.org/Static-Pages/Trend-Data-(Adults)/Whos-Online.aspx for an example of this trend.

There are a number of driving factors that influence why and how consumers as well as health professionals elect to use Web 2.0 technologies and applications. Understanding these factors is imperative if the maximum potential benefit for health promotion is to be achieved. The first key factor is understanding the knowledge, skills, values, and attitudes that are associated with individuals who use technology (computers, mobile digital devices, and the Internet) as a media for accessing and sharing information. Horrigan (2007), in his research, identified ten classifications of adults who use technology. These classifications ranged from *omnivores,* who are individuals using multiple devices to access Web 2.0 functionality to its fullest, to *indifferents,* who are individuals making limited use of cell phones or Internet access and finding the activity bothersome (Horrigan, 2007). This study reflects the wide range of knowledge, interests, and skills among the general population that health care professionals and organizations must incorporate when creating health care applications via social media and websites.

In 2009, the American Recovery and Investment Act was passed offering incentive payments to eligible health care providers to adopt technology within a health care setting (DHHS, 2012). This incentive program encourages the integration of various technology devices, such as EMRs and barcode scanners, at point of care in the clinical setting, and the integration of online technologies such as Web 2.0 to reach out to patients in the community.

The technologies, methods, and procedures for securing personal health and contact information is the second factor underlying the effective use of Web 2.0 technologies. Accessing confidential information from a mobile application within a cell phone or electronic tablet may allow the information to be downloaded to the actual device for future use when Internet access is not available. What happens when the device is stolen or accessed by another individual? What security measures are in place on the mobile device to prevent an unauthorized user from accessing personal data? A solution is offered by Oh (2011) who suggests using an alternative storage site called a "Cloud" to store confidential information. Cloud servers have been proposed by some as being a safe and more secure means to share information, as well as being a way of sharing services over the Internet (Cloud Computing, 2007). One would access the cloud via a web-browser, view content, and then exit without the data downloading to the mobile device. The concept of cloud storage is further explained in Exhibit 4.1.

The third key factor is the quality of information and level of interactivity offered by various websites. Based on one's profession and health-related interest, there are a variety of Health 2.0 sites available for access. For example, RT Connections (http://rtconnections.com/) is a website that focuses on improving clinical and professional practice for nurses. In 2011, RT Connections's blog was noted as one of the top 50 blogs by the Online LPN to RN organization, reflecting the level of interaction and quality of discussions that occur on the website (Online LPN to RN, 2011). RT Connections shares educational offerings, upcoming events, tips for nursing students and new nurses, and quick reviews of scholarly articles that would support nurses in their role. Other nursing Health 2.0 sites include A Nurse Practitioner's View (http://npview.blogspot.com/), 21st CenturyNursing (http://21stcenturynursing.blogspot.com/), the Nursing Ethics blog (http://nursingethicsblog.com/) and Center to Champion Nursing in America (http://championnursing.org/blog).

A study conducted by Nicholson Kovac, Inc., explored the use of social media among nurses (PRWeb, 2010). The study found 87% of nurses access the Internet for business or professional reasons, approximately 83% access websites for health care information, 41% explore manufacturers for products and services, 11% use Twitter, 77% visit Facebook, and 25% have visited LinkedIn. Interestingly the study showed that if nurses reviewed blogs, it was for educational or professional needs and, more

---

Exhibit 4.1 *Understanding Cloud Storage*

Cloud storage is a service model in which data are maintained, managed, and backed up remotely and made available to users over a network (typically the Internet). There are three main cloud storage models:

- Public cloud storage services, such as Amazon's Simple Storage Service (S3), provide a multi-tenant storage environment that's most suitable for unstructured data.
- Private cloud storage services provide a dedicated environment protected behind an organization's firewall. Private clouds are appropriate for users who need customization and more control over their data.
- Hybrid cloud storage is a combination of the other two models that includes at least one private cloud and one public cloud infrastructure. An organization might, for example, store actively used and structured data in a private cloud and unstructured and archival data in a public cloud.

importantly, that 65% of nurses plan to engage in social media for professional purposes (PRWeb, 2010).

Examples of physician websites that support physician communication and interaction include Sermo (http://www.sermo.com/), Doximity (https://www.doximity .com/), Ozmosis (http://ozmosis.com/), PeerCase (http://www.peercase.com/), and OrthoMind (https://www.orthomind.com/login). Although these sites offer different levels of communication, not all are secure sites that offer the same quality of interaction. For example, Sermo defines in their terms of use page that they may mine conversations for business and competitive needs (Bowman, 2011). Mining of conversations can lead to legal or ethical issues if personal health information is shared unintentionally by physicians. See Chapter 8 for additional information on targeted advertising and the market for this type of data.

A collaborative study between QuantiaMD (https://quantiamd.com/), a web-based community, and Care Continuum Alliance, an organization promoting a healthier population, was conducted to explore how physicians are currently using social media and how they can integrate social media into their practices (Modahl, Tompsett, & Moorhead, 2011). The study found 87% of physicians have used a social media/network site for personal needs (mainly through Facebook) and 67% have used one for professional reasons. The researchers believe these clinicians are key to connecting social media to medicine. In addition to quality and security factors, one needs to consider the legal, ethical, and moral obligations of a social media website. Chapter 9 includes a full discussion of these issues. Modahl et al. (2011) also found in their study of physician views on social media, only 11% (n = 439,829) of physicians were familiar with one or more online patient communities and 66% (n = 290,287) of these physicians believe they have a positive to very positive impact on patients.

Unfortunately, not all sites may be seen as noteworthy to all health care professionals. For example, Yin (2010) presents the *GuitarGirl RN* blog, which, when viewed, presents stories shared by an emergency room (ER) nurse that reflect funny or critical comments or experiences within the ER. A blog of this nature may not be as educational or rewarding as a blog designed to advancing one's knowledge or assisting one in improving current practice. In contrast, *Manage My Practice* is a blog run by Mary Whaley who is a practice administrator who offers information that assists physician practices to deal with changes regulated by various current mandates such as Medicare (Yin, 2010). Finding a blog that meets the needs of the individual is critical. Following and using blogs for personal or professional needs must be approached with caution by each individual. Three things impact which sites people find most useful or helpful:

- Level of computer and/or information literacy skills
- Needs of the person seeking health information or support
- Marketing skills of the site owner

Using mobile applications, web-based online communities, or other forms of online information-sharing platforms raises concern about how information or data that are shared is being used by patients and other consumers. PatientsLikeMe was the first social networking site to publically announce that the use of information shared on its site would be aggregated to assess the impact of taking lithium on patient outcomes (Lewis, 2011b). Although the investigation was not conducted following traditional research protocols, the outcome data offered real-time information that could possibly influence participants decisions related to their use of this medication (Lewis, 2011b).

Health care organizations must also consider what the financial implications will be to create, design, and maintain a presence in the virtual world, whether through blogs, wikis, or their own websites. How will information be maintained or updated? Who will review or approve postings if two-way discussions are encouraged? What are the legal ramifications in creating social networking sites associated with the organization? Literacy levels are also a critical factor that impacts use of social media using technology. In Chapter 1, you were introduced to various types and levels of literacy. Understanding that each individual is different with varying levels of literacy will assist health care professionals and organizations in how they utilize social media to reach patients or a community of consumers.

PROMOTING HEALTH 2.0 THROUGH SOCIAL MEDIA

Proactively promoting health and encouraging a healthier lifestyle is a primary goal of health care professionals. Providing services to promote health and treat illness is the primary initiative driving health care organizations. Health care professionals and institutions use technology and social media to achieve these goals. The following section presents specific tools, devices, and applications that health care organizations and professionals are using in achieving these goals.

Wikis

Many professionals are using wikis to build quality health care information resources for patients, consumers, and other health care professionals. Types of information resources that are being shared support peer-to-peer collaboration, patient education on specific diseases, professional support in caring for patients with specific diseases, or sharing of intelligent tools (such as questionnaires or surveys) that can be used to assess patients with a certain disease. An excellent example is Medpedia (http://www.medpedia .com/). This wiki, which advances medicine by connecting people and information, is accessed by medical professionals, patients, and organizations to enhance their level of health-related knowledge. Medpedia provides access to tools, news items, articles, clinical trials, alerts, and health communities with open discussions among several individuals on various topics. Examples of health communities within Medpedia include dementia, breast cancer, diabetes, emergency medicine, and medical ethics. Although most of the information is accessible for free, creating a profile that requires certain personal contact information is required for receiving feedback on questions posed.

Blogs

A health-related blog is a social media tool health professionals use to manage specialized information and share open discussions on various topics or situations. For example, case studies of events in health care delivery may be presented with in-depth discussions for all to read. The blog has the capability to interface to email, Facebook, Twitter, RSS, and Apple and Android platforms. A search engine is usually provided to assist in finding specific information, and ideally the site is certified by the HONcode (the Health On the Net Code of Conduct; http://www.hon.ch/home1.html) confirming that the quality of information is trustworthy. Most interestingly, a blog is usually maintained by a group of volunteer health professionals. Guests to the website are not required to register and do not have to submit personal contact information.

In 2005, Dr. Drew Rosielle created a blog designed to organize articles on palliative care (http://www.pallimed.org; Pallimed, n.d.). His blog is another example of how health care professionals are turning to social media to promote the exchange of health information in a virtual environment. Today, this blog has expanded and collects media that discuss hospice and palliative care issues. The blog is designed for interdisciplinary professionals working within a hospice and palliative setting, but consumers, patients, and families are welcome to view content as well.

Video Sharing

One social media tool whose growth is exploding is video sharing, which enables the exchange or offer of health information with and to a variety of professionals and consumers. The American Nurses Association (ANA) has developed a "Nursing Video Gallery" to share information illustrating key issues and health needs supported by the organization. Examples include influenza immunization needs, welcoming student nurses into the profession, and presenting issues significant for the profession (American Nurses Association, 2011).

In an attempt to bring health information to communities, the National Network of Libraries of Medicine (2011) created a blog that links award-winning videos on community health issues. The number one video in 2011 was titled "James and the Peanut Allergy" accessible at http://www.youtube.com/watch?v=VoCAizDEKlM and produced by University of Utah (National Network of Libraries of Medicine, 2011). This video presents a young boy's discussion about the seriousness of his peanut allergy. The video is only one of many videos consumers can view via YouTube. In fact, some videos are produced by patients for patients to assist them in accepting or dealing with certain health conditions. For example, there is a video titled "Dialysis Treatment Procedure" accessible at http://www.youtube.com/watch?v=E8Uj-C1-HyU. This video was produced by a patient in end-stage renal failure undergoing hemodialysis. The patient and her spouse share their weekly experiences and discuss how they accept and approach dialysis sessions as a date night in order to make it into a positive experience for them. When educating patients, it is important to point out that videos can be produced by anyone and do not necessarily contain accurate, current information unless they are from a trusted site or source.

Mobile Devices

Mobile devices are another type of digital device used to promote Health 2.0 by sharing and accessing health information virtually. As discussed in Chapter 3, many health care organizations are turning to mobile phones to assist in improving communication within their institutions. Today health care professionals and consumers are turning to "mobile applications," for they believe them to be faster and more useful (Amcom Software, 2011). Mobile applications or mobile apps are unique programs individuals can download for various functionality or needs. Today, with the increased use of smartphones and electronic tablets, health care professionals will be looking for the most recent mobile health care solutions that will assist them in performing their role as a health care professional. Incorporating mobile apps is one of the most promising and well-received tools assisting health care organizations in reaching their intended community or patient population. See Chapter 3 for more information on mobile devices.

Texting (SMS)

Communicating using short messages service (SMS) is one way of connecting quickly to a large population. SMS has become a common mode of communication among most teenagers and adults. Unfortunately the use of SMS within a health care setting can be a concern. A study that surveyed nurses found those who use a mobile phone or personal digital assistant (PDA) at work list "texting" as the main application used, followed by email and Internet access applications (PRWeb, 2010). In 2006, a study was conducted to assess the effect of nurses using SMS and Internet to assist patients with diabetes self-management (Kim, Kim, & Ahn, 2006). Patients using text messaging or the Internet were to share their daily glucose levels. Nurses in return would send SMS to the patients offering recommendations. A mean decrease of 1.1% in HbA1c level was noted at the end of 12 weeks (Kim et al., 2006). In 2006, the Royal College of Nursing developed a guide for nurses working with children and young people in how to use text messaging safely and effectively. They identified three levels for using text messaging:

- Simple—service provider initiates, such as a reminder for an appointment.
- Specific—an individual signs up for a service and receives programmed responses, referred to as "automated," or the individual initiates a specific question of which a nurse responds, referred to as "personal."
- Serious—an individual self reports a concerning event such as abuse or a life threatening situation (Royal College of Nursing, 2006).

Extending professional nursing services using SMS requires considerable planning. First, one must identify if the service is needed or is it a current trend? Is the service beneficial to all including the consumer, or is it a marketing tool? Finally, accountability of nurses needs to be carefully thought through with clear processes and guidelines established that have been approved by legal services and other authorizing groups.

Ultimately using SMS may open a door to send gentle reminders related to health initiatives such as obtaining pneumonia and influenza vaccinations. Two businesses leading the market in promoting health IT pathways through texting are Google and Microsoft (Kibbe & McLaughlin, 2008). Other innovators that are following their paths include MinuteClinics, Intels, and local stores such as Wal-Mart, Giant Eagle, and Walgreens (Springer Publishing, 2011). Soon, all consumers will be receiving SMS messages as reminders to pick up prescriptions or have their blood pressure checked.

Digital Gaming Devices

Another popular form of technology that is being used by health care professionals and consumers to promote a healthier lifestyle is digital gaming devices. These devices utilize various types of gaming strategies to attract the attention of individuals. A digital gaming device incorporates activities such as dancing, yoga, and boxing to promote healthier lifestyles. Exergaming is a term that was coined to define the use of video games that require the user to participate in physical activity to play the game as a method of promoting a healthier lifestyle (Healthgamers, n.d.). The devices are currently being used in various health settings as well as in consumer homes for family activities. The American Council on Exercise (ACE) is a nonprofit organization that has been in existence for over 25 years. The ACE researches various exercise regimens in an attempt to promote physical activity using safe products (Healthgamers, 2010).

ACE shares their findings and relevant information via a blog called Healthgamers, which can be accessed at http://www.healthgamers.com/2010/research-theory/the-most-heart-healthy-wii-games/.

One of the most popular gaming devices used to promote a healthier lifestyle is the Wii game. In 2008, ACE explored the benefits of Wii Sports (electronic games structured around sports activities such as tennis, bowling, and boxing) and Wii Fit (electronic activities structured around physical fitness exercises such as running and free steps). They concluded that both systems promoted physical activity, which leads to burning of calories; unfortunately the total amount of exercise was not sufficient enough to meet the requirements of the American College of Sports Medicine (Healthgamers, 2010). However, these researchers did support the use of the digital electronic games with the belief that some exercise is better than no exercise. From nursing homes that use Wii bowling for wheelchair-bound adults to families that challenge one another using electronic dance mats, digital gaming devices are a unique way to offer consumers of all ages, in all environments, visual activities to improve one's level of physical activity. Yengin (2011) states "digital game environments allow users to gather ideas by allowing them to gain virtual experiences as opposed to real life events."

Regardless of whether social media is being used for personal needs, personal professional needs, or for marketing of a health care organization's services, all individuals need to understand how to evaluate social media content for quality, accuracy, and safety. The National Center for Complementary and Alternative Medicine (NCCAM) (2011b), which is part of the NIH within the DHHS, has created a four- page document called CAMbasics accessible via URL http://nccam.nih.gov/health/webresources/D337.pdf. The document is an easy to read tool that offers clear and concise information on how to evaluate web-based health resources. Content is easy to read and offers key questions one needs to ask, such as who runs the site, who pays for the site, what is the purpose of the site, and what information sources are used on the site. The tool also offers suggestions as to when to talk with a qualified provider to discuss your interpretations of content found on websites (NCCAM, 2011a). There are multiple published tools available to assist individuals in assessing the validity and quality of social media sites. These resources include the National Cancer Institute (2011), National Network of Libraries of Medicine (n.d.), National Library of Medicine (2010), and National Institutes of Health (2010). LaRue (2011) created a quick and easy tool titled "SPAT," which is an acronym that stands for Site, Publisher, Audience, and Time. The tool is designed for easy memory recall and has gone through extensive scientific testing to verify its validity (LaRue, 2011).

SUMMARY

Advancing into a new era of health care delivery using innovative technology will require time, education, and a commitment by clinical professionals to better understand patient needs. Being proactive in using social media and networking within one's practice is the first step. This type of preliminary activity may include using social media to educate patients, monitor patient adherence to self-care and drug compliance, offering advice, or simply to advertise services offered within one's practice or health care environment. Advancing one's organization and practice to incorporate digital devices that promote physical activity for all patients and consumers is the next step in promoting Health 2.0 to be widely accepted.

DISCUSSION QUESTIONS (PLEASE SUPPORT YOUR RESPONSES)

1. Identify three reasons why health care organizations would use social media. Select one reason and discuss why it is important from a consumer and health care professional point of few.
2. View two videos found on the Internet (one produced by a qualified health professional and one by a consumer). Compare and contrast the quality of information shared. Would you recommend the videos to other health care professionals or patients? Why or why not? What legal and ethical considerations would a nurse consider when taping a health video?
3. Share a mobile application that promotes wellness to consumers. How would you promote the use of mobile applications within your health care organization?
4. After reviewing a blog and wiki designed to support health professionals in exchanging health information, identify what concerns you would have for consumers who access the websites, but are not licensed practitioners?
5. How would you educate your patients and fellow clinicians in evaluating social media websites for safe and reliable information?

EXERCISES

Exercise 1: Surfing for Health 2.0

Purpose: *The purpose of this exercise is to explore various health care institutions' websites in order to understand their marketing strategies and to explore how they utilize social media to attract consumers.*

Objectives
1. Explore services offered at a health care institution by viewing their website.
2. Select a health care provider by searching a health care institution's website.

Directions
1. Identify two health care organizations located within your community.
2. Search the Internet to find the websites for each organization.
3. Compare and contrast how each organization uses social media to market to the community. Include the answers to these questions:
   - What services are offered virtually?
   - What health information is accessible?
   - Are search features included within their website?
   - Is it easy to navigate displayed content or is it overwhelming to the individual?
4. Once you have taken time to review each website, would you choose one facility over the other to seek person-to-person assistance for a medical condition?
5. Share your responses in a two- to three-page paper.

Exercise 2: Nursing and Social Media

Purpose: *The purpose of this exercise is to explore current social media sites that are specific to nursing. This means the site supports the collaborative needs of nursing professionals or the site is hosted by nursing professionals supporting consumers' health information needs.*

Objectives
1. Explore the difference between social media sites supporting health care professionals' needs versus consumers' health needs.
2. Describe the type of information shared between nursing professionals and between nurses and consumers.

Directions
1. Surf the Internet and identify two social media sites that are specific to nursing. You need to select one site that supports collaborative needs of nursing professionals and the other site that is hosted by nursing professionals supporting consumers' health information needs (e.g., you can visit RT Connections at http://rtconnections.com/ or the Nurses Nurse at http://www.thenursesnurse.com/).
2. Review the information provided on each site and compare the quality of the content based on literacy levels.
3. In a two-page paper share your thoughts on how a consumer would or would not benefit from reading the information found on the social media site geared for interprofessional collaboration.

Exercise 3: Self Assessment

Purpose: *The purpose of this exercise is to complete a self-assessment to better understand what type of technology user you are.*

Objectives
1. Understand the different types of technology users.
2. Utilize a self assessment tool to assess an individual's technology skills.

Directions
1. Access the Pew Internet and American Life Project's self assessment tool at http://www.pewinternet.org/Participate/What-Kind-of-Tech-User-Are-You.aspx.
2. Complete the 14 questions on the website (none require personal contact information).
3. Once you have completed the quiz, review the definition of the type of technology user you are then review the other types (and their definitions) that are listed on the webpage.
4. Share in a two-page paper what type of technology user you are (share the definition provided on the site), if you believe the tool is an appropriate instrument to use in assessing one's technology ability, and if you believe the survey tool reflects your ability to use technology successfully? Explain why or why not.

Exercise 4: Exploring Disease-Specific Social Networking Sites

Purpose: *The purpose of this exercise is to explore what type of social networking sites currently exist to support a specific condition or diagnosis and to identify a social media tool or platform that will meet a specific population's health information needs.*

Objectives

1. Conduct an assessment of existing social media sites that share health information specific to one diagnosis.
2. Select a social media tool or platform that will meet a specific population's health information needs.

Directions

1. Choose a medical condition you are familiar with such as diabetes, hypertension, or cancer.
2. You have been asked by the Chief Nursing Officer to strategically plan how nursing can meet the needs of this population through social media.
3. Surf the Internet to identify ten social networking sites and social media tools that currently exist to support this population.
4. Develop an Excel spreadsheet that lists all the sites found and their URLs; note type of tools, services offered, information available, and the number of users on each site.
5. Identify what type of social media tool or platform you will recommend to support this growing population. This means, will you recommend a mobile app, a blog, SMS notifications, or a new website specifically related to the patients with the diagnosis?
6. Share in a two-page paper what social media platform and tool you will use and why. Discuss one advantage and one disadvantage of the sites you visited.

Exercise 5: Assessing Technology Usage in Other People

Purpose: *The purpose of this exercise is to distinguish between the different levels of technology users and explore how each level would benefit from social media activities.*

Objectives

1. Assess an individual's level in using technology.
2. Identify activities involving social media that are appropriate to the individual's level.

Directions

1. Access the paper titled "A Typology of Information and Communication Technology Users" at http://www.pewinternet.org/~/media//Files/Reports/2007/PIP_ICT_Typology.pdf.pdf.
2. This is a 65-page paper, but you only have to read the first five pages (summary of findings). On the second page, a table is presented that describes 10 groups of users.
3. Interview a coworker or friend using the self assessment tool presented in Exercise 3.
4. In a two-page paper, explain what type of technology user the person is using one of the ten groups presented in this paper. Explain how this user differs from the other nine. Share what type of social media activities you would and would not encourage the individual to use to promote a healthier lifestyle.

REFERENCES

Amcom Software. (2011). *Ten predictions for 2012 on smartphones in hospitals.* Retrieved from http://www.amcomsoftware.com/gwf/?id=NTc5&name=Amcom+Website:+Ten+Predictions +for+2012+on+Smartphones+in+Hospitals++

American Nurses Association. (2011). *Nursing video gallery.* Retrieved from http://ana .nursingworld.org/FunctionalMenuCategories/AboutANA/WhatWeDo/Nursing-Video-Gallery .aspx

Bowman, D. (2011). 6 physician social networks at a glance. *FierceHealth IT Weekly News for Health IT Leaders.* Retrieved from http://www.fiercehealthit.com/special-reports/ 6-physician-social-networks-glance

Cleveland Clinic. (n.d.). *Discover the power of today.* Retrieved from http://my.clevelandclinic.org/ default.aspx

Cloud Computing. (2007). *Search cloud computing.* Retrieved from http://searchcloudcomputing .techtarget.com/definition/cloud-computing

Government Printing Office. (2011). *Department of Health Human Services.* Retrieved from http:// www.gpo.gov/fdsys/pkg/FR-2011-08-10/html/2011-20296.htm

Healthgamers. (2010). *The most heart healthy Wii games.* Retrieved from http://www.healthgamers .com/2010/research-theory/the-most-heart-healthy-wii-games/

Healthgamers. (n.d.). *Glossary.* Retrieved from http://www.healthgamers.com/glossary/

Horrigan, J. (April 2007). *A Typology of information and communication technology users.* Washington, DC: Pew Internet & American Life Project. Retrieved from http://www.pewinternet.org/~/ media//Files/Reports/2007/PIP_ICT_Typology.pdf.pdf

Institute of Medicine. (2009). *Global health.* Retrieved from http://www.iom.edu/Global/Topics/ Global-Health.aspx

Kibbe, D., & McLaughlin, P. (2008). The alternative route: Hanging out the unmentionables for better decision making in health information technology. *Health Affairs, 27*(5), w396–w398 .doi:10.1377/hlthaff.27.5.w396

Kim, H., Kim, N., & Ahn, S. (2006). Impact of a nurse short message service intervention for patients with diabetes. *Journal of Nursing Care Quality, 21*(3), 266–271.

LaRue, E. (2011). *SPAT: Website evaluation tool.* Retrieved form http://www.spat.pitt.edu/

Lewis, N. (2011a). Facebook app reminds transplant patients to take meds. *Information Week Healthcare.* Retrieved from http://informationweek.com/news/healthcare/patient/231500152

Lewis, N. (2011b). Will social media tools transform clinical research? *Information Week Healthcare.* Retrieved from http://www.informationweek.com/news/healthcare/patient/229402603

Medpedia. (n.d.). Retrieved from http://www.medpedia.com/

Modahl, M., Tompsett, L., & Moorhead, T. (2011). *Doctors, patients and social media.* Retrieved from http://www.quantiamd.com/q-qcp/DoctorsPatientSocialMedia.pdf

National Cancer Institute. (2011). *FactSheet: Evaluating health information on the Internet.* Retrieved from http://www.cancer.gov/cancertopics/factsheet/information/internet

National Center for Complementary and Alternative Medicine. (2011a). *Evaluating web-based health resources.* Retrieved from http://nccam.nih.gov/health/webresources/#ttt

National Center for Complementary and Alternative Medicine. (2011b). *NCCAM Facts-at-a-glance and mission.* Retrieved from http://nccam.nih.gov/about/ataglance/

National Library of Medicine. (2010). *Evaluating internet health information: A tutorial from the national library of medicine.* Retrieved from http://www.nlm.nih.gov/medlineplus/webeval/ webeval.html

National Library of Medicine, & National Institutes of Health. (2010). *Medline plus guide to healthy web surfing.* Retrieved from http://www.nlm.nih.gov/medlineplus/healthywebsurfing.html

National Network of Libraries of Medicine. (2011). *Bringing health information to the community.* Retrieved from http://nnlm.gov/bhic/2011/05/16/youtube-health-videos/

National Network of Libraries of Medicine. (n.d.). *Evaluating health websites.* Retrieved from http://nnlm.gov/outreach/consumer/evalsite.html

Oh, J. (2011). *5 key considerations for hospitals to ensure mobile device security.* Retrieved from http://www.beckershospitalreview.com/healthcare-information-technology/5-key-consider

Online LPN to RN. (2011). *Top 50 blogs every online nursing student should read.* Retrieved from http://onlinelpntorn.org/2011/top-50-blogs-every-online-nursing-student-should-read/

Page, D. (August, 2011). *2011 most wired innovator awards. Hospitals & Health Networks.* Retrieved from http://digital.hhnmag.com/(S(1kkon455rdglmk55b23qn355))/Default.aspx

Pallimed. (n.d.). Retrieved from http://www.pallimed.org/2005/03/about-us.html

Pew Internet & American Life Project. (February, 2011a). *Spring tracking survey.* Retrieved from http://www.pewinternet.org/Static-Pages/Trend-Data/Whos-Online.aspx

Pew Internet & American Life Project. (May, 2011b). *Peer to peer healthcare.* Retrieved from http://pewinternet.org/~/media//Files/Reports/2011/Pew_P2PHealthcare_2011.pdf

Pew Internet & American Life Project. (May, 2011c). *The social life of health information.* Retrieved from http://www.pewinternet.org/~/media//Files/Reports/2011/PIP_Social_Life_of_Health_Info.pdf

PRWeb. (2010). *New study highlights social media use among nurses; comprehensive report also sheds light on social media behaviors of physicians.* Retrieved from http://www.prweb.com/releases/Nicholson_Kovac/Healthcare_Study/prweb3646144.htm

Royal College of Nursing. (2006). *Use of text messaging services: Guidance for nurses working with children and young people.* Retrieved from http://www.rcn.org.uk/__data/assets/pdf_file/0010/78697/003035.pdf

Springer Publishing. (2011). *The Springer Publishing 2011 Nursing ebook & smartphone survey.* Retrieved from http://springerpub.com/content/downloads/Springer-Publishing_2011_Nursing_eBook-Smartphone_Survey.pdf

UPMC Extra. (2007). *MyApps helps physicians, staff work from any UPMC computer location.* Retrieved from http://extra.upmc.com/070420/MyApps.htm

U. S. Department of Health & Human Services. (2007). *Testimony by Robert Kolodner, M.D. on interoperable IT.* Retrieved from http://www.hhs.gov/asl/testify/2007/10/t20071101e.html

U. S. Department of Health & Human Services. (2010). *Final rules to support meaningful use of EHRs.* Retrieved from http://www.hhs.gov/news/imagelibrary/video/2010-07-13_press.html

U. S. Department of Health & Human Services. (2012). *Overview: American Recovery and Reinvestment Act of 2009, Implementation summary.* Retrieved from http://www.hhs.gov/recovery/overview/index.html

Yengin, D. (2011). Digital game as a new media and use of digital game in education. *The Turkish Online Journal of Design, Art and Communication, 1*(1), 20–25. Retrieved from http://www.tojdac.org/tojdac/HOME_files/v01i103.pdf

Yin, S. (2010). 10 healthcare bloggers we're thankful for. *Fierce Healthcare Daily news for Healthcare Executives.* Retrieved from http://www.fiercehealthcare.com/special-reports/10-healthcare-bloggers-were-thankful

CHAPTER 5

Consumer-Centered Virtual Health Communities

Irene Joos

LEARNING OBJECTIVES

At the completion of this chapter the reader will be able to:

1. Define virtual health communities.
2. Analyze a virtual health community using the typology presented in this chapter.
3. Discuss the role of health professionals when working with groups of patients or consumers.
4. Establish and maintain a blog related to health.
5. Describe the process of developing and posting video or slide shows on social media sites.
6. Create a podcast related to health information.
7. Compare video conferencing services.

TERMS

Collective intelligence	Virtual communities
Participatory engagement	Web conferencing
Typology	Webcast
User-generated content	

Three tenets guide Health 2.0 discussions. The first tenet is the concept of a more participatory engagement by the consumer in their own health care. The second relates to data as the key for making vital health care decisions. The third tenet refers to harnessing the collective intelligence of the Internet (Hesse et al., 2011; O'Reilly, 2005). The web has quickly evolved from the static pages of the early web to interactive tools we now call Web 2.0, including social media tools that enable collective and individual engagement. Hesse et al. (2011) listed 7 key questions or implications for health practitioners and researchers:

- How many consumers are using these participative technologies?
- Does "toxic" information available on an unfiltered web threaten patient outcomes?

- How can the health care team diffuse the damage of "toxic" information?
- What impact will expanded online access have on improving health decision-making?
- What aspects of Web 2.0 will lead to improved community and individual health or advance our understanding of treatment plans?
- What design characteristics are effective when constructing participative sites?
- What impact do the positive aspects of design have on improving the quality of online communities? (p. 2)

The key questions for this chapter are: To what extent are virtual health communities engaging patients in their health care decisions? What roles are nurses playing or should nurses play in working with patients/consumers through social media? Which of these tools promise more engagement or better consumer outcomes? To engage the reader in answering these questions, this chapter defines virtual communities and related terms, provides directions and guidelines for using Web 2.0 tools when working with groups of patients or other consumers, and examines blogging and webcasts as two representative tools. This chapter examines virtual health communities from the perspective of a patient or consumer.

VIRTUAL COMMUNITIES DEFINED

While there is no one universal definition of a virtual community, there are some common threads in many of the definitions. In his classic book, *The Virtual Community: Homesteading on the Electronic Frontier* (2000), Rheingold defines virtual communities as "social aggregations that emerge from the Net when enough people carry on those public discussions long enough, with sufficient human feeling, to form webs of personal relationships in cyberspace" (p. xx). Rheingold goes further to say that "People in virtual communities use words on screens to exchange pleasantries and argue, engage in intellectual discourse, conduct commerce, exchange knowledge, share emotional support, make plans, brainstorm, gossip, feud, fall in love, find friends and lose them, play games, flirt, create a little high art and a lot of idle talk" (p. xvii). Boetcher, Duggan, and White (2002) define an online or virtual community as "a gathering of people, in an online space where they come, communicate, connect, and get to know each other better over time." They go on to say that people join virtual communities to socialize, collaborate, and discuss issues or causes. Porter (2004) defines a virtual community as "an aggregation of individuals or business partners who interact around a shared interest, where the interaction is at least partially supported and/or mediated by technology and guided by some protocols or norms." She then describes three types of communities: communities of commercial orientation, of interest, and of fantasy.

Common threads emerging in these definitions include:

- Frequent interaction with the many members of the community,
- A common single-defining focus or interest,
- A social identification that attracts and retains members, and
- A service that fulfills a need.

An aggregation of people is not necessarily a community; it is only a collection of individuals unless these people have something in common and interact with each other on a regular basis. When the term "virtual" is added, the interaction relies on some form of web technologies or common online platform. Some would argue that the Internet is a virtual community, but many disagree, as it lacks some of the essential components of a community, which are more focused and share something in common other than their virtual nature (Song, 2009). The Internet uses many platforms (search sites, social networks, commercial web pages, blogs, databases, etc.) for many purposes (buying, selling, information seeking, communication, etc.); a virtual community shares a common platform like a social network, wiki, or blog site, and has a common interest point, purpose, or focus. In this book, a virtual community is defined as a gathering of individuals who share a common interest, focus, or need, who use an Internet platform to frequently interact with each other, and who identify with the predefined community, which provides a sense of belonging or ownership. Virtual health communities are those that focus on

- Healthy lifestyles or health promotion;
- Diagnosis, treatment, and knowledge sharing around specific conditions;
- Marketing health expertise, like the Mayo Clinic blogs and podcasts;
- Support for people experiencing the same health problem;
- Promotion of research and funding for specific health problems through patient organizations (Guillamon, Armayones, Hernandez, & Gomez-Zuniga, 2010); and
- Sharing or continuing education for health professionals.

Typology

Porter (2004) proposed a typology of virtual communities in her article "A Typology of Virtual Communities: A Multi-Disciplinary Foundation for Future Research." This typology has two levels: the establishment level and the relationship orientation level. The establishment level includes organization-sponsored and member-initiated communities. Commercial or noncommercial organizations initiate and sponsor organization-sponsored virtual communities. Developers design these virtual communities to meet the mission or goals of the sponsoring organization. Examples of these types of virtual communities include Aids.gov (http://aids.gov/), which not only provides educational materials, but uses social media tools like blogs and podcasts to engage the audience; the Mayo Clinic Expert blogs (http://www.mayoclinic.com/health/blogs/BlogIndex), where patients can follow and participate in blogs about specific conditions; and the Joint Commission's Health care wiki (http://wikihealthcare.jointcommission.org/bin/view/Home/WebHome) for health care professionals.

Founders or community members who share a specific area of interest establish and maintain member initiated communities; many other members participate in these member-initiated communities. These members may be people looking for assistance in maintaining a healthy lifestyle, patients with specific medical conditions, or family members of patients with health issues. Examples of these types of communities include Shot of Prevention (http://shotofprevention.com/) and the *Slightly Alive* blog (http://slightlyalive.blogspot.com/).

The second typology level involves the relationship orientation (Porter, 2004); that is, who is interacting with whom within the relationship and the purpose or reason for the relationship—social, task-oriented, fantasy, and/or communication within a virtual world community. Organization-sponsored communities encourage relationships between members and the sponsoring organization, while member-initiated communities encourage social or professional relationships among members.

A systematic typology provides a framework for describing, classifying, and examining virtual communities. It is a valuable aid in conducting research into the effectiveness of virtual communities as well as framework for analyzing and implementing a virtual community as a tool in health promotion.

Community Attributes

Community attributes are the characteristics of a community and can be used to describe the unique nature of that community Porter (2004) presents the Five Ps as attributes of a virtual community:

- Purpose
- Place (technology interaction)
- Platform (design of interaction)
- Population interaction structure (pattern of interaction)
- Profit model (return on interaction).

Using a systems approach, Joos proposes the use of three attributes to describe the unique characteristics of a virtual community.

> *Purpose*—Why was this community established? What is the purpose of this virtual health community? The purpose can be related to information sharing and support around a host of health related issues. Examples of assessment questions that could identify the purpose of a health-related virtual community include: Is the purpose for information sharing around a specific disease condition like diabetes, cancer, and so on? Is it to provide support for people with congenital disorders or chronic conditions? Is it support for patients and family going through the same crisis? Is the purpose to share information concerning what works and what doesn't in promoting a healthy lifestyle? Is the purpose to create an online reference or resource for others with the same challenge? The clearer the purpose, the more effectively one can design the structure of the community.
>
> *Structure*—Structure refers to the organization of the community to facilitate performance of its functions. Porter (2004) refers to structure as place and platform while others include the concept of sponsors. Questions to ask here are: What is the location of the interaction (place)? This takes on the form of bounded space, like a URL, and sense of place, like belonging to a specific social media site like Facebook or LinkedIn. How is communication structured? Are there limits to the number of people who can join the community? Can anyone join and contribute? Does the technical platform support synchronous and/or asynchronous communication? How many individuals can interact on a synchronous basis at the same time?
> Who is sponsoring the virtual community and what are their motivations? Is there a profit motive? Who is maintaining the virtual community on a day-to-day basis? Groups and organizations sponsor many virtual health communities that target consumers. This can be desirable if it involves health professionals in monitoring the site and correcting misinformation, or this can be less than desirable if the only purpose is to market a product such as herbal remedies for increased energy, increased sexual interest, and anything else that "ails" you.

Function—Function refers to what the virtual community actually does to achieve or meet its purpose. One might consider functional concepts like boundaries, acceptable rules of behavior or conduct, sustainability, and relationships or interactions. Some key questions here might include: What are the rules of conduct for this virtual community? What happens when one member violates the rules? Can you be a member and not actively participate in the discussions or support, that is, is it acceptable to lurk? What regulations might come into play? Who can interact with whom? What keeps this virtual community alive and well? Are there key members that make this virtual community work? What role do they play? What do members gain from belonging to this community?

Health-related virtual communities are growing rapidly in number and scope. An important area for future nursing research involves identifying the attributes of virtual health communities that effectively promote the health of individuals and communities. Are some attributes more important to the effectiveness than others? Are there attributes that can be identified as risk factors for an unhealthy community? Evolving concepts that will help identify these attributes include:

Collective intelligence—According to Dictionary.com, "a phenomenon in sociology where a shared or group intelligence emerges from the collaboration and competition of many individuals" (Collective Intelligence, n.d.). This is a snapshot of what patients are doing or thinking as it relates to some aspect of their health care where they share and discuss their conditions, treatments, and so on. Collective intelligence is not a new term; what is new is the means of communicating data and the potential reach of that data.

Participatory engagement—Participatory engagement is a cooperative health care model that actively involves the patient and/or patient caregiver as an integral part of the full range of care continuum. This participation generally involves a patient with access to the web, access to data/information relevant to the patient's health care needs, and ability to share or engage in the decision–making process.

HEALTH CARE PROFESSIONAL ROLES

In 2010, the American Nurses Association published the newly revised ANA Nursing: Scope and Standards of Nursing Practice. These standards form the foundation for nursing practice in all settings, roles, and specialties. Underlying these standards are five tenets. The second of these tenets states, "The registered nurse establishes partnerships with persons, families, support systems, and other providers, utilizing in-person and electronic communications, to reach a shared goal of health care" (American Nurses Association [ANA], 2010, p. 4). This tenet suggests that nurses with other health care professionals are charged with the responsibility of understanding and utilizing virtual communities as another tool in their goal of promoting heath. There are several reasons nurses should take a leadership role in this responsibility:

- The nursing profession is the largest segment of the health care work force.
- Consumers are increasingly accessing the Internet and social media sites to seek information and support in managing their health and understanding health issues (Pew Research Center, 2009).

- An increasing number of nurses are using social media sites for professional reasons—seeking jobs, or finding information related to medical conditions and treatments.
- Many health care institutions, organizations, and schools of nursing have a social media presence.
- Traditional means of health promotion and behavioral changes are not always successful (Ressler & Glazer, 2010).
- Many health care delivery systems have an established website and are beginning to establish virtual health communities.
- Social media opens new access to vulnerable and underserved communities.

With more consumers and patients accessing health care information, nurses must understand the technology, the online resources available, and how patients are using social media sites. Within the world of expanding virtual communities, nurses must assume a leadership and advocacy role in helping to develop and share timely health care information with patients, consumers, families, and communities.

Roles

When discussing the role of nurses in use of social media, there are four basic role concepts that are of importance: role conception, role expectation, role behavior, and role gap (Collaboration Health Care, n.d.).

> *Role conception*—describes what nurses believe to be their role in accordance with course work, nurse practice acts, and what is experienced in the actual practice of nursing. These are nurses' beliefs about the behaviors, rights, and obligations that are foundational to practicing as a nurse. Do evolving patterns of electronic communication within society now support the reality that the role concept of nurses includes working in social media?

> *Role expectation*—describes what patients, consumers, other nurses, administration, and other health professionals expect nurses to do as they practice nursing. Do patients, consumers, and other health care professionals expect nursing involvement in social media as part of their practice? What do institutions that employ nurses say about use of social media in nursing practice? These are key questions to ask in defining how nurses should function within virtual communities.

> *Role behavior*—the activities that a nurse actually performs when providing care. When nurses are using social media as a tool in the provision of care and the promotion of health, what actual behaviors should be expected of nurses in this role?

> *Role gap*—exists when there is a difference between nursing expectation and role behavior. Role behaviors are the actual behaviors or actions of nurses in their role as nurses. Is there a gap between expectations and behavior as to nurses' involvement in virtual health care communities? For example, do current employee policies support or discourage a nursing role with social media?

The expanding roles of nurses in today's health care system are changing expectations. The result is a role gap between historical roles and increasing demands for new activities and responsibilities. Given the economic climate today, institutions expect nurses to be a major resource in providing efficient, effective, quality care. The key buzz words are outcomes and value. To meet these mandates, nurses must:

- Be innovative in delivering aspects of care and collaborate with others to make it happen. This may mean working with public health agencies, hospitals, consumers, and other health care providers to use social media to its fullest advantage.
- Communicate and coordinate various aspects of care, from living a healthy lifestyle to issues of death and dying and everything in between. It is no longer sufficient to see the patient out of the hospital. Nurses now oversee patient safety at home, and, when possible, prevent readmissions. Social media has the potential to help make this happen. Nurses need to extend their services to the home environment through use of social media.
- Educate health care consumers. Consumers expect more than a handout or printed piece of paper. Some of this education must be in the form of multimedia/ demonstration-type educational materials. Nursing education must include the use of social media sites and engagement of consumers in virtual communities in the nursing curriculum. Nurses must also play a role in educating the consumer on how to safely use these virtual community sites and how to evaluate the information that they obtain on the Internet.
- Be a change agent in bringing healthy virtual health communities to the table as the country discusses health care reform.

Nurses must embrace these new roles with social media while keeping in mind privacy; confidentiality; patient rights; ethical, moral, and legal considerations; and professionalism. These new roles extend to all nurses: acute care, outpatient, home health, school, long-term care, and future practice settings. All nurses should explore the virtual extension of their services to individuals in the hospital, the community, or within community living environments. Nurses can consider the use of these virtual communities while patients are still in the health care setting.

Patient

Historically, health care professionals have been accustomed to consumers who were passive recipients of care. Health care professionals told patients what was expected and it was up to them to either comply or not. Today, patients are demanding and playing an increasingly active role in designing their plan of care. The health care environment is moving toward a patient participatory focus. This change can often be seen during the initial visit of a patient with a health care provider. Patients are coming prepared to their provider's office with content to discuss or review. When a new diagnosis is made or new medication prescribed, the number of questions and issues to be discussed can be expected to increase. This change can in many ways be traced to the use of the Internet as an information resource. Families noting alternative forms of treatment often join the patient in their search for more complete information about their diagnosis and treatment.

The use of media can be expected to continue when patients are hospitalized. When a patient is admitted, the patient may receive materials to read about their diagnosis and treatment, instructions to watch a video on the hospital TV channel, or a procedure to review on an iPad provided by the hospital. The health care professional may then return to answer their questions or in some cases give them a short quiz to ascertain what they need further help with understanding. The role of the consumer now includes active participation in being a care navigator, family benefits manager, information manager, and legal manager. How will the nurse help the patient with these changing roles? Virtual communities and the role nurses take with them may provide some of the answers.

CONSUMER-ORIENTED VIRTUAL HEALTH COMMUNITIES

While research related to the effectiveness of virtual health communities is non-conclusive, consumers are indeed using these virtual communities to seek information and support on a variety of health issues (Eysenbach, Powell, Englesakis, Rizo, & Stern, 2004). Consumers are increasingly requesting discussion forums as part of their patient-support services, and organizations such as Kaiser Permanente and Johns Hopkins are complying with that request (Priya, 2011). Others find that supportive groups can negate the effects of stress for some types of problems, like infertility among women (Welbourne, Blancard, & Boughton, 2009). Hoch and Ferguson (2005) listed the following items that they discovered while monitoring Braintalk (a community of neurology patients and caregivers) in their article, *What I've Learned from E-Patients*:

- Patients want to know about their disease and treatments,
- A community like BrainTalk (http://www.braintalkcommunities.org/) is more comprehensive than many physicians and specialists, and
- A growing number of patients are empowering themselves.

The article identifies several advantages of participating in virtual health communities:

- Provision of information and advice from others undergoing similar health problems,
- Exchange of emotional support,
- Positive psychosocial outcomes and enhanced well-being from frequent postings that focus on gaining insight into their struggles,
- Development of a sense of community, and
- Adherence to treatment.

Additional advantages include participation 24/7 at the convenience of the consumer, no physical border limitations, and a sense of anonymity.

The major cited disadvantage is a concern for misinformation, but as Hoch and Ferguson (2005) monitored the BrainTalk site, they found that other members of the community frequently correct the 6% of misinformation found on BrainTalk. Additional disadvantages reflect literacy and technical issues. They include the requirement to read, write, and type; the need to access the Internet and related technology; the time-consuming nature of participation; and the possibility of losing touch with the real world by spending so much time in the virtual world.

Examples of Virtual Health Communities

The virtual communities included in this section are not an exhaustive list of such communities, but are representative samplings of these types of sites. Some are reputable sites; others are questionable. They include wikis, blogs, and websites sponsored by both individuals and organizations. These sites and related links were current as of the writing of this book. There is no significance to the order in which they are presented.

As you explore these sites, use the typology and attributes previously presented to ask if they meet the critical factors (interaction or engagement, sense of community, and frequent use) that create a healthy virtual health community. Determine the purpose or need this site might serve. If the site is established by a sponsor, determine the goals of the sponsor. Identify who could benefit from the site and what benefits they might obtain. Determine if there are any warnings or risk factors that should be included in patient education materials related to these sites.

> *CFVoice (corporate sponsor, website;* http://www.cfvoice.com/index.jsp?— CFVoice is an online community for people of all ages living with cystic fibrosis (see Figure 5.1). The website says that it "is a place for motivation, inspiration and connection to the CF community." Novartis Pharmaceuticals sponsors this site and it contains many podcasts and videos for patients of all ages as well as their caregivers. There are also games for young patients and recipes for families. This is an example of an organization-sponsored site for learn- ing about the disease and how others are coping with it. Novartis has started a new site: MyCFConnection at http://www.mycfconnection.com/index.jsp? At this site users can share their experiences in a true user-centered approach (see

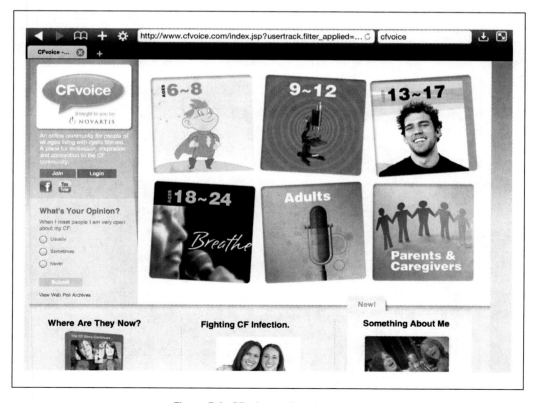

Figure 5.1 *CFvoice main web screen.*

Figure 5.2). There are many sites like this one, covering a range of topics on chronic diseases. Notice the selection at the bottom of the screen to identify a user as a patient, caregiver/family member, or health care professional.

Empowering Consumer Health (***individual, new wiki***; http://empowering consumerhealth.wikispaces.com/)—This is an example of a new wiki that is attempting to empower consumers by providing information about health (see Figure 5.3). It is consumer-run, with at the time of this publication only three members. Note the list of topics that one can write under; users may also create new topics. The question for this example is: Will they have a sufficient mass of contributors to keep it going? Will there be sufficient updates to make it worth being a member of this wiki? Since it is relatively new and there is no indication of who these three people are, would you trust the information on this site? Can you see when someone last updated it?

Diabetes wiki (***individual, wiki***; http://diabetes.wikia.com/wiki/Diabetes_ Wiki)—This site is an example of a wiki that raises questions and concerns (see Figure 5.4). There are a variety of topics about diabetes, but there is no indication of who runs this site, who belongs, when the pages were updated, and what resources support the content. While there are some cute pictures, the content is sparse. The navigation has many dead-end pages that require users to use the back button to return to their original place. This wiki host, known as wikia, is popular as a gaming and entertainment wiki. Should patients use this site? When selecting a hosting site, why would you select this hosting site?

CaringBridge (***nonprofit organization, website***; http://www.caringbridge.org/)— This website offers free personal and private websites to provide a place for people experiencing major health issues to connect with family/friends and receive

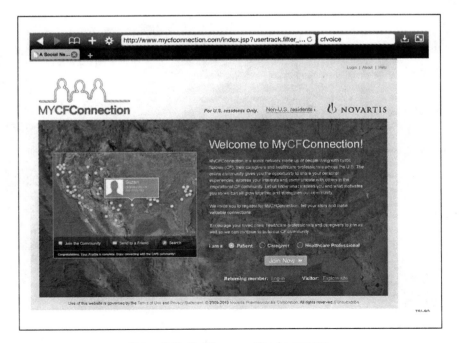

Figure 5.2 *MyCF connection homepage.*

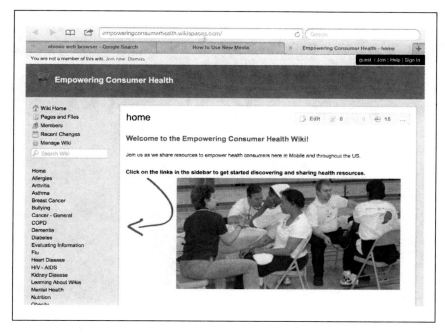

Figure 5.3 *Empowering Consumer Health homepage.*

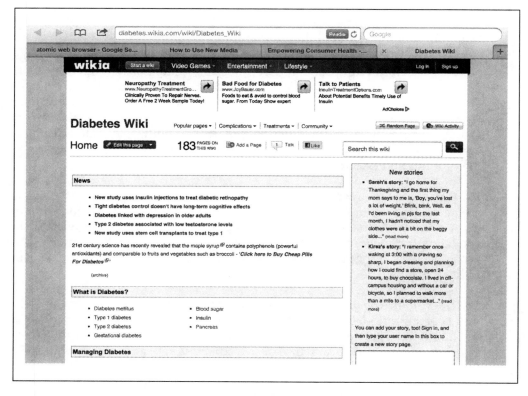

Figure 5.4 *Diabetes wiki homepage.*

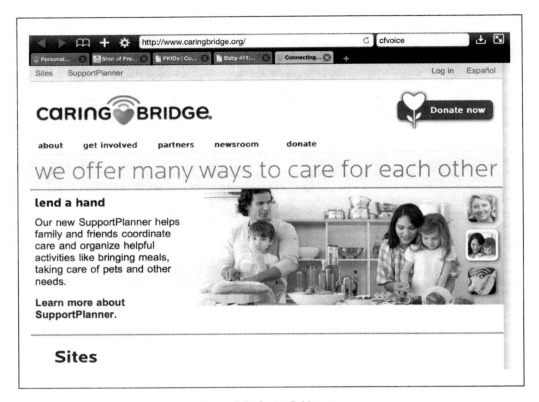

Figure 5.5 *CaringBridge.org.*

the support needed to make their journey easier (see Figure 5.5). Visitors to the private site can leave messages of love, hope, and compassion in the guestbook. It is supported totally by contributions. Patients provide their health updates on their private website. Does this type of site serve a purpose? Check out their statistics on the About CaringBridge page—half-a-million people connect through their site each day and they have more than 1 billion visits to consumer-created personal websites. Now, examine their ratings and awards pages as to their ratings and rewards.

Shot of Prevention (*individual, blog*; http://shotofprevention.com/)—This is a blog run by two mothers and the Executive Director of Every Child by Two (see Figure 5.6). It addresses making decisions about immunizations of children, providing comments and contacts on legislation, research findings, global citizenship issues, and dealing with schools and doctors. It is a good example of an individual blog.

PKIDS (*private organization, website*; http://www.pkids.org/)—The mission of this organization, Parents of Kids with Infectious Diseases, is to educate the public about infectious diseases, how to prevent infectious diseases, how infectious diseases are spread, and the latest in advances in treatment (see Figure 5.7). Started by two mothers who had trouble finding babysitters for their children with an infectious disease, it provides social media tools to help families deal with children living with preventable infectious diseases by providing a forum for discussions and support. There is also a link to ask the advice nurse!

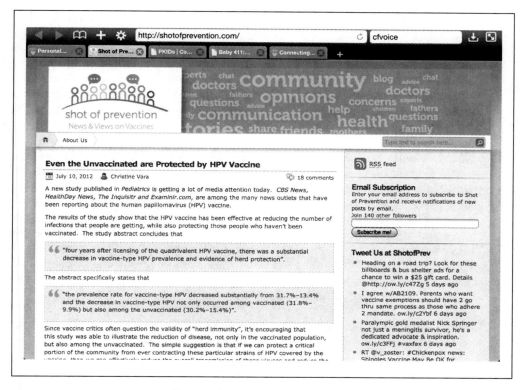

Figure 5.6 Shot of Prevention *blog.*

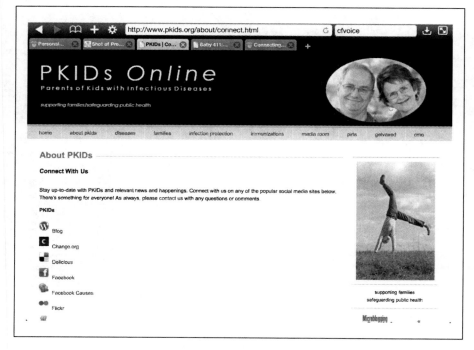

Figure 5.7 *PKIDS homepage.*

Baby 411 (organization, website; http://windsorpeak.com/sites/baby411/ blog/)—By the title of this website one might assume this is a site about learning how to take care of your new baby (see Figure 5.8). In reality, the authors of a book by the same name, Ari Brown, MD., and Denise Fields, MOM., are using this site to market their book and a new book called *Expecting 411.* While there are some interesting blogs and alerts on this site, one has to purchase the book to obtain the full range of information that the book contains. The website provides selected information from the book.

The M.E. and CFS Information Page and the Slightly Alive blog (individual, website and blog; http://www.cfids-me.org/index.html#Info4 and http:// slightlyalive.blogspot.com/)—This site (see Figure 5.9) includes an informational website with a link to a blog that covers a condition that is difficult to diagnose. It chronicles a PhD-prepared social scientist's experience with her disease, treatment, and attempts to find out more about what was going on with her health. There are many links to research sites and conferences addressing this issue— ME/CFS (Myalgic Encephalomyelitis/Chronic Fatigue Syndrome). Questions to ask are: Do the links work? Do they send the user to reputable sites? Can one verify that this information is accurate?

As can be seen from these examples, there is a wide range of virtual health communities available. Using the typology and attributes previously presented, one can

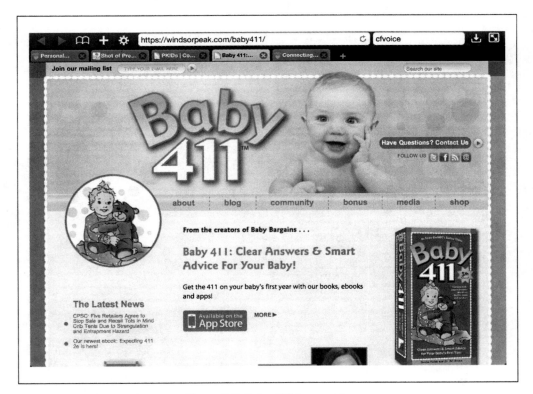

Figure 5.8 *Baby 411 homepage.*

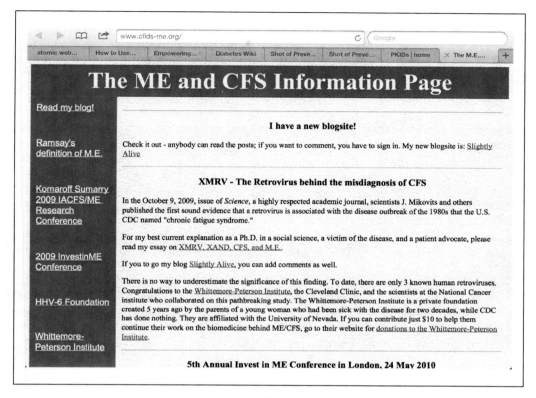

Figure 5.9 *ME and CFS information page.*

determine what educational content nurses might include to guide consumers in selecting appropriate virtual communities. In addition, one can identify what they as nurses might contribute to the community.

BUILDING A VIRTUAL HEALTH COMMUNITY

Boetcher et al. (2002) identify several steps for building a virtual community:

- Identify your community purpose or goal,
- Decide on the interaction tools to use to achieve the purpose and serve the target audience,
- Decide how to structure the space,
- Decide how to host or facilitate the virtual health community,
- Build it,
- Attract consumers, and
- Nurture it.

Once the purpose or goal is identified, start thinking about the tools, hosting, and design of the social media site. Discussed next are three tools for building virtual health communities and a few resources for learning how to use those tools.

Blogging

Chapter 2 sets forth a general introduction to the blogging social media tool. It includes pointers for starting a blog. A few additional pointers specific to health-related blogs include:

- Do the research. Read other blogs on similar topics to see what is working and what already exists. Use Technorati (a blog search engine mentioned in Chapter 2) to find relevant blogs to review.
- Ask what you liked and didn't like about the blogs that you reviewed. How effectively does the blog promote the health of the members? How will you handle comments or misinformation in your blog? How will you promote the blog to the people most likely to benefit from the blog? How can you make the blog easy to use or navigate?
- Support your posts with resources or links.
- Be careful in the use of medical terms and jargon. Make sure you pay attention to the reading level of the targeted consumers.
- Keep posts reasonable in length. People don't like to read dissertations in blogs.
- Format posts following good publication guidelines. For example, use a consistent template or format, grab the reader's attention with catchy headlines or pictures, use subtitles for ease of reading, and write at a level appropriate to this audience (Centers for Disease Control and Prevention [CDC], 2011).

Blog Resources

The following few resources should be useful when learning how to blog. Remember that the nature of the Internet is to constantly change. Learn to search for resources that help you to learn how to use a blog. Most blogging sites have a help section. There are also additional websites with tutorials and videos to help bloggers learn how to blog. The important point is to learn how to find and use tutorials and help guides when necessary. These examples use Blogger and WordPress, but there are also similar types of help for LiveJournal and TypePad.

Blogger Help

Blogger Tutorial (http://www.blogger.com/tour_start.g). This is a simple tutorial by blogger.com about what a blog is and how to get started.
List of Tutorials for Blogger (http://www.simplebloggertutorials.com/2009/07/simple-blogger-tutorials-list.html). This is a great site that lists many tutorials on how to use Blogger. It includes subtopics like basics, templates, tips and tricks, widgets, and so on.
Teacher Training Videos (http://www.teachertrainingvideos.com/blogger/index.html). This is a demo on learning how to use Blogger. The left side has a list of the available videos. It features screen captures as someone demonstrates the keystrokes to complete various tasks.

WordPress Help

WordPress.Org. (http://codex.wordpress.org/Main_Page). WordPress comes in both a .com (hosted) and .org (you host) version. This site, WordPress Codex, provides many tutorials on using WordPress and considers itself the online manual for WordPress.

Free WordPress Training (http://freewptraining.com/learn-wordpress-with-free-easy-step-by-step-training). There are a host of training videos at this site.

WordPress101-TutorialVideos (http://www.webbusinessreviews.com/wordpress-101-tutorials.html). This site provides some basic tutorials to help make the most of WordPress.

Health Care Blog Help

CasesBlog—Medical and Health Blog (http://casesblog.blogspot.com/2008/02/how-to-write-medical-blog-and-not-get.html). This site provides seven tips for writing medical blogs and a video on how to get started with Blogger.com.

CDC's Guide to Writing for Social Media (http://www.cdc.gov/socialmedia/Tools/guidelines/pdf/GuidetoWritingforSocialMedia.pdf). This document provides a lot of examples of do's and don'ts for writing for social media like blogs and tweets. It also includes social network sites and web pages.

Vascular Medicine: Evidence Based Vascular Medicine Review (http://www.angiologist.com/10-tips-for-a-successful-medical-blog/). There are a few tips on how to make your health blog stand out from the rest of them.

Health Works Collective (http://healthworkscollective.com/node/30402). This page focuses on how to market your health care blog.

Podcasts

General information about podcasting was in Chapter 2. Anderson (2009) states that "… the number of podcasts is growing related to consumer health" (p. 120). Health care providers need to understand what consumers are doing with podcasts and to contribute to quality podcasts targeted to consumers. While podcasts are a great tool for disseminating information, they are not an interactive, participatory tool. Their advantage is their convenient format for listening and learning on the go. Links to podcasts are on blogs, websites, and wikis. The CDC (2011) lists eight best practices for podcast production:

- Define the purpose—target audience, message, and communication goal.
- Create audience-relevant content—use appropriate consumer-related terms and language.
- Consider length—consider the topic and attention span of the audience; shorter is generally better. Where appropriate, divide into a series to keep any one podcast at 5 to 10 minutes.
- Develop and post a transcript of the podcast—this helps consumers who would like to refer to the material later in print form. Some may also prefer to follow along with the printed word while listening to the podcast.
- Develop a release schedule and post frequently—this applies to podcasts in a series. This may also keep your audience returning.
- Utilize cross-marketing—post links to the podcasts on websites, social networking sites, and so on.
- Provide additional information—provide additional resources the consumer may investigate, but make sure the content of the podcast stands alone.
- Connect with the audience (p. 14).

Equipment necessary for creating podcasts depends on whether the podcast contains video, audio, or both. For an audio podcast the recorder will need a computer with a sound card, speakers, and an Internet connection; headphones with microphone; software to record the sound, like Sound Recorder, Windows Movie Maker, Audacity, or Garageband; and software that permits saving the podcast as or converting it to an MP3 (audio only) format file. For video podcasting, the recorder will also need a video camera or webcam plus movie editing software like Windows Movie Maker, iMovie, or Camtasia Studio, and a file format converter for MPEG-4 (audio and video) files. Once the podcast is complete, a hosting site like YouTube, PodPress, iTunes, or Amazon S3 will be needed. There are many podcast hosting sites depending on the nature and intended audience for the podcast. Some examples include the World Health Organization's, website (http://www.who.int/mdeicacentre/multimedia/podcasts/en/), the CDC (http://www2c.cdc.gov/podcasts/browse.asp), and YouTube (http://youtube.com) under health and diseases, as well as regional health care facilities.

Podcasting Resources

Several resources for learning how to podcast include:

CDC's Audio Script Writing Guide (http://www2c.cdc.gov/podcasts/AudioScriptWritingGuide.pdf). This document provides general and script writing guidelines.

Podcast Answer Man (http://podcastanswerman.com/learn-how-to-podcast/). While the creator of this resource is marketing his services, there are a lot of simple video tutorials at this site.

The Ultimate Guide to Podcasting (http://www.cumbrowski.com/podcastingguide.asp). This guide contains resources as well as an online tutorial with screenshots. There is a wealth of information for the beginner as well as for more advanced podcasters.

What You Need to Make Your Own Podcast (http://radio.about.com/od/createyourownpodcast/u/What-Equipment-Software-Hardware-Tips-You-Need-To-Create-And-Make-Your-Own-Podcast.htm). This website is sponsored by About.com and includes legal issues related to podcasting as well as information about what is necessary and some tips and tricks.

Learning Guide: Podcasting (http://www.wyomingextension.org/wiki/index.php5?title=Learning_Guide:Podcasting). Hosted by the University of Wyoming Extension organization, this material covers requirements, resources, and references.

Web Conferencing (Webinar)

A webcast is a media presentation broadcast as a live video feed over the Internet to a large number of users and a small number of presenters using streaming technology

(MediaPlatform, 2010). This differs from podcasts, which users download to a device with streaming media playing as it downloads. Sponsors of webcasts can, however, save webcasts for later streaming. Commercial and private individuals use webcasts to get their message out in an inexpensive mode. Individual users can use social media forums like YouTube, BrightTALK, or Mediasite. Sponsors generally use webcasts as a broadcast medium, not as an interactive medium.

Web conferencing, sometimes called a webinar, is an interactive meeting conducted over the Internet, generally in real time, with 50 or less attendees. Web conferencing permits the sharing of the conference content with remote locations. Web conferencing is useful for meetings, training, lectures, and short presentations. It can also be suitable to hold office hours or to have interactive sessions with patients. These are more interactive in nature than webcasts and can include questions and answers, polling, and full participation with the audience. Web conferences can include:

- Slide shows
- Live video
- Real-time audio either over the phone or Internet
- Recording of the web conference
- White boards for annotation of discussions
- Text chat
- Screen sharing.

Web conferencing is generally a server-side service, meaning that participants connect to the web conference through a browser with a phone and webcam. Some common ones include Connect, Collaborate, Skype, Live Meeting, GoToMeeting, BigBlueButton, and WebEx. Check with your institution for what might be available for hosting and interacting with consumers in a web conferencing format.

As with any of the social media used in virtual communities, planning and preparation are critical to the use of this media. What is necessary is a computer or wireless device connected to the Internet, an audio connection through the computer or phone, and possibly a webcam. Roseberry (n.d.) suggests the following preparation for conducting a web conference:

- Plan ahead—look for time zone conflicts, notify participants of the date, time, duration, web address, login information, and any firewall potential issues.
- Web camera adjustments—make sure the presenter is on center and that the head is not cut off, focus the camera for a clear picture, and make movements slow or risk a blurry image.
- Microphones, speakers, and headphones—watch for sound feedback and adjust the microphone appropriately. Sound carries, so avoid extraneous movements like shuffling papers, sounds from a radio or TV, or other types of background noise, and, of course, no chewing. Headset phone models are the best so the presenter doesn't tire holding the phone.
- Appearance—dress for success. Consider appropriate business attire.
- Lighting—make sure lighting is sufficient so that the presenter is not in the dark, in a shadow, or bothered by glare.
- Test out the software before the conference. Practice helps here.
- Presentation—practice and practice. Stay on the topic and on time. Keep questions on the topic. Smile and act naturally.

Web Conferencing Resources

Web Conference Preparation Checklist (http://www.rotary.org/RIdocuments/en_doc/training_web_conference_prep_checklist_en.doc). This document is prepared by The Rotary International Organization and is a word document outline for what the presenter needs to do starting at 2 months before the web conference through to after the web conference.

How To Successfully Prepare for a Web Conference (http://www.incommconferencing.com/blog/How-To-Successfully-Prepare-for-a-Web-Conference.htm). This is provided by a consulting firm offering services related to web conferencing.

Various Vendors. Various vendors offer resources on their websites specific to their product. For example, Adobe Connect (http://www.adobe.com/products/adobeconnect.html) Blackboard's Collaborate (http://www.blackboard.com/Platforms/Collaborate/Overview.aspx), Cisco's WebEx (http://www.webex.com/), Citrix's GoToMeeting (http://www.gotomeeting.com/), and so forth.

SUMMARY

Virtual health communities have created a means for patients to further develop better understanding of and behavior toward treatment and health practices. This chapter presented a definition and typology for examining virtual health communities. It discussed the role of the nurse in virtual health communities along with several tools for facilitating virtual health communities. Given the potential legal issues with use of social media, the health care provider should refer to Chapter 9.

While consumers' use of virtual health communities is increasing, research on the extent to which this use impacts health outcomes is still in its infancy (Bastida, McGrath, & Maude, 2010; Frost & Massagli, 2008; Richardson et al., 2010). This is one area of research where nurses could make a difference in moving consumers toward the Health 2.0 agenda (Crespo, 2007).

DISCUSSION QUESTIONS

1. How do you define a community? How does that definition differ and how is it the same when you talk about virtual health communities? Support your responses with an appropriate resource.
2. When assessing a virtual health community that you might recommend to a consumer or patient, what are the critical components one should evaluate in that community? What would you tell them about joining and participating in a virtual health community?
3. What role do you see for nurses in virtual health care communities? Justify and support your answer.
4. A patient who is being discharged from the hospital has a very limited support system at home. The patient has heard of some online support services for adults with cancer and asks you to recommend a few. Provide the patient with one or two

recommendations. Explain why you chose those two and eliminated others. How did you go about finding reputable virtual communities? What else would you tell this patient about participating in virtual health communities?

EXERCISES

Exercise 1: Virtual Health Communities Defined

Purpose: *The purpose of this group exercise is to utilize a crowdsourcing process to develop a definition of the term "virtual health community."*

Objectives
1. Develop a working definition for a virtual health community.
2. Use a wiki server to work together with classmates to develop and refine the definition.
3. Produce a podcast to share the resulting definition.

Directions
1. One student creates the group wiki and invites all group members to join it. Alternatively, the faculty may create the group wikis and assign students to different groups.
2. Each student finds one podcast, video, and reference to share with the group that will assist the group in determining the key concepts inherent in defining a virtual health community. Think about how one defines a community and how virtual communities are the same or different.
3. The group develops a working document that is refined and edited to produce the final definition. This should also include a rationale for the components of the definition.
4. Using the final definition, the group produces a podcast to share its definition of a virtual health community.

Exercise 2: Assessment Form for Evaluating a Virtual Health Community

Purpose: *The purpose of this assignment is to develop a form that nurses can use in assessing virtual health communities. This assessment form could then be published on a resource site for nurses who are helping their patients find reputable virtual communities to join, or provided to patients to use when deciding which virtual communities to join.*

Objectives
1. Develop an assessment form for evaluating virtual health communities.
2. Use the form to evaluate a virtual health community.

Directions
1. Reread the material in this chapter dealing with definitions, typology, and attributes of virtual communities.

2. Read the Chen and Chang (2010) article, "Identifying Crucial Website Quality Factors of Virtual Communities" available at: http://www.iaeng.org/publication/IMECS2010/IMECS2010_pp487-492.pdf. Ask yourself what parts of these quality factors should be a part of your assessment form.
3. Find at least 3 other references (do not use any from the reference list) that define virtual communities.
4. Develop a template in Word with the evaluation features. This means the categories and questions you would use to gather information about a virtual health community. You might also want to have a feature at the end for the user to input yes or no, or to use a rating scale with some evaluative comment about this community.
5. Use this form and evaluate a virtual health community. Alternatively, you can use these sites to determine if this meets the requirements:
   - ReachOut.com at http://us.reachout.com/
   - Slightly Alive blog at http://slightlyalive.blogspot.com/
6. Submit your form and completed assessment as directed by the professor.

Exercise 3: Monitor a Virtual Health Community

Purpose: *The purpose of this exercise is to provide you with an experience in monitoring a health-related virtual community and to spark discussion on the role of the nurse in such a site.*

Objectives
1. Monitor a virtual health care community for a few weeks.
2. Discuss the role of the nurse in working with that site.

Directions
1. Select a health-related site where patients may post their questions or support each other. This can be an organizational or individual site.
2. Check into the site three times a week. Create a table in Word that you can use to keep track of the following:
   - Keep a record of how many posts appear and how many different people are posting.
   - Identify the nature of the posts, i.e. questions, responses, and content.
   - Make an evaluation of the accuracy of the information shared.
   - Identify the possible role of the nurse on this virtual health community.
   - What impact might a nurse's presence in this community have on the nature of the information and interaction of the consumers?
3. Share a summary of your findings with your classmates.

Exercise 4: Validating Content on a Virtual Health Community (Individual)

Purpose: *The purpose of this exercise is to validate information from a website/blog written by an individual who is experiencing a specific disease condition.*

Objectives

1. Compare the critical content on a website/blog to information published on known reputable websites.
2. Evaluate whether you would recommend that site to a patient with that condition.
3. Discuss the role nursing might take with rare or hard-to-diagnose conditions.

Directions

1. Go to http://www.cfids-me.org/index.html#Info4 and http://slightlyalive.blogspot .com/. Select content found on the website and blog that you believe is critical in understanding this condition.
2. Validate or dispute the selected information by using bibliographic databases like CINAHL, Medline, etc. and reputable health care information websites like WebMD, CDC, NIH, and so on.
3. Create a document that presents your comparison of the accuracy of the information on the website/blog with the information from the more established source.
4. Make a recommendation based on your analysis about the accuracy of the information on the website/blog.
5. Discuss what role you see for a nurse on this website/blog.

Exercise 5: Creating and Maintaining a Blog

Purpose: *The purpose of this exercise is to learn how to create and maintain a blog while paying attention to what attracts and keeps readers and participants. This is a blog with the purpose of informing and interacting with consumers around a health topic.*

Objectives

1. Create a blog following the guidelines presented in this chapter and Chapter 2.
2. Use a help guide, tutorials, or videos to learn how to design and add content to a blog.
3. Evaluate a classmate's blog.

Directions

1. Use blogger.com or WordPress unless otherwise instructed by your professor.
2. If needed, check out some of the blog resources to learn how to create and design your blog. Pick a resource for the specific program you are using.
3. Decide on the focus for your blog—healthy living, working with teenagers, specific disease conditions, surgery, or so forth.
4. Design the layout of your blog based on your intended audience. Set the blog to private and invite your classmates and professor.
5. Add content to the blog and enhance it with pictures, links to podcasts, or videos related to the content. Add a widget that keeps track of traffic on the blog.
6. Read and comment on two classmates' blogs for 4 weeks.
7. Add two posts over 4 weeks to your blog.
8. Evaluate a classmate's blog and provide the classmate with constructive suggestions for improvements, good resources, and so forth.

Exercise 6: Creating a Podcast

Purpose: *The purpose of this exercise is to learn what is involved in the creation of a podcast or video by creating either a voice or video podcast.*

Objectives
1. Plan a health-related podcast following appropriate guidelines.
2. Record and upload a podcast.
3. Critique a classmate's podcast.

Directions
1. Review any books, articles, help guides, or videos to learn how to podcast.
2. Select a topic for your podcast. Select something that is relevant to your practice
3. Determine your target audience.
4. Plan what you will convey. Consider the elements that can enhance it or ruin it. Consider things like volume, background music/noise, background appearance if a video, length, and so forth.
5. Select your setup: computer, microphone, software, and so on.
6. Record your podcast and save/convert to an acceptable file format.
7. Create an account on YouTube and upload your podcast. Share that URL with your classmates and professor.
8. View a classmate's podcast and provide the classmate with constructive critique. Your classmates and you might want to use a wiki and come to a consensus on the criteria the class will use for the critique and convert it into a critique check list.
9. Discuss what you learned from creating this podcast experience.

Exercise 7: Creating a Podcast from a PowerPoint Presentation

Purpose: *The purpose of this exercise is to research how one would convert an existing PowerPoint presentation into a Podcast. There are many ways of doing this, depending on your computer setup and what works easiest for you.*

Objectives
1. Convert a PowerPoint presentation into a podcast.
2. Upload the podcast to a podcast hosting site.
3. Enhance your blog with a link to your podcast.
4. Critique a classmate's podcast.

Directions
1. Review articles, help guides, videos to learn how to convert a PowerPoint presentation into a podcast. Make sure to use resources that relate to the equipment you will be using i.e. Mac or PC. Here are two that can get you started:
   http://office.microsoft.com/en-us/powerpoint-help/turn-your-presentation-into-a-video-HA010336763.aspx and http://www.labnol.org/software/tutorials/convert-powerpoint-video-upload-youtube-ppt-dvd/2978/.

2. Plan what you would like to say about each slide.
3. Adjust the design of your slides. Presentations with a lot of graphics in the design of the slides will increase the size of the presentation. A white background with color graphics takes up less space and still adds interest to the presentation.
4. Record your sound to the slides and add transitions/animations.
5. Save the presentation in a movie format. Microsoft has a feature to save it as wmv, but MPEG$_4$ (MP4) is more universal, so you may need to find a converter program for doing this like Authorstream.
6. Upload your Podcast to a video sharing site.
7. Provide a link to your Podcast your blog.
8. Use the critique sheet from Exercise 6 to critique a classmate's podcast.

Exercise 8: Comparing Web Conferencing Software

Purpose: *The purpose of this exercise is to experience comparing products that you might be asked to review regarding web conferencing and the related services.*

Objectives
1. Compare two web conferencing products and services.
2. Support your recommendation with additional resources.

Directions
1. Select two products and services for web conferencing.
2. Decide on the criteria you will use to compare the two products and services. Support these criteria with at least two resources.
3. Compare the two products and services using the criteria developed.
4. Use Word for your comparison. Start with a general introduction outlining reasons for using web conferencing, what this will do for the organization and the consumer, and a brief description of the two web conferencing products and services selected (this should include something about the company, address, contacts, etc.).
5. Use a 3-column table, with the first column the criteria and the second and third columns the products/services.
6. Place your evaluation comments in the correct cell.
7. Make a recommendation and justify the recommendation.
8. Submit to the professor.

REFERENCES

American Nurses Association. (2010). *Nursing: Scope and standards of practice* (2nd ed.). Silver Springs, MD: Nursesbooks.org

Anderson, M. (2009). The medium is the messenger: Using podcasting to deliver consumer health information. *Journal of Consumer Health on the Internet, 13,* 119–128. doi: 10.1080/15398280902896428.

Bastida, R., McGrath, I., & Maude, P. (2010). Wiki use in mental health practice: Recognizing potential use of collaborative technology. *International Journal of Mental Health Nursing, 19,* 142–148.

Boetcher, S., Duggon, H., & White, N. (2002). *What is a virtual community and why would you ever need one?* Retrieved from http://www/fullcirc.com/community/communitywhatwhy.htm

Centers for Disease Control and Prevention. (2011). *The health communicator's social media toolkit.* Retrieved from http://www.cdc.gov/healthcommunication/ToolsTemplates/SocialMediaToolkit_BM.pdf

Chen, L., & Chang, P. (2010). Identifying crucial website quality factors of virtual communities. In *Proceedings of the International MultiConferences of Engineers and Computer Scientists 2010.* Retrieved from http://www.iaeng.org/publication/IMECS2010/IMECS2010_pp487-492.pdf

Collaboration Health Care. (n.d.). *Role gaps in health care.* Retrieved from http://www.collaborationhealth care.com/library-and-resources/the-world-of-health-care/role-gaps-in-health-care.php

Collective Intelligence. (n.d.). *In Dictionary.com.* Retrieved from http://dictionary.reference.com/browse/collective+intelligence

Crespo, R. (2007). Virtual community health promotion. *Preventing Chronic Disease* [serial online]. Retrieved from http://www.cdc.gov/pcd/issues/2007/jul/07_0043.htm

Eysenbach, G., Powell, J., Englesakis, M., Rizo, C., & Stern, A. (2004). Health related virtual communities and electronic support groups: Systematic review of the effects of online peer to peer interactions. *BMJ, 328.* Retrieved from http://www.bmj.com/content/328/7449/1166.full

Frost, J., & Massagli, M. (2008). Social uses of personal health information within patientslikeme, an online patient community: what can happen when patients have access to one another's data. *Journal of Medical internet Research, 10*(3), e15. Retrieved from http://www.jmir.org/2010/3

Guillamon, N., Armayones, M., Hernandez, E., & Gomez-Zuniga, B. (2010). *The role of patient organizations in participatory medicine: can virtual health communities help participatory medicine accomplish its objectives?* Retrieved from http://www.jopm.org/evidence/reviews/2010/12/29/the-role-of-patient-organizations-in-participatory-medicine-can-virtual-health-communities-help-participatory-medicine-accomplish-its-objectives/

Hesse, B., O'Connell, M., Augustson, E., Chou, W., Shaikh, A., & Rutten, L. (2011). Realizing the promise of web 2.0: Engaging community intelligence. *Journal of Health Communication, 16*(Suppl. 1), 10–31. doi: 10.1080/10810730.2011.589882.

Hoch, D., & Ferguson, T. (2005). What I've learned from e-patients. *PLoS Medicine, 2*(8). Retrieved from www.plosmedicine.org

Mediaplatform. (2010). *Webcasting vs. web conferencing white paper: sorting out the difference between two related but different technologies.* Retrieved from http://www.mediaplatform.com/webcasting-software/wp-content/uploads/2010/12/Webcasting_vs_WebconferencingPaperFinal_10_131.pdf

O'Reilly, T. (2005). *What is web 2.0: design patterns and business models for the next generation of software.* Retrieved from http://www.oreillynet.com/lpt/a/7425

Pew Research Center. (2009). *The shared search for health information on the internet.* Retrieved from http://pewresearch.org/pubs/1248/americans-look-online-for-health-information

Porter, C. (2004). A typology of virtual communities: A multi-disciplinary foundation for future research. *JCMC, 10*(1), Article 3. Retrieved from http://jcmc.indiana.edu/vol10/issue1/porter.html

Priya, N. (2011). Evaluating patient experience in online health communities: Implications for healthcare organizations. *Health Care Management Review, 36*(2), 124–133.

Ressler, P., & Glazer, G. (2010). Legislative: Nursing's engagement in health policy and healthcare through social media. *OJIN: The Online Journal of Issues in Nursing, 16*(1), 11. doi: 10.3912/OJIN.Vol16No01LegCol01.

Rheingold, H. (2000). *The virtual community: homesteading on the electronic frontier* (Revised ed.). Cambridge, MA: The MIT Press.

Richardson, R., Buis, L., Janney, A., Goodrich, D., Sen, A., Hess, M., ... Piette, J. (2010). An online community improves adherence in an Internet-mediated walking program. Part 1: Results of a randomized controlled trial. *Journal of Medical Internet Research, 12*(4), e71. Retrieved from http://www.jmir.org/2010/4

Roseberry, C. (n.d.). *Before you participate in a web conference.* Retrieved from http://mobileoffice.about.com/od/webbased/bb/webconference.htm

Song, F. (2009). *Virtual communities: Bowling alone, online together.* New York, NY: Peter Lang.

Welbourne, J., Blancard, A., & Boughton, M. (2009). Supportive communication, sense of virtual community and health outcomes in online infertility groups. In *Proceedings of the Fourth International Conference on Communities and Technologies.* New York, NY: ACM.

CHAPTER 6

Personal Health Records (PHRs)

Debra M. Wolf

At the completion of this chapter the reader will be able to:

1. Explain the relationship and differences between the electronic medical record, the electronic health record, and the personal health record.
2. Understand the purpose and functionality of personal health records.
3. Explore providers of personal health records.
4. Utilize criteria to select a personal health record for personal use.
5. Discuss the legalities associated with personal health records.
6. Identify factors that hinder the adoption of personal health records.

TERMS

Electronic health record (EHR)	Personal health information (PHI)
Electronic medical record (EMR)	Personal health records (PHR)
Object-centered sociality	

Managing personal health information (PHI) is a task undertaken by every individual. PHI refers to any information that can be used to identify an individual's health status. Managing medical documents, medical appointments, health provider contact information, medication lists, past medical history, allergies, and insurance policies are just a few of the data elements that must be managed to maintain one's health. Some individuals have the responsibility of maintaining PHI for one or more family members. The process used to organize, store, and access PHI is important in maintaining and living a healthy lifestyle. A study conducted by Moen and Brennan (2005) found laypeople used four robust complex strategies to manage and store their PHI. The four strategies used to manage and store PHI included:

- Just-in-time information—is kept with an individual at all times, indicating importance or criticalness for an unexpected event (e.g., a paper list of medications stored in one's wallet).

▓ Just-at-hand information—refers to visible data or readily available data in a frequently "visualized" location (e.g., a posted calendar or papers on a bulletin board).

▓ Just-in-case information—refers to paper resources kept in files for future use (e.g., medical bills, discharge instructions, copies of test reports).

▓ Just-because information—refers to information related to a specific temporary condition that is either discarded or filed (e.g., previous directions on cast care or physical therapy exercises).

Historically, PHRs took many forms, from paper baby books (given by pediatricians on baby's first visit) to folders that house documents that validate some form of health care treatment, testing results, or payment. Interestingly, the term "Personal Health Log" first appeared in the literature in 1956 (Ragstedt, 1956) and the term "Personal Health Record" in 1978 ("Computerisation," 1978). Today, a Google search on the term "personal health record" would return over 53,900,000 results.

Multiple types of devices (computers, electronic tablets, secondary storage devices, and smartphones) assist individuals in sharing, managing, and using personal health information. The specific device selected will depend on individual preferences, their environment, their level of expertise in using technology, the type of information they need to store and the purpose for storing the information. Regardless of which device is selected, maintaining a record of past and current health information can be critical to maintaining a proactive approach to a healthy lifestyle.

Health care providers and health organizations are currently managing medical and health-related data through the use of electronic health records. The terms electronic "health" record (EHR) and electronic "medical" record (EMR) have been defined and used interchangeably by many groups, organizations, and publications. However, there is a clear difference between these terms as demonstrated by a review of definitions from a variety of key resources.

EMR refers to the electronic storage of health information by a licensed health provider who created, gathered, and manages a patient's data. An EMR is the digital version of a patient chart designed for a specific setting. The term EHR refers to aggregate electronic data from multiple sources for one individual that is used to manage one's overall state of health. The EHR is considered more powerful than an EMR because information is securely exchanged across a variety of health care settings and the data in an EHR goes beyond the clinical data in an EMR to focus on the full health status of the individual (U.S. Department of Health and Human Services [DHHS], Office of the National Coordinator, 2011).

Today the term EHR is used exclusively by the Office of the National Coordinator for Health Information Technology (ONC; Garrett & Seidman, 2011). The position of National Coordinator was created in 2004 through an executive order, and legislatively mandated in the Health Information Technology for Economic and Clinical Health Act (HITECH Act) of 2009 (The ONC for Health Information Technology, 2011, para. 1). The ONC is a "federal entity charged with coordination of nationwide efforts to implement and use the most advanced health information technology and the electronic exchange of health information. One of the major programs within this effort is termed 'meaningful use.'" The Medicare and Medicaid EHR Incentive Programs provide incentive payments to eligible professionals, eligible hospitals and critical access hospitals (CAHs) as they adopt, implement, upgrade, or demonstrate meaningful use of certified EHR technology (EHR Incentive Programs, 2012).

Heubusch (2010), when discussing the final rule on EHR standards and certification to meet meaningful use criteria, shared the statutory definition of a qualified EHR as: "an electronic record of health-related information on an individual that:

- Includes patient demographic and clinical health information, such as medical history and problem lists,
- Has the capacity:
  - To provide clinical decision support,
  - To support physician order entry,
  - To capture and query information relevant to health care quality, and
  - To exchange electronic health information with, and integrate such information from other sources" (Heubusch, 2010, para.12).

The American Medical Association (n.d.) confirms this statutory definition when presenting their meaningful-use glossary and requirement table. Interestingly, when presenting the glossary, the term EHR is used exclusively in the discussion with no mention of an EMR. The American Medical Informatics Association (AMIA) (2011), in a glossary of informatics-related terms, defines an EHR as "a repository of electronically maintained information about an individual's health status and health care, stored such that it can serve the multiple legitimate users of the record" (para. 22). Surprisingly, AMIA lists the term EMR in the glossary but does not provide a definition and refers the reader to the EHR definition.

As part of the ONC statutory definition, a qualified EHR must be able to exchange and integrate electronic health information with other sources including a PHR. The Department of Veteran Affairs (VA) has successfully demonstrated that information from an EHR and a PHR can be merged, supporting the collaboration between consumers and health care providers. My HealtheVet (https://www.myhealth.va.gov/index .html) is a PHR that assists veterans in actively participating and managing their overall level of health. In 2010, My HealtheVet had:

- 39 million visits,
- over 1 million registered users (accounting for 75% of their population),
- 199,000 people who were authenticated in person,
- 156,000 individuals who entered personal data into the PHR, and
- greater than 15.4 million prescription refills authorized since 2005 (Nazi, 2010).

With the increased usage of PHRs, and with more consumers taking an active part in managing their health care, the responsibility of gathering and managing PHI is shifting between the consumer and the health care provider. This chapter assists the reader in understanding the advantages, disadvantages, classifications, and providers of PHRs. Information is shared on how nurses can assist patients and consumers in selecting, using, and managing a PHR.

DEFINITIONS OF A PHR

Currently there is no statutory or mutually agreed upon definition for PHR, making collaboration, coordination, and policy development difficult to achieve (Fortin & Drazen, 2011; National Committee on Vital and Health Statistics, 2006). PHRs, also known as patient health records, are consumer-centric tools designed for individuals to maintain their own health information (Detmer, Bloomrosen, Raymond, & Tang, 2008; Joos, Nelson, & Smith, 2010). Although this definition is simple, to the point, and easy for a consumer to understand, there are other more comprehensive definitions written by various organizations that extend the overall meaning of a PHR. Three examples include:

- An electronic, universally available, lifelong resource of health information needed by individuals to make health decisions. Individuals own and manage the information in the PHR, which comes from health care providers and the individual. The PHR is maintained in a secure and private environment, with the individual determining rights of access. The PHR is separate from and does not replace the legal record of any provider (AHIMA Personal Health Record Practice Council, 2008, para. 3),
- An electronic Personal Health Record ('ePHR') that is universally accessible, layperson comprehensible, and a lifelong tool for managing relevant health information, promoting health maintenance and assisting with chronic disease management via an interactive, common data set of electronic health information and e-health tools. The ePHR is owned, managed, and shared by the individual or his or her legal proxy(s) and must be secure to protect the privacy and confidentiality of the health information it contains. It is not a legal record unless so defined and is subject to various legal limitations (HIMSS, 2007), and
- An electronic record of health-related information on an individual that conforms to nationally recognized interoperability standards and that can be drawn from multiple sources while being managed, shared, and controlled by the individual (DHHS: Office of the National Coordinator, 2008; p 15).

The following section presents an overview of PHRs currently available for consumers and health care providers. Considerations in choosing a PHR; the advantages and disadvantages of using a PHR; and the legal, ethical, and social concerns regarding PHRs will be discussed.

CLASSIFYING PHRs

There are numerous ways one can obtain or create a PHR. With the accelerated adoption of computers, individuals are using text applications and/or electronic spreadsheets to store health information on their own personal hard drives, CDs, or USB drives. In 2006, the Kaiser Permanente Institute for Health Policy (Kaiser), AMIA, the Robert Wood Johnson Foundation (RWJF), and the Agency for Healthcare Research and Quality (AHRQ) held a roundtable discussion to explore the potential of PHRs. Detmer et al. (2008) summarize three types of PHRs that were discussed at the roundtable:

- **Standalone or free-standing models**. Standalone models can be paper, computer based, or free-standing apps on ones' personal digital device. These models place the responsibility of maintaining and updating the health information on the individual. With changes to one's health status, medications, or diagnoses, individuals must be diligent to update their files on their data storage devices. Individuals should also make backups of the data. Unfortunately a drawback to this model is the limited access other individuals or health professionals will have to the information. The owner will be required to share printouts or the actual device with others. Accuracy and completeness may be questioned by health care providers.

▪ **Integrated, interconnected, or networked web-based models**. These models allow multiple entries of data from a variety of sources including the patient. Insurance agencies, health providers, pharmacies, and outpatient testing laboratories can view, enter, change, or exchange information. This model assists in decreasing the amount of manual entry of information, duplication of information, and access time in searching for data. This PHR increases accuracy of information since the patient can view and correct misinformation as needed. Overall, the model allows for an all-inclusive view of one's health status.

▪ **Institution-specific, web-based, or tethered models**. Health care institutions operate and own these models. Although the health record contains information regarding the patient, the patient may only be given limited access to certain areas. Unlike the standalone model, the provider controls this model. A major advantage of this model is the additional functionality the model offers, such as email communication with health care providers, online scheduling of appointments, and prescription requests.

Cronin (2006), in her review of PHRs, found the most popular PHRs were Internet/web-based, which required an individual to register through a web interface and obtain a username and password. The second most popular PHR was maintained on one's personal computer.

PHRs can also be classified in terms of the Health Insurance Portability and Accountability Act of 1996 (HIPAA) Privacy Rule. PHRs that are provided by health care providers and health plans covered by HIPAA are protected by HIPAA privacy regulations. Alternatively, PHRs that are not offered by HIPAA-covered entities do not have this protection (DHHS: Office for Civil Rights, n.d.). The privacy policies of the PHR vendor govern how information in the PHR is protected or in some cases not protected. Additional information on how the HIPAA Privacy Rule may apply and support the use of PHRs can be found at http://www.hhs.gov/ocr/privacy/hipaa/understanding/special/healthit/phrs.pdf.

PROVIDERS OF PHRs

In 2006, the AARP, Policy Institute conducted an examination of 24 PHRs that were available to consumers (Cronin, 2006). The study identified that 50% ($n = 12$) of the PHRs were introduced between 2004 and 2005, with the oldest PHR being introduced in 1999. The study acknowledged that "the vast majority of companies were independent, privately held, or small companies. In most cases such companies were not subjected to the HIPAA privacy law. Two of the companies (WebMD and CapMed) were publically traded. The only nonprofit owner was MedicAlert" (Cronin, 2006). Surprisingly, the study revealed that more than 33% of the companies were initiated by physicians.

There are two general categories for PHRs; the first is disease specific, meaning the PHR is designed for individuals with similar conditions or needs such as MyHIN (www .MyHIN .org). The other is a general format that is designed for general use by patients with multiple conditions such as Microsoft HealthVault (http://www.microsoft.com/en-us/healthvault/). Below is a representative listing of current PHRs that are available for consumers. In each case the URL is provided. The reader is encouraged to check each of these sites and note the overall style of the website, the privacy policies, the functions and services described, and cost. The reader is also cautioned that these companies should also be vetted before any of the PHRs listed here, or on any other site, are recommended to patients for use.

Mobile Device PHRs

911 Medical ID (http://www.911medicalid.com): This is a portable personal health record that stores information for ease of transfer whenever needed. The company created a "fold-out USB flash drive" that connects to any computer. The device is also available as a medallion that could be worn around one's neck. The website states the product comes with a 2-year warranty with a one time nominal charge of $39.99. The company also provides portable personal record storage devices for property and financial information. They even make a MY PET e-Safe device that attaches to a pet's collar. The pet device is a USB drive that has a removable cap (the cap remains attached to the pet's collar at all times). When the USB drive is removed from the cap, it can be used with any computer.

CheckUp (http://www.checkupsoftware.com/): This company offers software one can download onto a personal/private computer to manage and store information. The website offers a free trial offer for 30 days. If one decides to purchase the system, the cost is $29.95 with unlimited technical support and software updates.

TrEHRT (http://www.TrEHRT.com): This application assists travelers to access their personal health information via their mobile phone. The consumer enters their personal health information over the Internet at the company's website; the consumer's information is then downloaded to a mobile phone via a mobile app. One negative aspect is that the app supports a minimal data set. When using mobile apps for PHI, one needs to confirm that the Internet site (for data entry) and data storage are secured and protected. This company is based in Taiwan and is not subject to any U.S. regulations and laws.

Disease Specific Standalone Web-Based PHRs

Navigating Cancer and Blood Disorders (https://www.navigatingcancer.com/): Navigating Cancer and Blood Disorders is a web-based platform that offers cancer patients the ability to organize their care; create a secure record of treatments, such as medications, surgeries, radiation, and chemo; and store information concerning past medical experiences. The program helps patients to track side effects and prepare for office visits. In addition, Navigating Cancer offers multiple resources from trusted experts and other patients with similar diagnoses. The individual user has complete control on who views, alters, or edits their information. The PHR allows family and friends to view certain information in an attempt to follow one's progress (if granted by the owner of the PHI). There is no charge for using Navigating Cancer and Blood Disorders' PHR.

MyHIN (www.MyHIN.org): MyHIN is an online personal health record for patients with hydrocephalus that was launched in 2003. The PHR was designed by health care professionals who care for patients with hydrocephalus. The cost is $24.99 for the first year, then $39.99 thereafter. The privacy policy clearly states information is not shared unless one signs a separate permission slip authorizing the release of information. The policy does clarify what data are collected and sold. The policy states "We may share aggregate demographic information with our partners and sponsors. This is not linked to any personal information that can identify any individual person" (MYHIN, 2012, p. 1).

General Standalone Web-Based PHRs

Microsoft HealthVault (http://www.microsoft.com/en-us/healthvault/): This PHR is one of the most well-known, freestanding, web-based PHRs. This PHR strongly supports the use of mobile apps to allow a higher level of interoperability. In addition to the free standing PHR, Microsoft has partnered with a number of health care institutions to offer a tethered PHR. For example, Mayo Clinic partners with Microsoft HealthVault to offer their patients and community members access to their PHR. This access also allows various health care providers to view the PHI when authorization has be provided. The program is titled Mayo Clinic Health Manager (https://healthmanager.mayoclinic.com/). The Mayo Health Manager connects to Microsoft's HealthVault, allowing individuals to update and store information as needed.

Follow Me (http://www.followme.com/): This was created in 2000 by a mother caring for a child with hydrocephalus who wanted to keep her child safe regardless of where both of them were located. One of the benefits of this company is the ability to customize its platform to meet specific populations' health needs. Follow Me offers three types of products based on this flexibility. First, they offer a general standalone PHR. Second, they provide a framework for customizing a PHR to specific organizations or populations. For example, small businesses or health professionals in private practice can customize the template to meet their population's needs. Third, they offer customized PHRs that are designed for specific populations. An example of one customized PHR is MiVIA (www.mivia.org). This PHR was designed to support migrant farmers. The flexibility of having customization features within a PHR template supports groups of individuals with similar interests. A second example is the MyHIN PHR already described.

WebMD (http://www.webmd.com/phr): Is a free web-based PHR that allows individuals to manage their information on the Internet with access from anywhere in the country as long as Internet service is available. The privacy policy located at http://www.webmd.com/about-webmd-policies/about-privacy-policy on this site is very extensive, consisting of 11 sections and several subsections. When printed in Times New Roman size 12 font, the policy is 18 pages. Part 10 of the policy states they will inform individuals if there is a change to the privacy policy or if disclosures of personal identifiable information will occur. Interestingly further down in the policy, in italics, the policy reads that users will be informed of changes by postings to the website. This type of communication requires an individual to actively watch the websites for updates on a regular basis. When reviewing their privacy statement, they identity eTRUSTe (http://www.truste.com/) as a privacy solution provider and URAC (https://www.urac.org/accreditation/), a health care accreditation agency, as accrediting their site.

HealthFrame (http://www.recordsforliving.com/HealthFrame/): HealthFrame is a PHR that can be used to manage a family's health information. The product is available at a one-time cost of $39.99. This product offers the purchaser the ability to print medical cards that contain health information and can be carried in one's wallet for quick access. As frequently as medications change or new conditions are diagnosed, users can reprint their medical cards as needed. The privacy policy, which can be viewed at http://www.recordsforliving.com/Company/PrivacyPolicy.aspx, is an interesting contrast to WebMD, starting with the fact that it is half a page.

Health Care Provider PHRs

UPMC HealthTrak (https://myupmc.upmc.com/): University of Pittsburgh Medical Center offers individuals access to portions of their health information online through use of the Internet. The system allows individuals to request appointments and prescriptions as well as to view their medical history and test results. Currently there is no fee for these services.

MyChart (http://my.clevelandclinic.org/online-services/mychart.aspx): Cleveland Clinic is one of the providers that offer its patients access to their medical records. What is unique about this accessibility is that individuals can authorize a non-Cleveland Clinic physician access to their personal health information via the web-based platform.

Insurance Providers PHRs

Medicare PHR Choice (http://www.medicare.gov/navigation/manage-your-health/personal-health-records/medicare-phr-choice.aspx): Since 2006, the Centers for Medicare & Medicaid Services has engaged in a number of pilot projects to encourage Medicare beneficiaries to use (PHRs). For example, since 2009 people living in Utah and Arizona have had the option of using a web-based PHR offered through Medicare. The advantage of this PHR is that Medicare will automatically add Part A and Part B claims directly into one's record. Medicare offers individuals the ability to choose from three PHR vendors, myMediConnect (http://www.mymediconnect .net/), NoMoreClipboard .com (http://www.nomoreclipboard.com/), and Health Trio (http://www .healthtrio.com/). To make the selection easy, Medicare offers a PHR comparison chart to assist in choosing a PHR. The chart can be viewed at http://www .medicare.gov/Publications/Pubs/pdf/Summary_Vendors_Medicare_PHR_ Choiceupdated_9.30.10.pdf.

My health manager (https://healthy.kaiserpermanente.org/health/care/consumer/my-health-manager): This is a PHR offered by Kaiser Permanente, a not-for-profit health plan provider since 1945, located in California. This PHR offers several options to exchange communication with providers, make appointments, view medical records, and fill prescriptions.

The PHRs shared in this chapter are only a small representation of PHRs that are available. Other vendors to explore include Peoplechart (http://www.peoplechart.com/), K.I.S. PHR (http://kismedicalrecords.com/), and iHealthRecord (http://medemphr .mymedfusion.com/). As the demand for PHRs grows, the market will continue to change with newer and more improved systems. Unfortunately, as the competition becomes greater, some applications may be discontinued. Two well-known companies who recently discontinued their PHRs included Revolution Health, a part of AOL, which closed its browsers in 2010 (FierceHealathIT, 2010), and Google Health, which will be closed as of January 2013. The discontinuation of PHRs by providers raises an important question, "should PHR providers offer a backup plan if they are no longer able to support current users?" Consumers need to understand how a PHR can assist them in being actively involved in managing their health, and more importantly, how a PHR can assist their providers in supporting their overall health. By understanding the advantages and disadvantages of PHRs, nurses will be better informed to assist consumers in selecting the appropriate PHR system.

THE ADVANTAGES AND DISADVANTAGES OF PHRs

There are major efforts by the federal government, insurance companies, and employers to establish PHRs. For example, as part of the Meaningful Use ruling, eligible professionals who are attempting to receive financial incentives for EHR adoption under CMS must meet certain criteria. Under these criteria, eligible professionals are required to "provide clinical summaries to patients for each office visit and on request, provide patients with an electronic copy of their health information" (American Medical Association, n.d., p. 6). PHRs are listed as one of the options that can be used to transfer or share patients' PHIs.

Sharing PHI in this manner is one of the major advantages of a PHR. Today, the VA (within their My HealtheVet PHR) and Medicare (within their MyMedicare.gov program, https://www.mymedicare.gov/) are sharing information in this manner. Individuals can access, view, transfer, and download their PHI by clicking an icon they refer to as the "Blue Button," located within their PHR or their home page.

Access to one's PHI supports an individual in having more control over their PHI and the freedom to share information with others. Nurses are in key positions to help patients understand these advantages and to educate them on what resources are available. Educating patients on the advantages such as convenience, security, and accessibility of PHI supports a higher level of communication with providers. This higher level of communication could ultimately assist in managing one's acute medical condition and overall health. A major advantage nurses can stress to patients is the immediate access to PHI in an emergency situation. Having a web-based PHR or mobile device PHR allows immediate access to PHI during a critical time when seconds could mean the difference between life and death.

As part of educating patients on the advantages of having a PHR, nurses need to also inform patients of potential disadvantages. Privacy and security are major concerns for protecting one's PHI. In addition, individuals need to be diligent in updating their PHRs on a regular basis. If new medications or diagnoses are not recorded, providers could misdiagnose or mistreat a patient leading to more medical complications. A list of additional advantages and disadvantages is presented in Table 6.1.

ROLE OF THE NURSE: CONSUMERS AND PHRs

Selecting and using a PHR can be a challenging task if consumers are not prepared or educated on the advantages and disadvantages they offer. Nurses can play a very

Table 6.1 *Advantages and Disadvantages of PHRs*

Advantages of PHRs	Disadvantages of PHRs
Supports individual self-management and engagement	Security concerns
Facilitates access and sharing of comprehensive health information	Maintenance of information (must be updated)
Improves communication between patient and health care team	Cost (purchase and maintenance)
Improves efficiency and continuity of care	Time requirements to obtain and use
Strengthens accuracy of information	Not intuitive to use
Manages individual and family information	Complex, difficult to use
Shares reminders or alerts	
Avoids duplicate tests	
Strengthens health promotion and disease prevention	

important part in assisting individuals in selecting the appropriate PHR that meets their needs. Nurses are prepared through educational programs and clinical experiences to assess patients' needs on a regular basis. Nurses routinely develop care plans that are patient centered and family oriented. Nurses have the opportunity to influence patients in making informed decisions. Offering educational material on the advantages and disadvantages of PHRs (see Table 6.1), sharing key points to consider when choosing a PHR (see Table 6.2) or just offering tips on using a PHR (see Exhibit 6.1) can be the starting point to helping individuals make the right decision on choosing the right PHR.

Thede (2008), in her article "Informatics: Electronic Personal Health Records: Nursing's Role," identifies that nurses need to be in the forefront of designing PHRs. Thede discusses the nurses' ability to assess and understand the health and information literacy needs of patients, which are important when selecting and using a PHR. Understanding these literacy needs will be critical in understanding how a PHR can support individuals' health needs and assist in choosing the appropriate PHR.

Helping patients identify what they need from a PHR is a challenge that nurses can assist with. Thede (2008) points out, "What we as health care professionals think they need may not be what consumers want or will use" (para. 9). Exploring how patients currently manage their PHI, and identifying the advantages or disadvantages of their current process, will assist the nurse in helping them choose a PHR that meets their needs and, more importantly, that also supports better communication with their health care providers.

The TIGER Initiative (n.d.) recommends that nurses be trained in using PHRs. Empowering nurses with the knowledge and skills to use PHRs will enable them to empower the patient and consumer to engage in using them. Adding content regarding PHRs into nursing curricula is essential in preparing nurses to empower their patients (The TIGER Initiative, n.d.).

Depending on the manufacturer, the owner, and the need, PHI data elements stored on PHRs can vary considerably. Regardless of which system one selects, there is a general list of information PHRs should include. Table 6.3 provides a summary of data elements that may be included in PHRs. Data entry into a PHR could occur in many fashions, from direct electronic entry (using a keyboard or a point and click process), to scanning of documents, to using a template that guides one through a series of yes or no questions, to direct importing of data from the EMR and/or EHR. The following section presents several attributes one needs to consider when selecting a PHR.

Table 6.2 *Considerations When Choosing a PHR*

Considerations	Details
Access to health information	Individual (partial or full access) Multidisciplinary health care providers (partial or full access)
Ability to correct or edit information put in by a health care provider	Has editing privileges to correct existing data and/or ability to add additional information
Interaction checking	Drugs, allergies, food
Ownership of data	Individual or provider
Who supplies information	Individual Multidisciplinary members
Additional functionality	Provider and consumer email communication Electronic scheduling opportunities Prescription refills
Type of information managed	Testing results Medical history Medications Insurance claims Reflects a lifetime of history Collection from all multidisciplinary health care providers Routine data monitored daily (such as diet, exercise, vital signs)
Security measures	Prevent unauthorized access Protection of personal health information Access to list of names who reviewed record Limitations to sharing information through exchange networks (requiring individual permission)
Manufacture of the system	Trusted reliable company New unknown entrepreneur Profit, non-profit, independently owned or privately held company
Terms and conditions policy	Legal rights and responsibilities
Privacy policy	Research affiliations Covered by the HIPAA Privacy Rule (http://www.hhs.gov/ocr/privacy/hipaa/understanding/special/healthit/phrs.pdf)
Seal of approval is visible	eTrust, CCHIT
Reviews available from others who use the product	Know of others who use the system
Journal or diary notes	Allows one to record conversations, directions, questions
Document uploading/storage	Supports the storage and access to scanned documents, images, etc.
Capable of exchanging health information	Supports interoperability for multidisciplinary health care providers

---

Exhibit 6.1 *Tips on Using a PHR*

1. Read the terms of service and the privacy policy very carefully before storing your data. Some non-HIPAA-covered PHRs may market your data.
2. Make sure your PHR allows you the right to delete your record.
3. If you're using a wireless connection, be sure it's encrypted (look for a small lock symbol in the upper right-hand corner of the screen).
4. Keep a printed copy of your PHR in case the records get deleted or altered.
5. Double-check the information on your PHR to make sure it is accurate and up-to-date.

Source: Gearon, C. (2010).

Table 6.3 *Data Elements Found Within a PHR*

Basic demographic data	Name, age, sex, address
Allergies	Food, drugs, etc.
Medication list	Current and past
Medical history	List of co morbidities such as hypertension, diabetes, etc.
Existing prostheses or devices	Dentures, limbs, heart pacers, etc.
Past hospitalizations	Surgeries and/or past hospitalizations, etc.
Medical providers (primary, specialist)	Contact information
Insurance information	Name, contact information, provider, and group number
Test results	Labs, scans, x-rays, etc.
Family history	Cancer, hypertension, etc.
Emergency contact	Name, relationship, contact information
Living will, health directives	Location
Immunizations	Child and adult
Social history	Alcohol and drug use

SELECTING A PHR

Availability of PHRs has grown over the past few years and is anticipated to grow even more over the next 10 to 20 years. This growth is the result of health information management transitioning from a provider-centric model to a patient-centric model (AHIMA, 2008). Selecting a PHR can be a difficult task if one is not familiar with PHRs. Regardless of whether one chooses a disease-specific PHR or a general PHR, there may be other resources available to an individual. For example, PHRs may be available through a) one's employer as an attempt to promote wellness; b) one's insurance company to also promote wellness and manage information; c) one's provider such as the VA; or d) through independent vendors such as Microsoft HealthVault (AHIMA Personal Health Record Practice Council, 2006).

In 2006, the AHIMA Personal Health Record Practice Council produced a report to help consumers select a PHR. The report highlighted multiple attributes that fall into seven categories that need to be considered prior to making a final decision. The report also offers a chart titled "Emerging PHR Attributes," which compares attributes identified by four groups (AHIMA, the AHIC Consumer Empowerment Work Group, Health Level Seven, and the Markle Foundation). A summary of PHR attributes is listed below:

▨ Content—includes data sets and information required such as,
   — PHI for a lifetime
   — Insurance information
   — Demographic information
   — Supports a standard vocabulary
▨ Sources—allows providers to download information and the holder to self-report symptoms,
▨ Features—data entered should be cited as to who entered the content and when; consumers own and manage the information,

- Functions—shares resources to information to make decisions; captures, stores, and processes data,
- Technical approach—meets interoperability needs, is portable, and accessed via a portal,
  - Individuals can enter data into the PHR and download data from the PHR onto a secondary device (memory stick, CD, etc.)
  - Allows transferring of PHI electronically to other providers' EHR
  - PHI is accessible for viewing via the Internet
- Privacy and security—information must be protected and secured, and
- Access—holder is in control of who has access; content is transparent (AHIMA Personal Health Record Practice Council, 2006).

A final consideration that impacts the selection of a PHR is the cost associated in obtaining the product. Although some PHRs are free, others may offer a free trial for a short period of time, followed by a monthly or yearly payment. Other PHR vendors charge a flat fee for a template or portable device. Fees can range from $25 a month, to a one-time fee of $14.95 to $74.95 for PHRs on digital devices or downloaded templates (Cronin, 2006). Dimick (2008) shared the results of a study conducted by the Center for Information Technology Leadership projected annual savings when using a PHR ranges from $13 billion (insurance-tethered PHR) to $21 billion (Interoperable PHRs) yearly. Third-party PHRs were expected to save $16 billion and provider-tethered PHRs up to $14 billion (Dimick, 2008).

Health care providers who are seeking to establish or initiate a PHR within their practice or office must give careful considerations to what system or vendor is selected. The Health Resources and Services Administration (HRSA), part of the U.S. Department of Health and Human Services (DHHS) has created a resource center for health facilities and health providers to better understand PHRs. The module contains five units of information that discuss PHR standards, current initiatives, and criteria that can be used to evaluate PHR systems (DHHS, n.d.). The five units of information include:

- Understanding PHRs—addresses basic questions such as what is a PHR, what are the benefits of a PHR, and what types of PHRs exist.
- Understanding PHR standards—shares the HL7 standards, explains a continuity of care record vs. document, and addresses standards for privacy and security.
- PHRs and health centers—shares examples of health centers that are implementing PHRs and the advantages of having a PHR.
- Current PHR initiatives—shares federal, industry, and open-source initiatives for PHRs.
- Evaluating, optimizing, and sustaining PHRs—shares challenges of adopting PHRs, long-term value of PHRs, and costs associated with PHRs.

PHRs: FACTORS THAT HINDER ADOPTION

As with any new innovative idea or type of technology there is always a cautionary response to those who challenge the idea or the functionality of the new systems. Marketing and advertising technology can be very challenging, especially when consumers and health care organizations are not knowledgeable of the benefits or opportunities the technology offers. Detmer, Bloomrosen, Raymond, and Tang (2008) identified multiple obstacles that may hinder the adoption of PHRs for the individual as well as a health care organization. The obstacles include:

- Issues of consumer confidence and trust
- The digital divide such as:
    - Racial and socio-economic disparity
    - Literacy disparities
- Obstacles in the health care system and culture such as:
    - Balancing physician and patient autonomy
    - Scope of work and responsibilities
    - Physician compensation and incentives
    - Liability risks
- Lack of technical standards for interoperability such as:
    - Data interchange standards
    - Common data sets and minimum data sets
    - Privacy and security standards
- Lack of health information technology (HIT) infrastructure
- Uncertain value realization and return on investment (ROI)
    - Cost associated with purchasing a packaged system
- Uncertain market demand.

When reviewing PHR websites for the number of individuals who use their products, information was difficult to obtain. When reviewing the literature, one study revealed the number of users (vendor self-reported) per PHR model varied from less than 1,000 users to 2.3 million users (Cronin, 2006). In 2009, the AHIMA conducted a survey to assess the current state of PHRs. The study concluded that 80% of respondents (providers) stated their organization can view PHRs in any format they receive (up from 71% in 2007), and 59% (up from 39% in 2007) of the organizations reported having developed policies and/or procedures in regard to reviewing the PHI patients brought to the provider. Unfortunately, 73% of consumers still provided paper copies of their PHR to a provider and only 19% used CDs to share their information (AHIMA, 2009).

One study found 7% of adults nationwide used their providers web-based PHR to obtain information (California Health Care Foundation, 2010). The Markle Foundation (2011) conducted a survey that revealed 10% of the public currently use a PHR, a 7% increase from 2008. Interestingly the study also found that 9% of providers offer their patients a PHR. The correlation between what is offered and what is being actively used is an area of research that could be considered to see if providers can influence their patients to use PHRs.

PHRs: ETHICAL, LEGAL, AND SOCIAL ISSUES

In 2006, the National Committee on Vital and Health Statistics (NCVHS) presented a report to the DHHS with several recommendations for PHR and PHR systems (National Committee on Vital and Health Statistics, 2006). The report recommended that standards be established for all PHRs to define: a) evolving terms and practices, b) privacy, c) security, d) interoperability, e) federal role, and f) research and evaluation. Currently there are no guidelines "that clarify the respective rights, obligations, and potential liabilities of consumers, patients, providers and other stakeholders in PHR systems" (National Committee on Vital and Health Statistics, 2006; p 20). This lack of guidelines creates multiple opportunities for various legal, ethical, and moral problems to occur.

Without clear roles and responsibilities established by the government, individuals must be careful when selecting a PHR to understand:

- Who owns the information?
- Who has access to the information?
- Who is responsible for maintaining and updating the system?

If critical decisions are being made based on information found or presented within a PHR, and that information is not up to date, there is the opportunity for error, misdiagnosis, or unnecessary testing to occur.

In 2010, Robert Wood Johnson Foundation (RWJF) funded a team to explore the ethical, legal, and social issues surrounding PHRs and applications (Cushman, Froomkin, Cava, Abril, & Goodman, 2010). Concerned with the growing popularity of PHRs, RWJF believed there needed to be a critical evaluation of issues that surround PHRs. The team organized their concerns around four themes:

- Privacy and confidentiality—regarding inappropriate third-party access and disclosure of PHI resulting in discrimination, embarrassment, and dignitary harms. Concerns arise when a minor's data transfers from a PHR to an institution's electronic medical record (EMR). A question shared to demonstrate these concerns asked "Should a perceived parental failure with respect to PHR data management—be it too much or too little data sharing—expose parents to social or legal liability?" (p. s52).
- Data security—as currently experienced within EHRs, the security concern is further raised within PHRs. The challenges presented center on the "segmentation of data into appropriate spheres" (p. s52). Protecting information at different levels within a PHR raises considerable challenges especially when transferring to a provider EHR or allowing other health care providers access to one's PHR.
- Decision support—questions raised focus on backup plans; error detection and management; faulty input; or errors in decision support built into PHRs. An example of this concern involves the use of authoritative logic within a PHR. If one receives an alert or message from their PHR suggesting an activity such as "exercise today" or "take this pill" and the system cannot detect the individual does not feel well, and an adverse event occurs, who is responsible?
- Legal-regulatory requirements—concerns center on the "expanding possibilities for PHR data misuse with respect to potentially stigmatizing disease, conditions and medications" (p. s53).

The advancement of PHRs combined with existing EHRs escalates the possibilities of personal health information being unprotected. The Health Information Technology for Economic and Clinical Health (HITECH) Act has extended four requirements of HIPAA privacy and security rules to vendors of PHRs and EHRs (Gordon, 2010). Only one extension addressing breach notification applies to PHRs. PHR vendors are now required to notify the Federal Trade Commission within 60 days if personal information was breached. Under the Health Breach Notification Rule (http://www.ftc.gov/os/2009/08/R911002hbn.pdf), vendors are also responsible for notifying the individual whose information was not protected.

Other medical liabilities that need to be considered include holding physicians liable "for more than the ordinary standards of care based on reasonable review of a standard formal PHR; for providing care based on incomplete or inaccurate information contained in a PHR; for the act of consulting with a patient who lives in a state other than that in which the physician is licensed" (HIMSS, 2007; p 9).

PHRs AND SOCIAL MEDIA

Merging software, integrating technology, and sharing functionality are processes that occur daily in the lives of individuals who use technology. But have individuals ever considered merging parts of a PHR with a social networking site? Sharing personal health information among friends within a virtual community is becoming popular. Patientslikeme (http://www.patientslikeme.com/) is one example of a social networking site where individuals share personal health information electronically with others they may never meet in person. Currently, Patientslikeme (n.d.) reports they have over 145,000 patients and 1,000 conditions. Social networking sites that focus on health and wellness are attracting thousands of people daily who seek to connect to people with whom they share a health concern. Stewart (2009) identifies this concept as "object-centered sociality," meaning people want to connect with other people who have "an object of common interest … that object may be a job, a hobby, or a medical record" (Stewart, 2009, para. 22). Sharing experiences, understanding what will or could happen with one's disease process, or just knowing there are other similar individuals offers reassurance that they are not alone.

Patientslikeme (http://www.patientslikeme.com/) and Curetogether (http://curetogether.com/) are two social networking sites that allow individuals to enter information or specific data elements regarding their disease and treatment such as drug dosages, side effects, and history of symptoms. Having the ability to explore and read what others with the same condition are doing may be comforting and may assist others to be more confident in what to expect, to better understand what is required or needed to maintain a certain level of quality in one's lifestyle. Another advantage of these social networking sites is the ability to mine the data to help find a cure for various diseases. Recently, Patientslikeme (2012) updated their privacy policy. The policy includes a bulleted list of the various types of data elements that members may elect to share including:

- Biographical information: photograph, biography, gender, age, location (city, state and country), general notes
- Condition/disease information: diagnosis date, first symptom, family history
- Treatment information: treatment start dates, stop dates, dosages, side effects, treatment evaluations
- Symptom information: severity, duration
- Primary and secondary outcome scores over time: ALSFRS-R, MSRS, PDRS, FVC, PFRS, Mood Map, Quality of Life, weight, InstantMe
- Laboratory results: CD-4 count, viral load, creatinine
- Genetic information: information on individual genes and/or entire genetic scans
- Individual and aggregated survey responses
- Information shared via free text fields: forum, treatment evaluations, surveys, annotations, journals, feeds, adverse event reports
- Connections to other people on the site: invited care team member, mentors, feeds, subscriptions (Patientslikeme, 2012, para. 4).

With continued advancements in PHR templates and social media functionality, patients will be able to interface their PHI directly from a PHR into a social media site to further connect or assist others in understanding their disease. Having clearly defined standards and policies on how this will occur is critical for the safety of all.

As independent PHR vendors continue to create platforms that are customizable such as FollowMe (http://www.followme.com/), virtual communities that share common interests regarding health and wellness may turn vendors such as FollowMe to design their own PHRs for their community members. Navigating Cancer (https://www.navigatingcancer.com/) is currently offering this integration. Not only do they offer individuals a tool to manage their PHI, they also offer a community of thousands of cancer survivors who share experiences, start discussions, and recommend resources to each other (Navigating cancer, n.d.).

SUMMARY

As part of the nurse's scope and standard of practice, nurses are responsible for assessing and educating patients as needed. Assessing both a patient's understanding and use of a PHR will soon become part of the routine assessment that is conducted when working with patients in all settings. Assessing the patient's understanding of a PHR will guide the nurse in determining the educational needs of the patient. For example, patients who are using tethered systems with brand names such as Mychart or Healthtrak may not fully understand these are PHRs. In the patient's mind these applications may simply be a communication tool for requesting an appointment, renewal of a prescription, or obtaining test results. By assessing the patient's knowledge, the nurse has a baseline for introducing the patient to the full functionality of the institution's PHR. At the same time, nurses can encourage patients to become more actively involved in monitoring and managing their own health by using the PHR. The nurse can also correct misunderstandings patients may have about their PHRs. For example, patients may assume the nurse has full access to the information in their PHRs and may skip details in their history during the assessment process. Explaining to patients who has access to the PHR and their role in controlling this access can help a patient more effectively use their PHR.

Nurses need to be proactive in educating patients to better understand the impact of PHRs and the value of having access to their PHI when needed. With the anticipated increase in PHR production, web-based, integrated, networked, and tethered PHRs will create a higher level of concern for all. With the rapid adoption of social media and networking sites, the protection of PHI shared electronically through PHRs raises multiple security and privacy concerns. The need for strong health policy agendas aimed at designing and implementing standards will be critical for the emerging PHR users to be confident that PHI is secure and protected.

DISCUSSION QUESTIONS

1. What form of PHR do you currently maintain? What format did your parents use when you were growing up? Share experiences of how your PHR has assisted you or your family during an emergency. Share how a PHR could further assist individuals during an emergency situation. Discuss the advantages and disadvantages.
2. What role and responsibilities do you believe nurses should have when patients present with a PHR to an acute health care setting or to a private provider visit?
3. Research the concept "object-centered sociality" on the Internet. Share an experience or situation that you had that further demonstrates this concept using social media.
4. Discuss the advantages and disadvantages of having PHRs interfaced into a social networking site.
5. Find ten individuals who do not use a PHR. Explore their rationale on why they do not. Synthesize their responses, present common findings, and discuss how you could influence them to consider purchasing a PHR.

EXERCISES

Exercise 1: Health and Wellness Social Networks

Purpose: *The purpose of this exercise is to offer the reader the opportunity to explore a social media site that focuses on health and wellness in order to evaluate the type of personal health information that is currently being shared or exchanged between members.*

Objectives
1. Identify the type of personal health information that is currently being shared on social networking sites.
2. Explore the ethical, moral, legal, and social issues that may occur regarding one's personal health information.

Directions
1. Identify two social networking sites such as or similar to Patientslikeme (http://www.patientslikeme.com/) or Curetogether (http://curetogether.com/). Contact the site administrator to request permission to observe one or more communities as part of a class assignment. You can use other sites that openly share personal health information among its members if no sign-in or registration is required.
2. Select one health community, condition, or disease process that is active on both sites and observe the interaction and type of information that is being shared.
3. Identify the number of members actively involved with the specific community, condition, or disease on both sites.
4. Review each site's privacy policy and terms and conditions of use statements.
5. Write a summary and post to the class blog describing:
   a. The differences between, 1) the two sites, 2) what information you observed being exchanged on each site, 3) their privacy policies, and 4) their terms and conditions statements.
   b. The ethical, moral, legal, and social issues that may arise.

Exercise 2: Selecting a PHR

Purpose: *The purpose of this exercise is to explore PHRs to manage and share one's PHI.*

Objectives
1. Select a PHR using a set of guidelines.
2. Define the level of privacy and security each site offers.

Directions
1. Review two PHRs from the list presented in this chapter. Select one PHR that is web-based and one that is specific to a secondary storage device such as a memory card or template that is downloaded to a computer's hard drive.
2. Using the considerations found in Table 6.2, compare the two PHRs and identify one you would recommend to patients and their family members.

3. Develop a PowerPoint presentation to educate patients and families on the advantages of the PHR you selected over the one you did not select. Explain why.

Exercise 3: Utilizing AHIMA Recommendations

Purpose: *The purpose of this exercise is to utilize recommendations established by an organization that is dedicated to assisting others in managing their personal health information for higher quality of care.*

Objectives

1. Utilize recommendations from the American Health Information Management Association (AHIMA) regarding the selection and use of a PHR.
2. Evaluate a PHR using the recommendations from the AHIMA.

Directions

1. Visit the AHIMA web site at http://www.myphr.com/StartaPHR/what_is_a_phr .aspx
2. Review "What is a Personal Health Record (PHR)"
3. Answer the following four questions using the content provided by the AHIMA (evaluate the PHR you selected in Exercise 2)
   a. What does your PHR contain?
   b. How is your health information used?
   c. How can you use your PHR?
   d. How does a PHR work?
4. Write a three-page paper sharing your views.

Exercise 4: Thinking Hypothetically

Purpose: *The purpose of this exercise is to hypothetically evaluate the role PHRs will have on current practice and the health care provider.*

Objectives

1. Reflect on how PHRs will impact current practice and the role of the health care provider.
2. Evaluate the role of health policy and government agencies in implementing standards guiding vendors of PHRs.

Directions

1. Read the article by Cushman, R., Froomkin, M., Cava, A., Abril, R., & Goodman, K. (2010). Ethical, legal and social issues for personal health records and applications. *Journal of Biomedical Informatics, 43,* s51–s55. doi:10.1016/j.jbi.2010.05.003. Retrieved from http://www.sciencedirect.com/science/article/pii/S1532046410000614.
2. Answer the four questions below (also found in the conclusions section of the article) offering an explanation for each response. Include in your response how health policy could be used to support your response.

    a. Is a PHR best viewed as a complement to the official health record?

    b. Is a PHR a substitute for an official health record required in emergency situations or as a backup for institutional EHRs?

    c. How much confidence during a routine visit should a health care provider place on the data found within a PHR the patient brought to the visit?

    d. What are the legal, professional, and social answers to these questions?

3. Share your responses via a podcast and upload to YouTube.com. Add a link to your blog so others can access the podcast.

Exercise 5: Defining PHRs

Purpose: *The purpose of this exercise is to collaborate with other health care professionals in developing a consensus on a definition describing PHRs.*

Objectives
1. Synthesize existing definitions into a single cohesive definition.
2. Collaborate with other professionals to explore the impact a consistent PHR definition will have on society.

Directions
1. Work comparatively with two other professionals (one health focused and one IT focused).
2. Review the numerous definitions presented in this chapter.
3. Locate an additional definition of PHR that is not discussed in this chapter.
4. Each individual is to work independently to synthesize all the definitions into one definition they feel strongly reflects their interpretations.
5. Present your definition to each of the other two professionals.
6. Use a wiki to post the three final definitions. Collaborate with the two other professionals in summarizing all three definitions into one.

REFERENCES

AHIMA. (2009). Current state of PHRs. *Journal of AHIMA, 80*(6), 59–60. Retrieved from http://library.ahima.org/xpedio/groups/public/documents/ahima/bok1_043762.hcsp?dDocName=bok1_043762

AHIMA Personal Health Record Practice Council. (2006). Helping consumers select phrs: Questions and considerations for navigating an emerging market. *Journal of AHIMA, 77*(10), 50–56. Retrieved from http://library.ahima.org/xpedio/groups/public/documents/ahima/bok1_032260.hcsp?dDocName=bok1_032260

AHIMA Personal Health Record Practice Council. (2008). Defining the personal health information management role. *Journal of AHIMA, 79*(6), 59–63. Retrieved from http://library.ahima.org/xpedio/groups/public/documents/ahima/bok1_038473.hcsp?dDocName=bok1_038473

American Medical Association. (n.d.). Meaningful use glossary, 2011–2012. Retrieved from http://www.ama-assn.org/resources/doc/hit/meaningful-use-table.pdf

American Medical Informatics Association. (2011). Glossary of acronyms and terms commonly used in informatics. Retrieved from http://www.amia.org/glossary

California Health Care Foundation. (2010). Consumers and health information technology: A national survey. Retrieved from http://www.chcf.org/publications/2010/04/consumers-and-health-information-technology-a-national-survey

Computerisation of personal health records. (1978). *Health Visitor, 51*(6), 227.

Cronin, C. (2006). Personal health records: An overview of what is available to the public. *AARP.* Retrieved from http://www.aarp.org/research/health/carequality/2006_11_phr.html

Cushman, R., Froomkin, M., Cava, A., Abril, R., & Goodman, K. (2010). Ethical, legal and social issues for personal health records and applications. *Journal of Biomedical Informatics, 43,* s51–s55. doi:10.1016/j.jbi.2010.05.003. Retrieved from http://www.sciencedirect.com/science/article/pii/S1532046410000614

DHHS: Office for Civil Rights. (n.d.). Personal health records and the HIPAA privacy rule. *Office of Civil Rights.* Retrieved from http://www.hhs.gov/ocr/privacy/hipaa/understanding/special/healthit/phrs.pdf

DHHS: Office of the National Coordinator. (2008). Defining key health information technology terms. The national alliance for health information technology report to the office of the national coordinator for health information technology. Retrieved from http://www.hhs.gov/healthit/documents/m20080603/10_2_hit_terms.pdf

DHHS: Office of the National Coordinator. (2011). EMR vs EHR—What is the difference? *Health ITBizz.* Retrieved from http://www.healthit.gov/buzz-blog/electronic-health-and-medical-records/emr-vs-ehr-difference/

Detmer, D., Bloomrosen, M., Raymond, B., & Tang, P. (2008). Integrated personal health records: Transformative tools for consumer-centric care. *BMC Medical Informatics and Decision Making, 8,* 45.

Dimick, C. (2008). A cost-benefit model for PHRs. *Journal of AHIMA.* Retrieved from http://journal.ahima.org/2008/11/17/a-cost-benefit-model-for-phrs/

EHR Incentive Programs. (2012). *Centers for Medicare & Medicaid Services.* Retrieved from http://www.cms.gov/Regulations-and-Guidance/Legislation/EHRIncentivePrograms/index.html?redirect=/ehrincentiveprograms/

FierceHealathIT. (2010). Revolution health kills its PHR. Retrieved from http://www.fiercehealthit.com/story/revolution-health-kills-its-phr/2010-02-01

Fortin, J., & Drazen, E. (2011). Personal health records: A true personal health record? Not … Not yet. *Computer Sciences Corporation.* Retrieved from http://www.csc.com/health_services/insights/61137-personal_health_records_a_true_personal_health_record_not_really_not_yet?ref=ls

Garrett, P., & Seidman, J. (2011). EMR vs EHR—What is the difference. Retrieved from http://www.healthit.gov/buzz-blog/electronic-health-and-medical-records/emr-vs-ehr-difference/

Gordon, M. (2010). HITECH extends privacy obligations to EHRs and PHR vendors. Retrieved from http://www.itbusinessedge.com/cm/community/features/guestopinions/blog/hitech-extends-privacy-obligations-to-ehrs-and-phr-vendors/?cs=38631

Heubusch, K. (2010). Meaningful use an EHR certification. *Journal of AHIMA.* Retrieved from http://journal.ahima.org/2010/09/02/meaningful-use-and-ehr-certification/

HIMSS. (2007). Personal health records definition and position statement. Retrieved from http://www.himss.org/content/files/phrdefinition071707.pdf

Joos, I., Nelson, R., & Smith, M. (2010). *Introduction to computers for healthcare professionals.* Sudbury, MA: Jones and Bartlett Publishers.

Markle Foundation. (2011). PHR adoption on the rise. Retrieved from http://www.markle.org/publications/1440-phr-adoption-rise

Moen, A., & Brennan, P. (2005). Health@home: The work of health information management in the household (HIMH): Implications for consumer health informatics (CHI) innovations. *Journal of the American Medical Informatics Association, 12*(6), 648–656.

MyHIN. (2012). Privacy policy. *MYHIN.* Retrieved from http://MyHIN.org/privacy.html

National Committee on Vital and Health Statistics. (2006). Personal health records and personal health record systems. Retrieved from http://www.ncvhs.hhs.gov/0602nhiirpt.pdf

Navigating Cancer. (n.d.). Navigating cancer and blood disorders. Retrieved from https://www.navigatingcancer.com/

Nazi, K. (2010). My HealtheVet personal health record. A PPT presentation from the Veterans and consumers health informatics office. Retrieved from http://www.queri.research.va.gov/meetings/eis/CIPRS-EIS-Nazi-MyHealtheVet.pdf

The Office of the National Coordinator for Health Information Technology. (2011). About ONC. Retrieved from http://healthit.hhs.gov/portal/server.pt/community/healthit_hhs_gov__onc/1200

Patientslikeme. (n.d.). Putting patients first. Retrieved from http://www.patientslikeme.com/

Patientslikeme. (2012). Privacy policy. Retrieved from http://www.patientslikeme.com/about/privacy

Ragstedt, C. (1956). Personal health log. *Journal of the American Medical Association, 160*(15), 1320. doi:10.1001/jama.1956.02960500050013

Stewart, D. (2009). Socialized medicine: How personal health records and social networks are changing healthcare. Retrieved from http://www.econtentmag.com/Articles/ArticleReader.aspx?ArticleID=56166&PageNum=3

Thede, L. (2008). Informatics: Electronic personal health records: Nursing's role. *OJIN: The Online Journal of Issues in Nursing, 14*(1). doi:10.3912/OJIN.Vol14No1InfoCol01

The TIGER Initiative. (n.d.). Consumer empowerment and personal health records: Recommendations from the TIGER consumer collaborative team. Retrieved from http://www.thetigerinitiative.org/docs/TigerReport_ConsumerEmpowermentAndPHR.pdf

U. S. Department of Health and Human Services. (n.d.). Personal health records. Retrieved from http://www.hrsa.gov/healthit/toolbox/HealthITAdoptiontoolbox/PersonalHealthRecords/index.html

CHAPTER 7

Telehealth

Debra M. Wolf

LEARNING OBJECTIVES

At the completion of this chapter the reader will be able to:

1. Define terms associated with telehealth services offered through innovative technology.
2. Explore the role of social media in telenursing.
3. Identify professional organizations supporting telehealth services.
4. Analyze how health care organizations use Web 2.0 and telecommunication to extend telehealth services.
5. Explore how innovative telehealth technology is used by consumers within the home environment.
6. Review standards and guidelines used to establish telehealth programs.

TERMS

Telecommunications	Telemonitoring
Teleconferencing	Telenursing
Telehealth	Teleprescence
Telehealth nursing practice	Teleradiology
Telemedicine	Telerehabilitation

*T*ransforming the spoken word into the written word can be traced back to prehistoric times, as evidenced by cave drawings. But in 1876, the exchange of information became a virtual reality thanks to Alexander Graham Bell and the introduction of the telephone (Jelen, McCord, & Pearson, 2000). Over the past decades, people have been exchanging information, including health-related information, in a variety of ways, using various technologies. One of these technologies, the Internet, began as a one-way communication of health information, or Health 1.0. Telehealth is a two-way dialog delivering health care at a distance. In many ways the development of telehealth represents the beginning of social media in health care, or Health 2.0.

153

Lessons learned in the development of telehealth and telenursing have major significance as the new tools of social media become standard protocols within health care delivery.

This chapter focuses on the virtual exchange of information between two entities regarding health related needs, also known as telehealth. The U.S. Department of Health and Human Services (n.d.) defines telehealth as the "use of electronic information and telecommunication technologies to support long-distance clinical health care, patient and professional health-related education, public health and health administration" (para. 1). The American Academy of Ambulatory Care Nursing (AAACN, 2011) defines telehealth as:

> the delivery, management, and coordination of health services that integrate electronic information and telecommunication technologies to increase access, to improve outcomes and contain or reduce costs of health care. Telehealth is an umbrella term used to describe the services delivered across distances by all health-related disciplines. (p. 42)

As demonstrated above, telehealth can be defined by multiple groups in multiple ways. Key to understanding telehealth and its related terminology is understanding in what context these terms are used. This chapter is not a comprehensive discussion of telehealth services, but rather the focus of this chapter is telehealth in the context of social media.

TELE DEFINITION AND RESOURCES

The prefix "tele" is defined as over a long distance (Cambridge Dictionaries Online, 2011). Placing the prefix tele in front of other words reflects activities and/or services that occur between two environments that are located in two different geographic locations. Thus, telecommunication occurs when "using the telephone, Internet, interactive video, remote sensory devices or robotics to transmit information from one site to another" (AAACN, 2011, p. 42). Telemonitoring is "the use of information technology to monitor patients at a distance" (Meystre, 2005, p. 1). Other frequently used terms to address health activities that occur over a distance include telecare, telehealthcare, telerehabilitation, telemedicine, and teleservices. Unfortunately, there is no formal consensus on what terminology should be used to describe the telehealth services at a national or international level (Martin, Kelly, Kernohan, McCreight, & Nugent, 2008). A list of commonly used tele terms is presented in Exhibit 7.1.

Tele Resources

Established in 1993, the American Telemedicine Association (ATA) is an international resource that advocates the use of advanced remote medical technologies (American Telemedicine Association [ATA], 2011a). The ATA outlines within their mission and value statement that what matters is promoting professional, ethical, and equitable improvement in health care through telecommunications and technology (ATA, 2011a). More importantly, what doesn't matter is defining the differences between telemedicine, telehealth, mhealth, remote health, and multiple other new

Exhibit 7.1 *Tele Terms and Definitions*

Telecommunications
"Use of the telephone, Internet, interactive video, remote sensory devices, or robotics to transmit information from one site to another" (AAACN, 2011, p. 42).

Teleconferencing
"Interactive electronic communication between two or more people at two or more sites, which make use of voice, video, and/or data transmission systems" (National Research Council, 1996, p. 248).

Telehealth
"The delivery, management, and coordination of health services that integrate electronic information and telecommunications technologies to increase access, improve outcomes, and contain or reduce costs of health care. Telehealth is an umbrella term used to describe the services delivered across distances by all health-related disciplines" (AAACN, 2011, p. 42).

The use of technology to address the health needs of others across a geographical area (our working definition).

Telehealth Nursing Practice
"The delivery, management, and coordination of care and services provided via telecommunications technology within the domain of ambulatory care nursing. Telehealth nursing is a broad term encompassing practices that incorporate a vast array of telecommunications technologies (e.g., telephone, fax, email, Internet, video monitoring, and interactive videos) to remove time and distance barriers for the delivery of nursing care" (Espensen, 2009, p. 5).

Telemedicine
"The use of electronic and telecommunications technologies to provide and support health care when distance separates the participants" (National Research Council, 1996, p. 248).

Telemonitoring
The use of information technology to monitor patients at a distance (Meystre, 2005)

"The use of audio, video, and other telecommunications and electronic information processing technologies to monitor patient status at a distance" (National Research Council, 1996, p. 248).

Telenursing
The nurses' use of technology to address the health needs of others across a geographical area.

The use of telecommunications and information technology for providing nursing services in health care whenever a large physical distance exists between the patient and nurse (Wikipedia, n.d.).

Teleprescence
"The use of robotic and other devices that allow a person (e.g., a surgeon) to perform a task at a remote site by manipulating instruments (e.g., lasers or dental hand pieces) and receiving sensory information or feedback (e.g., pressure akin to that created by touching a patient) that creates a sense of being present at the remote site and allows a satisfactory degree of technical performance" (National Research Council, 1996, p. 248).

Teleradiology
"Electronic transmission of radiological patient images, such as x-rays, CTs, and MRIs, from one location to another for the purposes of interpretation and/or consultation" (Webster's Online Dictionary, n.d.).

Telerehabilitation
"Application of evaluation, preventative, diagnostic, and therapeutic services via two-way or multi-point interactive telecommunication technology" (American Occupational Therapy Association, 2010, p. 1).

terminologies (ATA, 2011a). The ATA has eleven special interest groups (SIG) that range from Business & Finance SIG to Telehealth Nursing SIG to Home Telehealth & Remote Monitoring SIG (ATA, 2011b).

There are a variety of other associations that have been established to further support the advancement of health care within the telehealth world. In 2002, Congress formally established the Office for the Advancement of Telehealth (OAT; Clancy, 2005). The OAT is located in the Office of Rural Health Policy, located within the Health Resources and Services Administration (HRSA) at the U.S. Department of Health and Human Services, and promotes the use of telehealth technologies for health care delivery, education, and health information services. In 2010, the budget for OAT was $11.6 million (U.S. Department of Health and Human Services, n.d.). Since its inception, this federal agency has been one of the most active groups promoting the use of telehealth services within the Indian Health Service (IHS), which is a federally funded program for American Indians and Alaska Natives (Clancy, 2005). Examples of telemedicine clinical services offered through the IHS include tele-radiology, tele-retinal screening, tele-dermatology, tele-mental health, and tele-cardiology (Clancy, 2005). Exhibit 7.2 provides a list of OAT projects and funding efforts.

Exhibit 7.2 *Telehealth Programs and Grants Supported by the Office for the Advancement of Telehealth (OAT)*

The Telehealth Network Grant Program's primary objective is designed to help communities build the human, technical, and financial capacity to develop sustainable telehealth programs and networks. The Telehealth Network Grant Program supports 17 telehealth networks that are used to expand access to, coordinate, and improve the quality of health care services; improve and expand the training of health care providers; and expand and improve the quality of health information available to health care providers, patients, and their families. http://www.hrsa.gov/ruralhealth/about/telehealth/telehlthnetworks.html

The Licensure Portability Grant Program (LPGP) is a competitive grant program that provides support for state professional licensing boards to carry out programs under which licensing boards of various States cooperate to develop and implement state policies that will reduce statutory and regulatory barriers to telemedicine. http://www.hrsa.gov/ruralhealth/about/telehealth/telehealth.html

The Telehealth Resource Center Grant Program (TRC) is a competitive grant program that provides support for the establishment and development of Telehealth Resource Centers (TRCs). These centers are to assist health care organizations, health care networks, and health care providers in the implementation of cost-effective telehealth programs to serve rural and medically underserved areas and populations. http://www.hrsa.gov/ruralhealth/about/telehealth/telehealth.html

---

Since 1995, the American Academy of Ambulatory Care Nursing (AAACN) has recognized telehealth services as a critical part of the nursing profession (AAACN, 2011). In 2001, the AAACN published their first set of guidelines by and for nursing professionals who were visionary leaders in advancing the nurse's role in telehealth services. In 2011, the 5th edition of the AAACN Scope and Standards of Practice for Professional Telehealth Nursing was released. In this last edition, sixteen standards were defined. Six standards focused on telehealth nursing and the nursing process, referred to as the Standards of Clinical Practice, and ten standards focused on telehealth nursing behavior in the organizational and professional dimensions, referred to as the Standards of Professional Performance (AAACN, 2011). Exhibit 7.3 lists the topic of each standard.

Exhibit 7.3 *AAACN Standards of Practice for Professional Telehealth Nursing*

Standards of Clinical Practice
- Assessment
- Nursing diagnosis
- Identification of expected outcomes/goals
- Planning
- Implementation
- Evaluation

Standards of Professional Performance
- Ethics
- Education
- Research and evidence-based practice
- Performance improvement
- Communication
- Leadership
- Collaboration
- Professional practice evaluation
- Resource utilization
- Environment

AAACN defines the "scope of practice" for telehealth nursing as "clinical, organizational, and professional activities with individuals, groups and populations who seek assistance improving health and/or seek care for health-related problems" (AAACN, 2011, p. 6). The AAACN offers more clarity by sharing the definition of "telehealth nursing practice" as:

> the delivery, management and coordination of care and services provided via telecommunications technology within the domain of ambulatory care nursing. Telehealth nursing is a broad term encompassing practices that incorporate a vast array of telecommunications technologies (e.g., telephone, fax, email, Internet, video monitoring, and interactive videos) to remove time and distance barriers for the delivery of nursing care. (Espensen, 2009, p. 5)

For the purpose of this book, telehealth is being defined as the use of technology to address the health needs of others across a geographical area, and telenursing is being defined as the nurse's use of technology to address the health needs of others across a geographical area.

As professionals, nurses need to have a teleprescence that engages patients and consumers to use technology to advance their health needs. By taking advantage of innovations, nurses and other health professionals can support the needs of the served population. Translating these definitions of telenursing into actual nursing roles and activities is best appreciated by analyzing several examples of existing services, along with selected research studies that support the role of nurses in telehealth environments.

TELEHEALTH AND TELENURSING—EXAMPLES AND DATA

Telehealth is not a new method of meeting the health needs of individuals; in fact, the modern telehealth era can be traced back as far as the 1960s, when astronauts traveled into space. Various forms of technology were used by health professionals on earth to measure and monitor physiologic parameters of the astronauts while they traveled through space (Stokowski, 2008). Today, telehealth services can be administered in many different forms using various technologies. As discussed in Chapter 3, computers, camcorders, webcams, smartphones, electronic tablets, along with Web 2.0 functionality represent a variety of technological devices that support social media activities, further supporting telehealth services.

Telenursing and Telephone Call Centers

One of the earliest types of telenursing was referred to as "nursing telephone call centers." Originally, this type of service was utilized by health maintenance organizations to offer advice over the telephone and later to extend health services after hours (Grossman, n.d.). Today there are several types of nurse call centers utilized by consumers, some are privately owned and others are supported by health care organizations. These centers support patients' needs by having qualified nursing professionals available to answer consumer calls. One example is FONEMED (http://fonemed.com/), which is a limited liability corporation that currently covers 30 states throughout North America and the Caribbean. A second example is supported by a health care organization called Mary Greeley Medical Center. This system is called First Nurse Call Center (http://www.mgmc.org/services/emergency/first-nurse/).

In 2010, Purc-Stephenson and Thrasher conducted a meta-ethnography study to explore nurses' experiences with telephone call centers or telephone triage. Sixteen studies were found, dating from 1980 to 2008. The study identified five major themes reflecting issues and concerns of the telenurse. These concerns included:

- Gaining and maintaining skills
- Autonomy
- New work environment
- Holistic assessment
- Stress and pressure

Even though telenurses are held to the same nursing process and scope of practice as established by the American Nurses Association (ANA; 2010) as non-telenurses, their method of assessment and diagnosing is very different. Nurses who work in telephone call centers must learn to assess a patient through self reports, tone of voice, and an individual's response to questions (Stokowski, 2008). This level of skill requires an experienced nurse who has strong clinical and critical thinking skills (Stokowski, 2008).

Telenursing and Telemonitoring Services

Nurses who are employed in telemonitoring also require strong clinical and critical thinking skills, but have the advantage of additional data through the use of specialized equipment to monitor a patient across a geographical area. Home health nursing is one of the leading nursing services currently using telemonitoring. Telecommunication technologies such as webcams, speakers, and microphones are being used to support synchronized audio/video communication between nurses and patients in the home. Other types of telehealth technology or biometric devices such as blood pressure cuffs, stethoscopes, and pulseometers are being interfaced via a computer with Internet access. These devices support the monitoring of vital signs such as blood pressure, pulse, respiration, and oxygenation. In addition, weight, lung sounds, and glucose levels can be recorded. An example of a home health teleservice is the Lutheran Home Care & Hospice, Inc. (http://www.lutheranhomecare. org/home-health-telemonitoring/). This organization uses telemonitoring to assist individuals in their home to collect vital signs, which are transmitted to the facility's office where a nurse evaluates the data. If the nurse has any concerns, she will contact the patient with a follow-up call. A video demonstrating how telehealth and telenursing can enhance in-home care can be found at http://www.youtube.com/watch?v=MmKNv9detu8.

Although telemonitoring in the home is expanding, telenurses need to stay focused as to the ultimate goal of home health nursing. Assisting the patient and family in self monitoring to maintain a level of self care is the ultimate goal one wants to achieve (Shea, 2011). In most cases, patients should not become dependent on the telenurse to alert them of abnormal findings or become dependent on the nurse to take their vital signs.

Telenursing is a service that can be expanded into almost any area of health care. The ATA (2011c) identified several areas where telehealth nursing can exist: teleICU, teletriage, teletrauma, telestroke, telepediatrics, telemental health, telecardiology, telehomecare, telerehabilitation, and forensic telenursing. A 2005 study identified telehealth nurses in 49 of 50 states as well as in 36 countries worldwide (Grady, Schlachta-Fairchild, & Elfrink, 2005). Telenurses must realize, that an additional licensure to practice across state lines may be required. In non-federal settings, telehealth nurses must have a registered nurse license that complies with both state and federal regulations. In the United States, the nurse licensure compact (NLC) allows RNs to practice across compact members' state lines (National Council of State Boards of Nursing, n.d.).

Although more research is needed to better understand the impact of telehealth on patient outcomes, current studies have found favorable and unfavorable outcomes. A systematic review of the literature on home telehealth for patients with obstructive pulmonary disease compared to usual care, for example, found telehealth to reduce hospitalization rates and emergency room visits; unfortunately, mortality rates were greater in the telephone support group compared to usual care (Polisena et al., 2010). Further research should clarify if additional telemonitoring support would have changed these results.

Another study by Vinson, McCallum, Thornlow, and Champagne (2011) found a statistically significant relationship between patient satisfaction and timeliness of response when telehealth nurses addressed the endocrinology needs of patients within a hospital-based clinic. The authors suggest that telehealth nursing services also can support the chronically ill patient. Lastly, Konschak and Flareau (2008), through their personal experience and review of the literature, found that patients and health care professionals understand the value of telemonitoring programs and the benefits to their stakeholders. Table 7.1 lists several of the advantages and challenges when using telemonitoring to support telemedicine in the home environment, some of which Konschak and Flareau (2008) also recognized.

Table 7.1 *Advantages and Challenges of Telemonitoring in the Home*

Advantages	Challenges
Decrease in hospitalization rates overall	Patients may find technology to be intrusive
Decreased number of hospital days per encounter	Patients are unable to manipulate technology
Increase compliance in taking oral medications	Technology may be seen as not "caring"
Decrease in travel expenses and overall time requirements for patients	Additional costs up-front for equipment to be placed in the home
Extends provider's reach to treat patients in a broader georgaphical area	Technical issues with technology placed in the home
Increases nurse-patient ratio (advantage for administration)	Increased nurse-to patient ratio (disadvantage for staff)
Increase in nursing productivity	Poor nurse adoption of technology, resulting in higher turnover (initially)
Empowers patients	Initial educational needs of staff and patients
Decrease in rehospitalization rates	Need for new policies and guidelines
Decreased traveling time for patients and nurses	Lack of hands-on assessment
Offers earlier interventions	Less human personal contact
	Equipment failure

Telenursing and Social Media Considerations

As nurses advance their practice using various types of telehealth technology, social media will provide them additional tools and options for extending telenursing services to a wide range of patients. As nurses explore opportunities for using social media to advance their practice in telenursing, it is important to note that the ATA (2008) provides a framework of principles for nurses to develop this area of their practice which includes the following points:

▪ Policy—exploring nurse licensure portability such as Nurse Licensure Compact (NLC), establish guidelines and standards for practice, and advocate for legislation that supports telehealth nursing practice.
▪ Clinical—collaborating with ATA and other organizations that promote nurses in telehealth and telemedicine.
▪ Administrative—exploring technology to be effective for telenursing practice, provide adequate training and supervision of all clinicians using the technology, monitor cost effectiveness of nursing care via telehealth technologies.
▪ Education—incorporating telenursing and telehealth information into nursing curriculum.
▪ Research—conducting research to support evidence-based practice in telenursing.
▪ Ethical/legal—advocating for safe and effective technology to meet everyone's needs.

While social media is a tool for delivering telenursing services, it is, also, another tool for professional development. To further support telenurses and other telehealth professionals, social media sites such as The HUB, (http://www.americantelemed .org/i4a/pages/index.cfm?pageID=3795) sponsored by the ATA, facilitate networking, communication, and information sharing. Another social media site is the *Telehealth and Healthcare Social Media Daily* (http://telehealthhealthcaresocialmedia.blogspot.com/), which is a news blog that shares multiple resources to support all forms of telehealth services and professionals. Supporting the consumer in their home using telehealth technology by health care professionals is only one way in which telehealth services are being utilized. Health care organizations are also turning to social media and telehealth to support their patient population.

TELEHEALTH AND ORGANIZATIONAL SERVICES

Health care systems use telehealth technologies to extend their existing services in many ways. For example, health care providers use telecommunication technologies such as emails, wikis, blogs, video conferencing, and webinars to collaborate in a more productive manner across the United States and globally. Telehealth technologies connect departments to departments or facilities to facilities within a health care system. Health care organizations also use telemonitoring technologies to extend existing services to patients' homes through the use of sensors, webcams, videoconferencing, and telecommunications such as texting and emails. The following two sections provide examples of how organizations are using technologies to advance their telehealth services within their organization and to the patient home environment.

In the Health Care Setting

In an attempt to address the lack of pharmacists in a rural cancer center, visionary leaders turned to telecommunication to address their needs and create a process called telepharmacy services. Using telehealth technology, pharmacy technicians at remote community cancer centers were connected with pharmacists at coordinating centers to oversee mixing of intravenous chemotherapy and to review physician orders (Gordon, Hoeber, & Schneider, 2012). Within an 8-month period, approximately 27,000 miles of travel were averted by 47 patients, who accounted for 247 intravenous treatments.

Another example of telehealth is the use of telecommunication to connect specialized expert clinicians to other clinicians to treat and diagnose patients in a critical acute situation. In a study conducted by Demaerschalk, Raman, Ernstrom, and Meyer (2012) to assess if telemedicine (using telehealth technology other than telephones) versus the use of a telephone alone was a better method to treat patients with acute ischemic stroke in a rural underserved community, telemedicine was found to make correct decisions 96% of the time versus 83% via telephone. The researchers believe this 13% higher rate confirms that telemedicine is a viable tool for consulting with acute stroke patients.

As health care systems become more complex, services become more advanced, and clinician shortages continue, multiple hospitals are looking to outsource aspects of their services to privately owned companies using telecommunications. Since the early 2000s, some hospitals adjusted to staff shortages by turning to companies across the world and within the United States for specific services. An example of this is demonstrated by the shortage of U.S. radiologists and the inability of hospitals to meet the demand for 24/7 coverage, resulting in radiologists in Australia, India, Israel, and Lebanon reading scans of patients who live in the United States (Associated Press, 2004).

In 2003, the American College of Radiology (ACR) established a taskforce to explore international teleradiology (Van More et al., 2005). Key areas the ACR explored included legal, regulatory, reimbursement, insurance, and quality assurance. The purpose of the taskforce was to explore these areas and offer information that would be helpful to health care organizations as well as radiologists. In 2006, the American College of Radiology Council adopted a revised statement of the interpretation of radiology images outside of the United States (American College of Radiology [ACR], n.d.). The revisions contained a new paragraph focusing on "ghost" reporting, requiring health care organizations to inform patients of the outsourcing of radiology services through the use of teleradiology (ACR, n.d.).

With this guidance, outsourcing has continued using companies with both national and international locations. A current example of these outsourced radiology services is demonstrated by Teleradiolgy Solutions, located in Bangalore, India, accessible at http://www.telradsol.com/about_us.html. Dr. Kalyanpur, who manages the company, is a U.S.-licensed and credentialed radiologist with post-graduate work at Yale University (Associated Press, 2004). This company was initially established to provide hospitals in the United States with night shift radiology solutions such as reading of scans and x-rays films. Now the company offers Teleradiology to hospitals in Singapore and to hospitals in 20 countries globally. Teleradiology Solutions is accredited by the Joint Commission located in the United States.

Within the United States, ONRAD (2012), accessed at http://www.onradinc.com, is a private physician-owned radiology service that is accredited by the Joint Commission and offers teleradiology services 365 days a year and 24 hours a day. The website states that the company has American Board of Radiology certified teleradiologists who read electronic images in less than 30 minutes; this includes sending the preliminary and final report (ONRAD, 2012). Another U.S. company that offers teleradiology services is USARAD, accessible at http://usarad.com/mission.html, whose mission is to provide accurate, cost-effective radiology services to hospitals and outpatient clinics.

In rural acute care settings, health organizations are turning to telehealth centers to assist in caring for their critically ill patients. The term virtual ICU is used when ICU clinicians monitor critically ill patients who are miles away, often in rural settings. In 2011, the Veterans Affairs Medical Center in Minneapolis initiated a virtual ICU that serves as a control center for seven of their regional hospitals (Lerner, 2012). The virtual ICU is staffed by medical experts who offer specialized expertise. Currently, the virtual ICU oversees five smaller hospitals and is believed to have saved patients from potentially dangerous situations (Lerner, 2012). Lerner (2012) shares statistics from a hospital in Wisconsin that saw a 34% drop in the death rate of ICU patients after initiating a Virtual ICU.

These examples are just a few of the ways health care organizations are turning to telecommunications and telehealth services to address their current patient needs. Nurse leaders need to envision and prepare for how telehealth solutions can be integrated into current nursing practice to support quality outcomes and patient care. In the future, one can anticipate that social media will play an increasingly important role in delivering telenursing. Knowing that creating change and developing new models of care is never easy, nurses need to explore the work done to date in establishing telenursing and other telehealth initiatives in order to guide this process. Having an understanding of how others are being successful and embracing the technology will help lead to success. The following section demonstrates how health care organizations are using telehealth to extend their services to a patient's home environment in an attempt to improve one's overall quality of life.

In the Home Setting

One prominent health care system leading the integration of telehealth services in the home environment is the Veterans Health Administration (VHA). The VHA is a large integrated health care system within the U.S. Department of Veterans Affairs, offering health care services to 5.6 million patients a year (Darkins et al., 2008). In an attempt to meet the needs of the growing patient population with chronic diseases, the VHA introduced the Care Coordination/Home Telehealth (CCHT) program. The program uses various types of innovative technology to communicate and care for patients within their own home. The program combined health informatics, home telehealth services, and disease management support services into one service center. Devices such as videophones and video telemonitors are being used to support audio/video consultations (mimicking the traditional face-to-face encounters); biometric devices are being used to record and monitor vital sign data; and messaging devices are being used to question patients following disease management protocols (Darkins et al., 2008). The CCHT program provided each patient with a care coordinator who assessed the patient's overall condition while improving the patient's level of self-management. Within a four-year period, the program enrolled over 41,000 patients who reflected an 86% mean satisfaction with services provided (Darkins et al., 2008). Overall, the program was responsible for a 25% reduction in number of bed days of care and a 19% reduction in hospital admissions, with CCHT costing $1600 per patient per year (Darkins et al., 2008).

The extent to which telehealth or teleservices can support a variety of health care professionals in reaching patients is unlimited. Cason (2012), when exploring how the Affordable Care Act could benefit occupational therapy practitioners (OTP) and their patients, identified telehealth as the platform to promote national wellness and preventative initiatives. Cason identified four areas in which telehealth is being used by OTP. These areas include "developing skills; incorporating assistive technology and adaptive techniques; modifying work, home or school environments; and creating health promoting habits and routines" (Cason, 2012, p. 132). Cason believes the following are potential benefits of telehealth for OTP:

- Increased accessibility of services to clients who live in remote or underserved areas.
- Improved access to providers and specialists otherwise unavailable to clients.
- Prevention of unnecessary delays in receiving care.
- Decreased isolation for practitioners through distance learning, consultations, and research (Cason, 2012, p. 133).

The use of telecommunication, telemonitoring, and teleservices is not utilized by health care organizations alone, but is also utilized by consumers through social media resources. Manufacturers are designing innovative technology to meet the needs of consumers to live a healthy, independent lifestyle. The following section presents examples of how consumers are utilizing innovative technology and social media to address their needs while assisting or caring for senior family members.

TELEHEALTH TECHNOLOGIES AND CONSUMERS

One of the most common utilized services within the home environment is the use of emergency alert systems, which offer immediate communication with emergency services with the push of a button. The system is frequently used in an attempt to support independent living and provide 24/7 connection to emergency services. There are a variety of companies who offer this service, such as Philips Lifeline (http://philips.lifelinesystems.com/content/default), LifeStation (http://www.lifestation.com/brochure4.php?ConID=12&gclid=CK3ao onV364CFUPc4Aod_yh7ZQ), and First Response (http://www. firstresponsesystem.com/).

These systems consist of a personal pendant, bracelet, or belt clip worn by an individual, which is remotely connected through wireless frequency to a communication box that is wired to a telephone line. When activated by an individual, the system sends an immediate signal to the system provider, who then communicates through the phone system to the individual in need of assistance. If no contact can be made or if emergency services are needed, the provider then contacts emergency personnel and a predefined list of contacts.

Mobile apps, discussed in chapter 4, are also being used by consumers for telehealth services that promote a healthier lifestyle. For example, "Waterlog" (http://www. neatgeek.net/now-your-phone-reminds-you-to-drink-more-water.html) is a mobile app that can be downloaded to a smartphone or digital device. This app will assist individuals in tracking how much water they drink in a day, and if they forget to drink the predetermined amount, the app will remind them to drink more.

Another type of telehealth technology is MedSignals, an innovative technology designed to assist individuals in taking prescribed medication on a daily basis (MedSignals, n.d.). The technology is designed to be an interactive system to alert individuals to take their medication at prescribed times during the day (MedSignals, n.d.). The device has programmable compartments and uses voice announcements, beeps, LED flashes, and a display screen to communicate instructions on taking medications (MedSignals, n.d.). MedSignal's device (see Figure 7.1) sits in a cradle that uses a telephone line to upload information to a database that will assess one's efficiency in taking medications as prescribed. Mozes (2008) reported in a study funded by the National Institute on Aging, that patients ages 65 to 84 who used MedSignals had a decrease in the number of days they had an interruption in taking their medications from 12% to 6%.

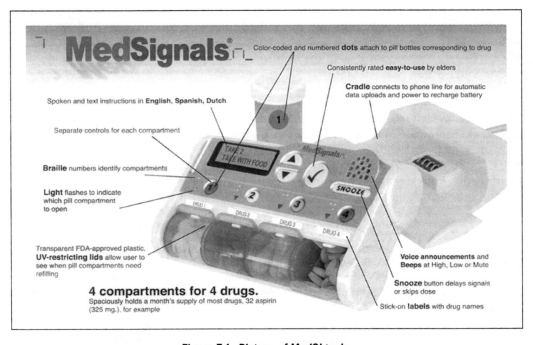

Figure 7.1 *Picture of MedSignals.*
Source: MedSignals®. Retrieved from http://www.medsignals.com/HowItWorks.aspx

Using personal emergency response systems, mobile apps, and electronic medication dispensers are the more common forms of telehealth technology being integrated into the home environment by consumers. Other forms of telehealth technology include the use of motion sensors and remote monitoring systems to assist individuals in caring for family members. Olsen (2008) presents a real case scenario where family living in Wyoming were able to check the status of an elderly relative living in Minnesota by viewing reports that appear daily on their home computer. The family installed a series of motion detectors that record specific times and locations of when and where the family member walks throughout the home. This type of monitoring system is expected to become commonplace in the future (Olsen, 2008).

Care Innovations is a newly structured company that emerged from a joint venture between GE Healthcare Intel Telehealth, and Independent Living Company (Intel, 2011). Care Innovations' purpose is to support healthy independent living for senior housing communities (Intel, 2011). One of the first products developed through Care Innovations is "QuietCare®." QuietCare is an advanced motion sensor technology that learns the daily activity patterns of an individual (Care Innovations, 2011). If an individual's activity pattern changes from their routine, or if there is an extended period of time when a motion sensor is not tripped, an alert is sent to caregivers to respond to a potentially urgent situation (Care Innovations, 2011).

These are a few examples of how telehealth services are now being utilized by consumers. A search of the Internet in May 2012, using the Boolean search string *telenursing AND* "social media" and the Google search engine, produced 9550 hits in .08 seconds. This number is expected to explode exponentially with more and more individuals turning to social media for nursing services and health-related needs. As consumers begin to mandate more access to telehealth services, nurses, other health care professionals, and health care institutions will need to establish a variety of telehealth programs to meet the growing consumer demand. The following section provides several considerations and resources that can be utilized in establishing a telehealth program.

ESTABLISHING A SUCCESSFUL TELEHEALTH PROGRAM

As health care organizations and consumers turn to innovative approaches such as telecommunication, motion detectors, and social media to advance a healthier lifestyle, nurses and other health care professionals need to explore the development of these new opportunities for extending their role or services.

Professional Organizations, Standards, and Guidelines

From 1993 to 2011, ATA, in its role as an organization advocating for telehealth services, developed nine sets of standards and guidelines (ATA, 2011d; see Table 7.2 for a full listing of the standards, guidelines, and URL addresses).

There are also several nursing organizations or associations who have established networks and resources to support the role of telenursing. The International Council of Nursing (http://www.icn.ch/networks/telenursing-network/) has created a "telenursing network" to support the educational and collaborative needs of nurses involved with telehealth technologies. The International Society for Telemedicine and eHealth (http://www.isfteh.org/working_groups/category/telenursing) provides a forum for nurses to share information and extend services worldwide using telehealth

Table 7.2 *ATA Standards & Guidelines*

Standard & Guidelines	Year	URL Address
Videoconferencing-Based Telepresenting Expert Consensus Recommendations	2011	http://www.americantelemed.org/i4a/forms/form.cfm?id=41&pageid=3919&showTitle=1
Telehealth Practice Recommendations for Diabetic Retinopathy	2011	http://www.americantelemed.org/i4a/forms/form.cfm?id=42&pageid=3920&showTitle=1
A Blueprint for Telerehabilitation Guidelines	2010	http://www.americantelemed.org/i4a/forms/form.cfm?id=37&pageid=3915&showTitle=1
Practice Guidelines for Videoconferencing-Based Telemental Health	2009	http://www.americantelemed.org/i4a/forms/form.cfm?id=24&pageid=3717&showTitle=1
Evidence-Based Practice for Telemental Health	2009	http://www.americantelemed.org/i4a/forms/form.cfm?id=25&pageid=3718&showTitle=1
Core Standards for Telemedicine Operations	2008	http://www.americantelemed.org/i4a/forms/form.cfm?id=40&pageid=3918&showTitle=1
Practice Guidelines for Teledermatology	2007	http://www.americantelemed.org/i4a/forms/form.cfm?id=39&pageid=3917&showTitle=1
Home Telehealth Clinical Guidelines	2003	http://www.americantelemed.org/files/public/standards/Home%20Telehealth%20Clinical%20Guidelines(1).pdf
Clinical Guidelines for Telepathology	1999	http://www.americantelemed.org/files/public/standards/ClinicalGuidelinesForTelepathology_withCOVER.pdf

Source: Retrieved from http://www.americantelemed.org/i4a/pages/index.cfm?pageid=3311

services. The College of Registered Nurses of Nova Scotia (http://www.crnns .ca/documents/TelenursingPractice2008.pdf) has developed a set of telenursing practice guidelines. In addition to providing the telenurse with a scope and standards of practice (see Exhibit 7.3), the AAACN (http://www.aaacn.org/cgi-bin/WebObjects/ AAACNMain.woa/wa/viewSection?s_id=1073743920) also offers telenurses additional services such as:

- Telehealth Nursing Practice Core Course On-the-Road
- Telehealth Nursing Practice Core Course on CD-ROM
- Telehealth Nursing Practice Essentials Textbook
- Telehealth Nursing Practice Special Interest Group
- Telehealth Nursing Practice Resource Directory
- Telehealth Nursing Practice Tool Kit

The Digital Imaging and Communications in Medicine (DICOM) organization, located at http://medical.nema.org/, is another example of an organization that offers standards one can review. DICOM is a division of NEMA, which is a trade association for the electrical manufacturing industry. The DICOM Standards Committee was established to "create and maintain international standards for communication of biomedical diagnostic and therapeutic information in disciplines that use digital images and associated data" (Digital Imaging and Communications in Medicine [DICOM], 2012, p. 4).

The Society of American Gastrointestinal and Endoscopic Surgeons (SAGES) is another example of a professional organization that offers assistance in developing a telehealth service. This professional association established guidelines for the surgical practice of telemedicine. These guidelines can assist in developing policies and procedures for safe practice. The guidelines can be accessed at http://www.sages .org/sagespublication.php?doc=21. These are just a few examples of organizations that offer established guidelines for telehealth services offered from institution to institution.

Krupinski et al. (2011), when reviewing telehealth programs, identified one telehealth program that became very successful. These authors believe that when preparing to establish telehealth services, organizations need to have a strong infrastructure, a variety of clinical services, a training/educational program, and a strong business model. The Arizona Telemedicine Network (ATN), part of the Arizona Telemedicine Program (ATP), has this type of infrastructure. ATN has the ability to link 170 different sites in approximately 70 communities within 55 independent health care settings, offering more than 60 telehealth clinical subspecialties (Krupinski et al., 2011). When exploring infrastructures, organizations need the capability to link various services within different geographical locations.

Education and Training

Education and training are two very important and time-consuming needs for any new program. When exploring a new telehealth program, an organization must understand the educational needs of the office staff, the clinical experts who will be using the technology, and, most importantly, the patients who will be receiving virtual services in their home. Krupinski et al. (2011) believe the providers must have the following knowledge and skills:

- A strong foundation in understanding how technology works.
- An opportunity to play with the equipment in order to achieve certain proficiency and comfort levels.
- A strong ability to troubleshoot issues or address problems when they arise.
- An understanding of how to socialize virtually with patients. For example, staff needs to understand the best way to make eye contact when performing a virtual consult using synchronized video teleconferencing.

Most successful organizations would agree that a strong business model is key to being successful. Depending on the services offered and programs available, a business model will vary from organization to organization. Understanding what one wants to achieve; what population one wants to attract; the legal, ethical, and moral considerations; and what others have done to achieve success in the same area are just a few questions that must be explored. Stroetmann, Dobrev, and Jones (2010), in a presentation to WoHIT regarding how to establish a business plan for telehealth, shared a list of essential elements that must be included in a business plan. The elements include services, sub-suppliers, social preference, direct competitors, supply channels, payers, business partners, regulations, indirect competitors, users, and business culture. The presenters believe one needs to understand the demand side (customers, payers, stakeholders) versus the supply side (including one's business, competition, and partner options). See Chapter 8 for more information on business models.

Within the health care arena, developing a new service or extending an existing service takes considerable planning, time, resources, and finances. Table 7.3 provides a list of resources that offer a multitude of information and guidance in what has worked successfully in telehealth and what guidelines one needs to follow or meet.

Table 7.3 *Resources Supporting Telehealth*

Name	URL Address
American Academy of Ambulatory Care Nursing—Telehealth	http://www.aaacn.org/cgi-bin/WebObjects/AAACNMain .woa/wa/viewSection?s_id=1073743920
American Telemedicine Association	http://www.americantelemed.org
California HealthCare Foundation—Telehealth	http://www.chcf.org/topics/telehealth
Center for Telehealth & e-Health Law	http://ctel.org/#
DICOM (Digital Imaging and Communications in Medicine)	http://medical.nema.org/
iTeleHealth Inc.—Telenursing	http://www.itelehealthinc.com/telenursing.htm
International Council of Nurses—Telenursing Network	http://www.icn.ch/networks/telenursing-network/
Medicaid Policies on Telehealth Services: A comparative analysis	http://www.mehaf.org/media/docs/resources/2006/06/01/ telehealth_ctel.pdf
Medicaid.gov (telemedicine)	http://www.medicaid.gov/Medicaid-CHIP-Program-Information/By-Topics/Delivery-Systems/Telemedicine.html
Nurses.info	http://www.nurses.info/media_telenursing.htm
Office for the Advancement of Telehealth	http://www.hrsa.gov/ruralhealth/about/telehealth/
SAGES (Society of American Gastrointestinal and Endoscopic Surgeons)	http://www.sages.org/sagespublication.php?doc=21
Telehealth Law History	http://www.connectedhealthca.org/policy-projects/ telehealth-model-statute/telehealth-law-history
Telehealth Ontario	http://www.health.gov.on.ca/en/public/programs/telehealth/
Telehealth Resource Centers	http://www.telehealthresourcecenter.org/
Telemedicine.com	http://telemedicine.com/
Telenursing Practice Guidelines	http://www.crnns.ca/documents/TelenursingPractice2008.pdf
VHA Office of Telehealth Services	http://www.telehealth.va.gov/

SUMMARY

The use of telehealth technology to advance a higher level of telehealth services can only be expected to expand. The ability to a) extend services to rural areas that lack access to specialized services, b) extend services to patients home, c) address patients needs virtually, and d) consult with other expert clinicians to make critical decisions at point of care is just the beginning. As the newer tools of social media continue to impact telenursing, nursing professionals will need to be visionary leaders embracing innovative approaches to helping each other; helping empowered, engaged consumers; and helping caregivers who themselves may be at a distance. This chapter has reflected upon numerous examples of how one can utilize innovative telehealth technology through social media to advance one's practice.

DISCUSSION QUESTIONS

1. Discuss how you can support the Telehealth Nursing SIG goal to develop guidelines for nursing curriculum development and integration regarding telehealth by including content related to social media. Their website can be found at http://www.americantelemed.org/i4a/pages/index.cfm?pageID=3327/.

2. As the caregiver of a 95-year-old coherent woman (who lives independently in her own home), discuss how you would support her independence virtually, including the use of social media. Share what telehealth services you would integrate into the home to assist with daily medications, glucose monitoring, and physical activity. Try to ascertain the cost of the services you would recommend.

3. Table 7.3 provides a list of resources that focus on telehealth. Select one resource and explore their website. Discuss the following: a) how would you utilize the resource to establish a telehealth service within your organization; b) what patient population would you focus on to extend services to their home environment; and c) with what professional services would you collaborate, using telecommunication and other social media to make point of care decisions?

4. Using various forms of technology within a home environment that supports telecommunication for independent living, discuss the advantages and disadvantages the consumer may experience. What resources will be needed to support the individuals?

5. You are the Director of a home health visiting nurse association. As you are preparing to initiate a new model of care involving social media, telemonitoring, and telehealth services, discuss how you would involve your staff in designing and preparing for the transition. Discuss how you would prepare your staff and patients for this transition. Identify what standards and guidelines you would use to assist you in the process, explaining why.

EXERCISES

Exercise 1: Debate on Standards

Purpose: *The purpose of this activity is to provide students with the experience of debating a practice standard while exploring the need for change due to the advancement of telehealth services.*

Objectives
1. Research standards of practice for telehealth nursing in ambulatory care.
2. Articulate a position on a standard of practice for telehealth nursing in ambulatory care.

Directions
1. Students will divide into two debate teams.
2. Each team will research the pros and cons of the American Academy of Ambulatory Care Nursing's (AAACN) current approach to the standards of practice for telehealth nursing in ambulatory care. In their research, each team should note how the current standards address the reality of social media.
3. Each team will select either the pros or the cons.
4. The first team will present their argument for or against the approach, followed by the second team.
5. Each team will then respond to the other's position.

Exercise 2: Selecting a SIG Supporting Telenursing

Purpose: *The purpose of this exercise is to understand the value and support organizations can offer when establishing a telehealth service.*

Objectives
1. Identify at least two SIGs that support telenursing.
2. Evaluate the benefit in working with an SIG that supports telenursing.

Directions
1. Visit the American Telemedicine Association website (http://www.americantelemed .org/i4a/pages/index.cfm?pageID=3327).
2. Select two of the eleven SIGs and develop a PowerPoint presentation that compares the overall mission, interests, goals, and activities of each group for the upcoming year.
3. Compare how the two SIGs have addressed the impact of social media and the development of Health 2.0.
4. Explain why you chose these two SIGs and how you see the group advancing health care in 2020.
5. Identify which SIG you would be willing to join and explain why.

Exercise 3: Exploring Nurse Call Centers

Purpose: *The purpose of this exercise is to explore existing nurse call center services that are available to support consumers' health-related needs.*

Objectives
1. Identify two nurse call centers used by consumers.
2. Define services offered through nurse call centers to meet consumers' health-related needs.

Directions
1. Search the Internet and locate two nurse call centers, if possible, within your local geographical area. FONEMED (http://fonemed.com/) and First Nurse Call Center (http://www.mgmc.org/services/emergency/first-nurse/) are two examples to consider.
2. Take some time and review both websites.
3. Answer the following questions:
   a. As a consumer, would you feel comfortable calling the center for your health-related needs? Explain why or why not.
   b. Is there a cost for the services offered? Do you feel there should or should not be a cost associated with using the services?
   c. Are the companies associated with a health care organization or are they privately owned? What are the benefits or disadvantages of using a company associated with a health care organization versus one that is independently owned?
   d. Compare and contrast the differences between the two centers.

e. Compare how these two centers are or are not using social media to support their services.

f. Identify which call center you would recommend to consumers and explain why.

4. Prepare a two-page paper sharing your responses

Exercise 4: Searching for TeleTerminology

Purpose: *The purpose of this exercise is to explore existing terminology used to describe telehealth services via the Internet.*

Objectives
1. Identify terminology used to discuss telehealth services.
2. Define common terms used to describe telehealth services.

Directions
1. If you were to search the Internet for the following terms: telemedicine, telehealth, telenursing, and telecommunications, estimate which term would have the most results/returns.
2. Now actually conduct a search on each term using a search engine. Was your initial answer correct? Explain why or why not.
3. Explore how various websites define these terms.
4. Determine if the advent of social media and its potential uses in telehealth require the development of new terms.
5. Develop your own definition of each term, including any new terms you have proposed in item 4.
6. Using a class blog, post your definitions for others to review. Offer one Internet site that supports each of your definitions.

Exercise 5: Telenursing and Social Media

Purpose: *The purpose of this exercise is to understand how telenursing is using social media to meet the health needs of consumers.*

Objectives
1. Identify different social media tools used by telenurses.
2. Evaluate the type of services offered by telenurses through social media sites.

Directions
1. Conduct a search on YouTube.com using the term "telenursing"
2. Identify the number of results that were returned. Did you expect to find more or less? Explain why or why not.
3. Select two of the results and watch the entire video presentation.

4. Answer the following questions:
   a. What type of social media tools or activities are presented in the video?
   b. Does the video clearly state that certified telehealth nurses will be taking the calls?
   c. Does the video share what accrediting bodies approve their services?
   d. Does the video identify what telehealth standards or guidelines are used to establish the program?
   e. Would this video help you in developing a telenurse service within your institution?
   f. Does the video identify what types of technological devices are needed to support the telehealth services?
5. Post to a class blog the two videos you selected. Share your responses to the questions above.

REFERENCES

American Academy of Ambulatory Care Nursing. (2011). *Scope and standards of practice for professional telehealth nursing* (5th ed.). Pitman, NJ: Author.

American College of Radiology. (n.d.). *ACR Council adopts revised statement on the interpretation of radiology images outside of the United States.* Retrieved from http://www.acr.org/SecondaryMainMenuCategories/BusinessPracticeIssues/Teleradiology/ACRCouncilAdoptsRevisedStatementontheInterpretationofRadiologyImagesOutsideoftheUnitedStatesDoc1.aspx

American Nurses Association. (2010). *Nursing: Scope and standards of practice* (2nd ed.). Washington, D.C: Author.

American Occupational Therapy Association. (2010). Telerehabilitation. *American Journal of Occupational Therapy, 64*(6), S92–S102. http://dx.doi.org/10.5014/ajot.2010.64S92

American Telemedicine Association. (2008). *Telehealth nursing: A white paper developed and accepted by the telehealth nursing special interest group.* Retrieved from http://www.americantelemed.org/files/public/membergroups/nursing/TelenursingWhitePaper_4.7.2008.pdf

American Telemedicine Association. (2011a). *About ATA.* Retrieved from http://www.americantelemed.org/i4a/pages/index.cfm?pageID=3281

American Telemedicine Association. (2011b). *Telehealth nursing SIG.* Retrieved from http://www.americantelemed.org/i4a/pages/index.cfm?pageID=3327

American Telemedicine Association. (2011c). *Telehealth nursing fact sheet: ATA telehealth nursing SIG.* Retrieved from http://www.americantelemed.org/files/public/MemberGroups/Nursing/Fact_Sheet_FINAL.pdf

American Telemedicine Association. (2011d). *Telemedicine standards & guidelines.* Retrieved from http://www.americantelemed.org/i4a/pages/index.cfm?pageid=3311

Associated Press. (2004). *Some U.S. hospitals are outsourcing work: Shortage of radiologists spurs growing telemedicine trends.* Retrieved from http://www.msnbc.msn.com/id/6621014/ns/health-health_care/t/some-us-hospitals-outsourcing-work/

Cambridge Dictionaries Online. (2011). Retrieved from http://dictionary.cambridge.org/dictionary/british/tele

Care Innovations. (2011). *Care innovations quietcare.* Retrieved from http://www.careinnovations.com/products/quietcare-assisted-living-technology

Cason, J. (2012). Telehealth opportunities in occupational therapy through the affordable care act. *The American Journal of Occupational Therapy, 66*(2), 121–136.

Clancy, C. (2005). *Testimony on telemedicine activities at the department of health and human services.* Retrieved from http://www.hhs.gov/asl/testify/t050518a.html

Darkins, A., Ryan, P., Kobb, R., Foster, L., Edmonson, E., Wakefield, B., & Lancaster, A. (2008). Care coordination/home telehealth: The systematic implementation of health informatics, home telehealth, and disease management to support the care of veteran patients with chronic conditions. *Telemedicine and e-Health, 14*(10), 1118–1126. doi:10.1089/tmj.2008.0021

Demaerschalk, B. M., Raman, R., Ernstrom, K., & Meyer, B. C. (2012). Efficacy of telemedicine for stroke: Pooled analysis of the stroke team remote evaluation using a digital observation camera (STRokE DOC) and STRokE DOC Arizona telestroke trials. *Telemedicine Journal and E Health, 18*(3), 230–237. PMID: 22400970.

Digital Imaging and Communications in Medicine. (2012). *Strategic document*. Retrieved from http://medical.nema.org/dicom/geninfo/Strategy.pdf

Espensen, M. (Ed). (2009). *Telehealth nursing practice essentials*. Pitman, NJ: American Academy of Ambulatory Care Nursing.

Gordon, H., Hoeber, M., & Schneider, A. (2012). Telepharmacy in a rural Alberta Community Cancer Network. *Journal of Oncology Pharmacy Practice, 18*(3), 366–376. PMID: 22378811.

Grady, J., Schlachta-Fairchild, L., & Elfrink, V. (2005). Results of the 2004-2005 International telenursing survey. *Telemedicine and e-Health, 11*(2), 197.

Grossman, V. (n.d.). *History of telephone triage*. Retrieved from http://www.rnceus.com/triage/triageframe.html

Intel. (2011). *GE and Intel's telehealth and independent living company is operational today*. Retrieved from http://newsroom.intel.com/community/intel_newsroom/blog/2011/01/03/ge-and-intels-telehealth-and-independent-living-company-is-operational-today

Jelen, A., McCord, S., & Pearson, J. (2000). The telephone in Wisconsin. *The Wisconsin Mosaic: Information Infrastructure*. Retrieved from http://comminfo.rutgers.edu/~dalbello/FLVA/infrastructure/infoinfra/telephone/index.html

Konschak, C., & Flareau, B. (2008). New frontiers in home telemonitoring: It's already here. Where are you? *JHIM 22*(3), 16–23.

Krupinski, A., Patterson, T., Norman, C., Yehudah, R., ElNasser, Z., Abdeen, Z., ... Freedman, M. (2011). Successful models for telehealth. *Otolaryngologic Clinics of North America, 44*, 1275–1288. doi:10.1016/j.otc.2011.08.004

Lerner, M. (2012). Remote 'eye in the sky' keeping tabs on VA hospital patients. *StarTribune/Wellness*. Retrieved from http://www.startribune.com/lifestyle/wellness/140512933.html?page=all&prepage=1&c=y#continue

Martin, S., Kelly, G., Kernohan, W. G., McCreight, B., & Nugent, C. (2008). Smart home technologies for health and social care support. *Cochrane Database of Systematic Reviews, 4*. Art. No.: CD006412. doi:10.1002/14651858

MedSignals. (n.d.). *MedSignals: How it works*. Retrieved from http://www.medsignals.com/HowItWorks.aspx

Meystre, S. (2005). The current state of telemonitoring: A comment on the literature. *Telemedicine Journal and E Health, 11*(1), 63–69. Retrieved from http://www.ncbi.nlm.nih.gov/pubmed/15785222

Mozes, A. (2008). Electronic pillbox helps seniors stick to drug regimens. *HealthDay News for Healthier Living*. Retrieved from http://www.medsignals.com/MediaAwards.aspx

National Council of State Boards of Nursing, (n.d.). Nurse Licensure Compact. Retrieved from https://www.ncsbn.org/nlc.htm

National Research Council. (1996). *Telemedicine: A guide to assessing telecommunication for healthcare*. Washington, DC: The National Academies Press. Retrieved from http://www.nap.edu/openbook.php?record_id=5296&page=R1

Olsen, E. (2008). High-tech devices keep elderly safe from afar. *New York Times*. Retrieved from http://www.nytimes.com/2008/05/25/us/25aging.html?_r=1&pagewanted=1

ONRAD. (2012). *Teleradiology solutions*. Retrieved from http://www.onradinc.com/services/teleradiology

Polisena, J., Tran, K., Cimon, K., Hutton, B., McGill, S., Palmer, K., & Scott, R. (2010). Home telehealth for chronic obstructive pulmonary disease: A systematic review and meta-analysis. *Journal of Telemedicine and Telecare*. Retrieved from http://jtt.rsmjournals.com/content/16/3/120.abstract

Purc-Stephenson, R. J., & Thrasher, C. (2010). Nurses' experiences with telephone triage and advice: a meta-ethnography. *Journal of Advanced Nursing, 66* (3), 482. doi:10.1111/j.1365-2648.2010.05275.x

Shea, K. (2011, October). Guest editorial: Home health telemonitoring: Don't forget the goal of self-care. Issues, impacts and insights column. *Online Journal of Nursing Informatics (OJNI), 15* (3). Retrieved from http://ojni.org/issues/?p=861

Stokowski, L. (2008). *Healthcare anywhere: The pledge of telehealth*. Retrieved from http://www.medscape.com/viewarticle/581800

Stroetmann, K., Dobrev, A., & Jones, T. (2010). *Establishing the business case for telehealth services: Success factors and lessons learned*. Retrieved from http://www.worldofhealthit.org/sessionhandouts/documents/PS3-3-Stroetmann.pdf

U.S. Department of Health & Human Services. (n.d.). *Telehealth*. Retrieved from http://www .hrsa.gov/ruralhealth/about/telehealth/

Van More, A., Bibb, A., Campbell, S., Carlson, R., Dunnick, R., Fletcher, T., ... Thrall, J. (2005). Report of the ACR task force on international teleradiology. *Journal of the American College of Radiology* 2(2), 121–125. Retrieved from http://www.acr .org/SecondaryMainMenuCategories/BusinessPracticeIssues/Teleradiology/ ReportoftheACRTaskForceonInternationalTeleradiologyDoc3.aspx

Vinson, M. H., McCallum, R., Thornlow, D. K., & Champagne, M. T. (2011). Design, implementation, and evaluation of population-specific telehealth nursing services. *Nursing Economics,* 29(5), 265–272.

Webster's Online Dictionary. (n.d.). *Teleradiology*. Retrieved from http://www.websters-online-dictionary.org/definitions/Teleradiology#Wikipedia

Wikipedia. (n.d.). *Telenursing*. Retrieved from http://en.wikipedia.org/wiki/Telenursing

CHAPTER 8

Business Models and Health-Related Social Media

Ramona Nelson

LEARNING OBJECTIVES

At the completion of this chapter the reader will be able to:

1. Conceptualize health care delivery systems as an industry consisting of government, profit, and non-profit organizations, agencies, and businesses.
2. Explain the concept of a business model and the related sub-concepts.
3. Explore the implications of business models utilized by Health 2.0 companies and organizations.
4. Analyze the significance of Terms and Conditions and Privacy statements when used with Health 2.0 applications.

TERMS

Aggregators

Behavior targeting

Business model

Business strategy

Contextual targeting

First-party tracking

Freedom of Information Act (FOIA)

Geo targeting

Gray literature

Gross national product (GNP)

Initial public offering (IPO)

Leakage

Personal identifiable information (PII)

Publicly traded company

Super-cookies

Third-party tracking

Third-party tracking cookies

Clickwrap or clickthrough agreement

Browsewrap

Nurses are committed to providing cost-effective, quality care for communities, families, and individuals. Web 2.0 opens a new array of tools for delivering that care as well as challenges to ensuring the safety, privacy, and quality of the provided care. To effectively use Web 2.0 tools for one's own professional development, to extend the level of health-related services provided, and to educate patients about health-related social media sites, nurses and other caregivers need to understand business models and processes. In today's networked world of social media, nurses and other health care providers require an understanding of (1) health care as an industry or business, (2) ownership and business model concepts, and (3) business models used in the Health 2.0 industry.

In most cases, when patients, nurses, and other users access social networking sites and other Web 2.0 tools, it appears that these tools and services are provided for free. However, the social networking sites, wikis, blogs, and other applications all require hardware, software, and support personnel. The user may not pay a fee, but these applications and services are not provided without business costs and the potential for business income. This is true whether the company or organization providing the sites and applications are profit or non-profit. Just as one would check the source and credentials of individuals providing health information on the net, an educated user of a Health 2.0 site should evaluate who is providing the services as well as the motivation and business model of that individual or company.

For example, Facebook, which has recently become a publicly traded company, sought to raise $5 billion from its initial public offering (IPO), which placed the estimated market value for Facebook at $80 to $100 billion. In 2011, Facebook employed around 3,000 people, which calculates to an average revenue of $1.2 million per employee. This level of productivity is possible because the site's users effectively act as employees, adding content and value. The information added to the site by its individual users is their personal information. One of the key methods used by Facebook to generate income is selling advertisements that are targeted to the specific interests of its users based on the personal information that the users have posted (Daily Chart, 2012). This chapter focuses on translating the business model demonstrated in this example to Health 2.0 social media with the goal of understanding the implications of business models for patients, nurses, and other users of social media.

THE AMERICAN HEALTH CARE SYSTEM AS AN INDUSTRY

Health 2.0 is an evolving subsection within the larger health care industry. Most nurses think of health care as a service provided by health care providers, but patient care is just one part of this larger industry. Note the number of statistics related to the cost of health care and demonstrating this point. Using gross national product (GNP) as one measure, the health care industry is the largest single industry in the United States. In 2010, U.S. national health expenditures were over $2,593 billion. This translates to $8,402 per person. Of this amount, 84.3% or $2,444.6 billion was spent on personal care (Centers for Medicare and Medicaid Services, 2012). Figure 8.1 demonstrates how each of these health care dollars is divided. This figure is based on health care costs that are directly tied to health services and does not include other health-related costs such as nonprescription drugs, vitamins, or decisions to join a gym or to purchase books with health related advice. Health 2.0 industries focus on business opportunities related to these directly tracked costs as well as all the other revenue opportunities related to health and health care. In other words, the market for Health 2.0 applications is even larger than the numbers presented here would indicate.

The directly tracked costs for health care are covered through a combination of sources. Public and private insurance paid $1,870.8 billion of the total. The cost of providing a typical family of four with an employer-based insurance plan is expected to top $20,000 in 2012 (Dickler, 2012). The out-of-pocket portion of the total equals $299.7 billion. Table 8.1 demonstrates how these out-of-pocket monies were spent.

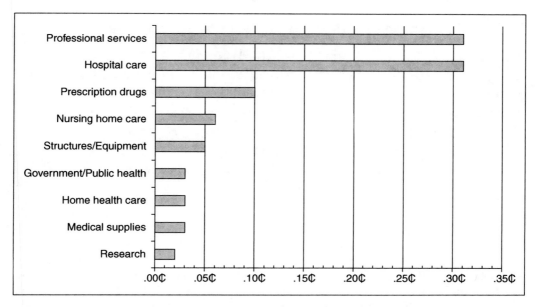

Figure 8.1 *Where each health care dollar is spent.*
Source of data: Hartman, M., Martin, A., Nuccio, O., Catlin, A., and the National Health
Expenditure Accounts Team. (2010).

Table 8.1 *Consumer Out-of-Pocket Health Care Expenditures in 2008*

Category	Expenditure
Health care total[1]	$138,527,000,000
Hospital care	21,120,000,000
In-patient care	12,209,000,000
Outpatient/emergency room care	8,912,000,000
Physicians' services	21,993,000,000
Dental services	30,741,000,000
Other professional services	11,170,000,000
Prescription drugs	42,962,000,000
Medical supplies	10,541,000,000

[1] Excludes health insurance premiums, nursing home care, nonprescription drugs, nonprescription
vitamins, and topicals and dressings.
Source: U.S. Department of Labor, Bureau of Labor Statistics (2010, March 25).

The remainder of these costs is covered by other third party programs (Centers for
Medicare and Medicaid Services, Office of the Actuary, National Health Statistics
Group, 2012). These numbers are so large most people have a hard time comprehending this amount of money. In addition, these costs are presented as money spent—not
as income.

But health care is an industry and the other side of this coin is that every dollar
spent for health care is a revenue source for the health care industry. Exhibit 8.1 lists
several examples of the types of businesses that are part of the health care industry.

Exhibit 8.1 *Examples of Business Types Within the Health Care Industry*

Biotechnology	Hospitals
Diagnostic substances	Insurance and health care plans
Drug delivery	Long-term care facilities
Drug manufacturers	Medical appliances and equipment
Drug-related products	Medical instruments and supplies
Health care practitioners	Medical laboratories and research
Health care information systems	Specialized health services
Home health care	

Health Care Industry Structure

At the top level, this industry can be conceptualized as a hierarchical system divided first into public or private subsystems. The private side, which is divided into profit and not-for-profit, is also referred to as the non-governmental side of the industry. The public side, which is sometimes referred to as the government side, is further divided into local, state, and federal government health care agencies. These agencies provide direct care in some cases, but they are also a major payer for health care services. Figure 8.2 illustrates the hierarchical structure of the health care system.

Although government agencies are a major section of the health care industry, they have some important differences from the non-governmental segment of the industry, including their liability and disclosure requirement. As government agencies are paid for by tax payers they are owned by citizens. While there are a number of legal exceptions, as a general rule government agencies cannot be held liable unless the government says it can be sued (NOLO Law for All, n.d.). In theory, since the government is owned by its citizens, suing a government agency is the same as suing yourself. This protection extends to the use of Health 2.0 applications provided to the government. For example, the 152 Department of Veterans Affairs medical centers are each represented on Facebook (United States Department of Veterans Affairs, 2011). But if Facebook wanted to sue the Department of Veterans Affairs, Facebook would need permission from the government.

However, in the private sector, liability is an important factor in structuring business decisions. The concept that the government is owned by its citizens also frames laws and legislation dealing with access to information. The United States Freedom of Information Act (FOIA) is the legislation providing public access to government records.

> FOIA carries a presumption of disclosure; the burden is on the government—not the public—to substantiate why information may not be released. Upon written request, agencies of the United States government are required to disclose those records, unless they can be lawfully withheld from disclosure under one of nine specific exemptions in the FOIA. (The Gelman Library, The George Washington University, n.d.)

On the non-government side of the health care industry, the presumption is that information is private unless there are specific reporting requirements. This can have a significant influence on what information is available to the public as well as the format

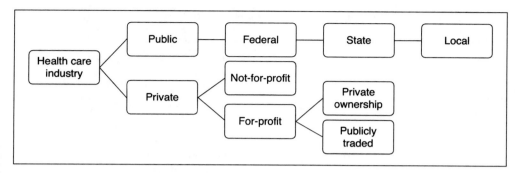

Figure 8.2 *Health care industry structure.*

for accessing that information. This has significant implications for what information a company must reveal about their business practices in their online privacy statement.

Government and non-government services also differ in their sources of income. For the government, taxes and fees are the primary source of income. The government can also take in funds for providing certain services for the community. For example, state-owned universities charge tuition. In Pennsylvania, liquor stores are run by the state government. Public transportation is subsidized by the government. In contrast, non-government agencies must be self supporting and a business model is used to frame the process by which these organizations generate income.

Business Model Concepts in the Health Care Industry

Non-government health care services are divided into non-profit and for-profit. Non-profit organizations are established to provide a community service. All income generated by a non-profit is returned to the organization. Non-profit organizations are not owned by individuals or stockholders and have different reporting requirements than for-profit businesses. In a for-profit business, the money that is left after expenses is income that is returned to the owners of that business. There is a further distinction between publicly traded for-profit companies and private for-profit companies. Any person, company, or institution that owns a share of a company is called a shareholder. In both private and publicly traded companies, the company is owned by the shareholders. A company is classified as publicly traded if the opportunity to purchase a share of the company in the form of stock is open to the general public. A private company usually has 100 or less shareholders and their shares of stock cannot be purchased by the public.

Publicly traded companies are traded on an open market and have different reporting requirements than private for-profit companies. An example of this reality is demonstrated by the information that is required in the prospectus for any publicly traded company. Where an individual business fits in the larger health care industry is determined by several other factors including: (1) the size of the organization or company, (2) the services or products offered, (3) the profit or non-profit status, and (4) the ownership of the business, including how that ownership is structured. With for-profit companies, there are four basic types of ownership possible with a number of variations of each type. Table 8.2 provides an overview of these four types with examples of Health 2.0-related businesses.

All businesses, including those focused on health care, must generate income or revenue to survive. The revenue pays expenses of the organization and maintains and grows the business. For example, in 2008 the top ten pharmaceutical companies took in

Table 8.2 Types of Business Ownership with Health 2.0 Examples

Type of Ownership	Description	Levels of Liability	Examples
Sole Proprietorship	Owned and operated by an individual.	The owner is personally liable for the actions and expenses of the business.	A private speaking and consulting business established by Dave deBronkart located at http://epatientdave .com/
General Partnership	Owned and operated by two or more individuals who have agreed to form a business together.	Each owner is personally liable for the actions of each of the partners and the total expenses of the business.	
Limited Partnership	Owned and operated by two or more individuals who have agreed to form a business together; however, one or more of the partners has a limited status and is not involved in the day-to-day operation of the company.	The limited partner(s) is only liable to the extent of his or her individual investment.	Patientslikeme was established as a private for-profit company founded in 2004 by two brothers and a long-term friend. A list of the investors can be seen at http://www .patientslikeme.com/ about/investors.
Limited Liability Company (LLC)	Similar to a sole proprietorship or partnership except the liability is transferred to the company.	Liability is limited to the company and the owner(s) are protected from personal liability.	Health 2.0 LLC located at http://www.health2con .com/ was co-founded by Matthew Holt and Indu Subaiya.
Corporation	A legal entity that is separate from the people who own it. There are several different types of corporations.	Liability is limited to the company and the owner(s) are protected.	WebMD Health Corp. located at http://www .wbmd.com/index .shtml is a publicly traded company listed on the NASDAQ Stock Exchange with the symbol WBMD.
Professional Corporations	Operated by licensed professionals, such as doctors and nurses.	Limited personal liability for business debts or claims against the corporation. However, professionals are still liable for their own actions and can be sued for malpractice.	Global Medical Networks, P.C., a California based professional corporation consisting of board-certified and fully licensed physicians. Additional information can be seen at http:// www.ringadoc.com/ about/
Subsidiary Corporation	A corporation that is totally owned by another corporation. This company is referred to as the parent corporation.	Liability is limited to the company and the owner(s) are protected.	Wellsphere located at http://www.wellsphere .com/ is wholly owned by the private company Health Central located at http://www .healthcentral.com/

a total of $301 billion in sales alone. This money was then used for a variety of purposes from research and development of new drugs to dividends for company shareholders. Much of health care is a labor-intensive industry with significant employment opportunities within the larger economy. The U.S. Department of Labor (DOL) reported that as of May 2011 there were 7,514,980 people employed in health care with an average annual salary of $72,730. Registered nurses were the largest occupation group, with nearly 2.4 million jobs, and an average salary of $69,110 (DOL, Bureau of Labor Statistics, 2012). An additional 3,954,070 people were employed in health care support in occupations such as nursing aides or assistants at an average salary of $27,370 (DOL, Bureau of Labor Statistics, 2012). A business model describes how a business generates income or makes money. The process of developing a business model is referred to as developing a business strategy. Web 2.0 applications are increasingly an integral part of the business model for many businesses including the businesses that make up the health care industry. In addition, a number of Health 2.0 businesses have been established. The concept of a business model is not usually applied to a government agency. However, many of the same activities that create a successful business model in private business, including use of Web 2.0 applications, can be applied to evaluate the effectiveness of government agencies and their programs.

Business models have been integral to trading and economic behavior since pre-classical times (Teece, 2010). However, the term "business model" first began appearing in the literature in 1975 (Zott, Amit, & Massa, 2011). A review of the literature demonstrates that the number of articles addressing this concept exploded after 1995. Various authors have proposed the extensive usage of the concept since the mid-1990s, and this may have been driven in part by the advent of the Internet (Amit & Zott, 2001).

While there are several different types of business models, all business models have five common attributes: (1) a product, (2), customers, (3) a process for producing the product, (4) a method for delivering the product, and (5) a process for attracting customers to the product.

Product

To generate income, a company must bring something of value, referred to as a product, to the market. Identifying the product and defining the market is the first step in building a business model. The product can be a tangible item such as medical equipment or medications; it can be a service such as providing a physical exam or EKG; or an intangible item such as emotional support or health care information. For example, key products offered by Health 2.0 companies can include access to others with similar challenges or health data contributed from patients. A nursing blog may include advertisements. Nurses are a trusted and respected group. Access to screen space that associates the business being featured in the advertisement with nursing is a product of value. The company being advertised is willing to pay for that access.

Any one business can bring a single product to the market or can offer a variety of products. In either case the business will focus on a segment of the market. For example, a pharmaceutical company will focus on developing and marketing drugs. The market is made up of willing buyers for the product who are the customers.

Customer

The customer is the individual(s) or company(s) interested in using/obtaining or buying the product. The market can be a small local population or it can be a worldwide market. The better the business understands the customer creating the market for their product, the more effectively the business can develop the product to meet the market need as well as target the product to their specific customer. For example, many people noticed that when conducting a search using Google the ads on the right-hand side of the screen reflect businesses in your area or your recent searches. If you do a search using the word pizza you are very likely to see advertisements for local pizza businesses. Your personal interest in pizza has been identified by the term you typed in a search engine. Being able to target an advertisement directly to a person who could be interested in that product is a major advantage for a business. Your personal interests, which can be separated from your personal identifying data, are the products that have been sold to the businesses displaying ads on your computer screen.

Process for Producing the Product

Having identified the product and defined the market, the business is ready for the second step in building a business model. The second step is to identify the resources and processes needed to produce the product. The resources can be both tangible and intangible. For example, computer equipment and software for setting up a Health 2.0-related website are tangible resources used to provide health care. The reputation of the site for delivering quality information can be an important intangible resource. One of the most important resources within any business is the people. The knowledge, skills, and attitudes will in the end determine if the other resources in that business are effectively used to create the product. For example, one should expect to see well educated experienced health care professionals closely associated with and/or employed by a Health 2.0 website designed for patients with specific health problems.

How the employees interact with each other in using the resources of the business define the processes for creating the product offered by that business. Web 2.0 tools and applications are increasingly part of the product development process. For example, wikis can be used to facilitate the development of patient-education materials, policy and procedure manuals, and educational materials for managing difficult clinical situations.

Method for Delivering the Product

It might seem obvious that the method for delivering the Health 2.0 product would be the Internet. But it is not that simple. First, the product must be packaged in a usable format. Castlight, which has been listed on *The Wall Street Journal*'s Top 50 Venture-Backed Companies for 2011, provides an example of this challenge. This company offers an online tool that gives patients cost and quality information for doctors, hospitals, and specific procedures based on **their** individual insurance plan. Hopefully, this information will improve the quality of care received while controlling costs. Packaging the product requires access to the specific health insurance benefits of each employee. As a result the product is only available to employees whose employers have a contract with Castlight. Packaging also requires a user-friendly intuitive interface for the employee to use in doing a search. Getting employees to log on, search the data, and then use this information in making decisions is the second challenge in actually delivering the product. The goal is to obtain 70% employee engagement. The oldest client has only been with Castlight for a year, so they are just beginning to analyze their ability to actually deliver their product (Bebinger, 2012). Telehealth, which is the focus of Chapter 7, provides several additional examples of delivering a Health 2.0 related product.

Process for Attracting Customers to the Product

The process of attracting customers is termed advertising. The goal with all advertising is to reach the highest number of potential customers for the lowest cost. Online advertising provides an excellent environment for reaching both these goals, and as a result has become a huge business. The Interactive Advertising Bureau and PricewaterhouseCoopers reported that U.S. Internet advertising revenue hit $7.3 billion in the first quarter of 2011 alone (*The Boston Globe*, 2011). This level of revenue has generated a number of related businesses and powerful interest groups.

In 2009, the Interactive Advertising Bureau reported that 80% of online advertisements used a targeted approach (Hugo, 2011). With a targeted approach the potential customer has been carefully selected to receive a specific advertisement based on factors such as their current or previous activities, demographics and/or location. Some common approaches (Web Ad Vantage, n.d.) include:

- Contextual targeting—The ads are supplied based on related content a user is currently viewing online. For example, if a patient would search Google for information on arthritis or search Facebook for arthritis-related groups, ads related to anti-inflammatory drugs and other treatments for arthritis would appear on the screen.
- Geo-targeting—The ads supplied are based on a user's geographic location. This is an effective approach for local businesses. For example, the search using the term arthritis can produce ads for local pain clinics and/or chiropractic services. To provide location-specific ads, the location of the user's computer must be tracked.
- Behavioral targeting—The ads are based on user behavior. Behavioral targeting uses a variety of online activities such as recent online purchases, searches, and browsing history, as well as demographic details such as age, gender, sexual orientation, medical history, and income.

A study sponsored by the Network Advertising Initiative (NAI) and conducted by Former FTC Consumer Protection Chief Howard Beales found that behaviorally targeted advertising is more than twice as effective at converting users who click on the ads into buyers (6.8% conversion vs. 2.8% non-targeted ads and secured an average of 2.68 times as much revenue per ad; Beales, 2010). While this approach is effective, it is also very controversial.

As early as 2000, well before social networking was established, targeted advertising was described as online profiling (Federal Trade Commission, Bureau of Consumer Protection, 2000). In February 2012, the Pew Internet and American Life Project released the Pew Internet Project survey dealing with search engines. Pew reported that 91% of online adults age 18 and older use search engines to find information on the web, including 59% of those who do so on any given day. Of this group, 91% say they always or most of the time find the information they are seeking when they use search engines. However, 73% of these search users indicated that they would not be okay with a search engine keeping track of their searches and using that information to personalize future search results because they feel it is an invasion of privacy. At the same time, just over half of the adults who use search engines (52%) report that search results have become more relevant and useful over time. These results might suggest that targeting is helping users find relevant information. At the same time, 68% of these users indicated that they are not okay with targeted advertising because they don't like having their online behavior tracked and analyzed (Purcell, Brenner, & Rainie, 2012).

The process of collecting and analyzing these data, often referred to as third-party tracking, is usually a separate industry, from advertising. Inherent in the concept of targeting is the reality that specific customer attributes are known and being matched to target specific ads to an individual. Key privacy concerns include: (1) what specific personal data have been collected; (2) what individuals and/or companies have access to that data; (3) how are these data being used; (4) can the individual find out what data have been collected; (5) are there any procedures for correcting errors in these data; and (5) do they have any control over what data are now being collected and have been collected in the past?

Social media, with the significant increase in personal identifiable information (PII), has escalated the concerns these questions represent. PII is defined as data that can be used to distinguish or trace a specific individual's identity either alone or when combined with other information (Krishnamurthy & Craig, 2009). The use of a third-party server, which is steadily increasing, provides content and advertisements for websites such as Facebook or Google+. Many of these third-party servers are aggregators, which track and aggregate user data across different sites, often via third-party tracking cookies. Leakage of PII occurs when an individual logs in to a social networking site and the social network includes their advertising and tracking code in such a way that the third-party aggregator can see and record the contents of the profile page for that individual. These PII data are then added to third-party aggregators files. Krishnamurthy and Craig (2009) surveyed 12 social networks. The sites surveyed included Bebo, Digg, Facebook, Friendster, Hi5, Imeem, LiveJournal, MySpace, Orkut, Twitter Xanga, and LinkedIn. Only Orkut did not leak PII to third party aggregators.

Business Models in Social Media

Most social media sites are free to the user. At the same time, a variety of business models are used (Loayza, 2009; Rappa, 2010) to underwrite the cost of providing these services as well as generating profit. For example, Facebook generated $1 billion in profit in 2011. In that same year EBAY earned over $8 billion. The potential market for Heath 2.0 companies is, of course, smaller than the market for a company such as Facebook, and in turn the profit is less. For example, WebMD earned a profit of $357.10 million in 2011. In addition, many health-related social media sites are not publicly traded and, as a result, specific financial data that documents the source and amount of income is not easily available. While the term business model is not usually applied to non-profit organizations, these approaches to generating income are used on both profit and non-profit social media sites. Business models most commonly seen in health-related social media sites include the following:

Advertising Model
There are a variety of approaches that can be used to introduce users to products on a health-related social networking site. With a content-targeted ad, an online support group for cancer patients would include banner ads for nutritional supplements. A breast cancer site might include ads for lymphedema-related products and treatment. A website designed to attract nurses could include ads for additional nursing degrees or continuing education. A more subtle approach can be even more effective. For example, with contextual advertising a continuing education unit on the nurse's role in treating lymphedema can include links to companies that sell compression sleeves. This provides the nurse with the latest information related to compression products and prices

at the same time the company obtains valuable advertising space. Another approach used mainly with video is to insert a 15 to 30 second ad before the video is shown and/or to include specific brands of products within the video.

Another subtle form of advertising involves the uses of sponsored links. For example, the Dr. Susan Love Research Foundation lists several companies on their website. If you go through the Foundation to purchase products from these companies, a portion of the money paid for the product is donated back to the Foundation. The first company listed is Amazon, which donates 5% of purchases through the Foundation site to the Foundation.

Infomediary Model

With this model the users of the social media site create information that can then be sold. For example, the social media company, PatientsLikeMe, includes the following statement on their site:

> We take the information patients like you share about your experience with the disease and sell it to our partners (i.e., companies that are developing or selling products to patients). These products may include drugs, devices, equipment, insurance, and medical services. Except for the restricted personal information you entered when registering for the site, you should expect that every piece of information you submit (even if it is not currently displayed) may be shared with our partners and any member of PatientsLikeMe, including other patients. We do not rent, sell or share personally identifiable information for marketing purposes or without explicit consent. Because we believe in transparency, we tell our members exactly what we do and do not do with their data. (PatientsLikeMe, n.d.)

In describing their business model they go on to say "We work with trusted non-profit, research and industry partners who use this health data to improve products, services and care for patients" (PatientsLikeMe, n.d.). One of the themes throughout this book deals with the changing relationships and beliefs between the various stakeholders within the health care industry. Using a *transparent approach*, this for-profit business can be described as partnering with patients to potentially improve the health care they receive by selling their data.

While PatientsLikeMe makes their business model very clear, other sites are often not so clear in their communication. The Caring4Cancer site includes the following statement in their Terms and Condition Statement:

> We may, however, make anonymous by removing or masking personal identifiers and/or aggregating publicly available information, your personal health information, and that of other registered users to provide such information in that form to third parties, but never in such a way that it violates your privacy. (P4 Health care, n.d.)

Another version of the infomediary model is in operation when the users review a product or service and these opinions are collected and sold. There are several websites that rate health care providers and institutions. The patient ratings are not objective data based on measurable criteria. For example, a surgeon with excellent knowledge and skill may lack strong communication skills and in turn receive low overall ratings from patients. How these ratings are interpreted and used can have a significant impact on this surgeon's employment. There are a variety of ways these opinions can be analyzed, packaged, and sold. The website HealthGrades.com includes the following statement in a list of approaches to packaging these types of data: "CPM has the only tool that uses physician psychographic profiles to help you understand how a physician thinks and behaves to create more impactful communications with better response" (HealthGrades, n.d.).

As the number of users increases, the amount and value of the data provided by the users of the site also increase. In 2011, HealthGrades,

> a leading provider of information to help consumers make an informed decision about a physician or hospital and CPM, the leading provider of customer relationship management solutions for hospitals ... announced a definitive agreement to merge the two companies. The combination will create a single online company with more than 200 million annual visitors, providing consumers the ability to find, select and connect with physicians and hospitals by accessing its comprehensive information about clinical outcomes, patient satisfaction, and patient safety. Together the companies will provide hospitals with an efficient and accountable digital media and relationship management platform with the unique ability to help hospitals differentiate their brands, build their physician practices, grow admissions, and improve the health of their populations. (HealthGrades, 2011)

Access Model
In this model, access to a specific group of users is the product provided by the company. The social media site SERMO (www.sermo.com) provides an example of this approach as demonstrated by the following quote on their website:

> The Business Model
> Sermo is free to practicing physicians. Revenue is generated as health care institutions, financial services firms and government agencies purchase Sermo Products to access this elite group of practitioners.
> For physicians, the two-sided Sermo marketplace provides a unique online environment in which clinical observations can be exchanged in real-time. They can build consensus on products and issues, take advantage of financial opportunities and improve patient care by working directly with colleagues and industry leaders.
> For Sermo clients, Sermo offers a revolutionary way to target and engage physicians on-demand by leveraging social media. In doing so, they can instantly capture real-world physician insights into treatments, medications and devices that support a broad range of objectives. (Sermo, n.d.)

The company, founded in 2005, has over 120,000 members (Sermo, n.d.), which is close to 20% of the active physician population in the United States.

Subscription Model
As the name implies, this model involves the user paying for the service. Sometimes the memberships are tiered with a free limited membership and a charge for higher

levels of membership. Angie's List, a for-profit publicly traded company, is an example of this approach. "Angie's List operates a consumer-driven service for members to research, hire, rate, and review local professionals for critical needs, such as home, health care and automotive services" (Angie's List Inc., 2011). The service is consumer driven. Members rate local businesses including health care providers. Members pay a fee to buy access to these ratings. The membership fees vary by location, length of the subscription, and specific package selected. In the Pittsburgh market, fees varied from a high of $125 plus $10.00 sign-up fee for four years of access to all ratings, to a low of $1.25 plus $10.00 signup fee for one month of access to the health-related service providers (Angie's List, 2012).

Businesses including health-related businesses do not pay to join. However they are offered a "premium" membership as well as additional services for a fee. For example, when a member contacts the call center for a referral, they will receive the names of businesses with a premium membership (Angie's List, n.d.). For the fiscal year ending in 2011, this company reported a profit of $64.52 million. Membership fees constituted 38% present of Angie's revenue, while products provided to the businesses made up the remaining 62% (Angie's List Inc., 2011). In other words the great majority of the income for this company is earned from the services provided to those whose basic membership is free; however, they are buying a number of the additional services offered by the company. On this site, the combination of business models where members pay for a subscription and businesses pay for access creates a potential conflict of interest between services for the Angie's list members and the businesses that are providing the majority of the income.

Product Model

This model involves selling an app, item, or product to the users of the website. This model is used equally in for-profit and non-profit sites. For example, health-related apps can be purchased on Facebook, while the American Cancer Society includes an online bookstore. Many non-profit health-related websites that provide social networking, blogs, and other social media opportunities sell jewelry and T-shirts with their name or logo.

Donation Model

The donation model is unique to non-profit sites but an important part of the business model for these sites. This model is usually used by non-profit organizations that offer social networking services in addition to a number of other services that are traditionally associated with brick-and-mortar agencies. The opportunity to donate is usually on the homepage or within one click. For example, both Goodwill (http://www.goodwill.org/) and the American Cancer Society (http://www.cancer.org/) include a tab with the words Get Involved. Clicking on this tab will take you to a screen that includes the opportunity to donate among a list of options. The American Heart Association (http://www.heart.org/HEARTORG/) included the word *Giving* on this home page.

The business model of an individual company may be clearly disclosed on their website or the user may be left to infer the business model from other documents posted on the website. In these cases, the most common documents revealing the business model are the Terms and Conditions as well as the Privacy statements. While very few people actually read these before actively participating with the Web 2.0 site, these documents have significant implications for users.

TERMS AND CONDITIONS AND PRIVACY STATEMENTS

Increasingly, a number of websites include a "Privacy Statement" and a statement of "Terms and Conditions." This is especially true for social media sites. The Privacy Statement describes how the site collects and uses private information. The Terms and Conditions statement describes how users may access and use the content and functions offered by the site. Each of these documents is a legal contract between the website company providing the social media services and the user of these services. These contracts take effect when that contract is signed. On the Internet these contracts can be signed in two ways. First, if the user is given an opportunity to read the document and must select an "accept" option to access the website or services, they have legally signed a clickwrap or clickthrough agreement. The user does not have to actually read the document for the contract to be enforceable. There are a wide range of variations on different websites in terms of how easy it is for a user to actually access and read these documents. The easier it is for the user to read the agreement before accessing the site, the more enforceable the contract. The Electronic Frontier Foundation includes a list of "best practices" for clearly presented clickwrap agreements (Bayley, 2009):

1. Conspicuously present the Terms of Service or Privacy Statement to the user *prior* to collecting any payment or data or making any changes to the users machine such as installing a cookie.
2. Ensure the document has a readable font that is not confined in a scroll box making it easy to read and navigate *all* of the terms. Provide an opportunity to print, and/or save a copy of, the document.
3. Offer the user the option to decline as prominently and by the same method as the option to agree.
4. Ensure the document is easy to locate online *after* the user agrees.

The second way a contract can be signed is termed browsewrap. These agreements bind the users by passive conduct such as continuing to use the website or proceeding past its homepage. As with clickwraps, the key issues are notice and opportunity to review the terms. Courts are especially skeptical where service providers do not place links and/or references to terms or privacy statements in conspicuous locations. However, some courts have ruled that browsewraps can be enforced under certain circumstances. The more a site calls the user's attention to the terms while browsing, the more likely a court will be to find it enforceable (Bayley, 2009).

One of the major limitations with these types of documents is that they are rarely read by any user. There are several reasons why this is true. First they are long, often several pages. In 2008, researchers at Carnegie Mellon University (CMU) estimated that the average user would need over 25 eight-hour days each year to skim over the privacy statements from the sites they visit (McDonald & Cranor, 2008). Today these documents are longer. In addition they are difficult and boring to read. Figure 8.3 provides an analysis of the reading levels for four common examples of privacy statements. This analysis was conducted by scanning each document in Microsoft Word 2010.

Exhibit 8.2 lists the types of information that one can expect as part of a Privacy Statement. Exhibit 8.3 lists the types of information that one can expect as part of a Terms and Conditions statement.

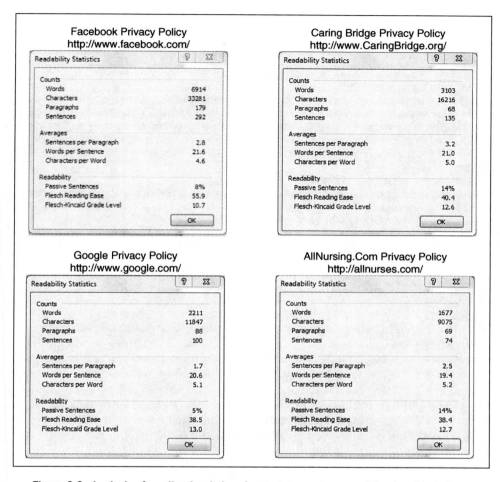

Figure 8.3 *Analysis of reading levels in privacy statements on social networking sites.*

Exhibit 8.2 *Expected Content and/or Sections in an Online Privacy Statement*

- Definition of terms including the definition of personal data.
- List of types of data collected such as personal and/or technical.
- List of personal identity data elements collected.
- List of the collected information that can be seen by the user.
- Description of how data are being collected. Is this done via cookies including super-cookies? Are data being collected by forms or automated scanning of content on the website?
- What third-party sharing of data is occurring and how are those data collected?
- What privacy agreements exist or do not exist with third-party companies?
- Are there other privacy statements that apply to the data collected by third-party companies?
- Options available for opting-in or opting-out of data collection and data sharing.
- Description of how all data that are collected are used.
- Provisions specific to collecting and using data from children.
- How are all data secured?
- Does the policy meet any recognized standards or have approval from any outside organization?
- Procedure for notification when changes are made.
- Contact for questions and concerns.

Exhibit 8.3 *Expected Content and/or Sections Found in Terms and Conditions Statements*

▧ Scope of the document or overview of document contents.
▧ Who is eligible to use the site?
▧ A list of behaviors that are required and a list of behaviors that are not permitted by all users.
▧ A list of behaviors that are required and a list of behaviors that are not permitted by select groups. For example, if the account is established by a business vs. an individual, are there additional rules?
▧ Statement on ownership, copyright, and use of material you post on the site. For example, who holds the copyright, to information, pictures, and other materials posted by users on the site?
▧ Relationship with third-party sites and developers.
▧ Liability limits of the website company.
▧ Rules and regulations specific to payments, refunds, and financial dealings between the user and the website company.
▧ Description of the procedure(s) for resolving disputes.
▧ Contact information for concerns and questions.

SUMMARY

Safely and effectively using social media and Health 2.0 applications requires that users understand the business model and motivation of the companies and organizations that offer these services. This is especially true for nurses and other health care providers who are responsible for providing patient education or are interested in extending health-related services using Web 2.0 functionality via social media tools. Patients and health care providers use these services because they provide information and meet human needs that are imperative for quality health care. However, one needs to understand the full cost of these services to make intelligent choices about how these services can best be used.

DISCUSSION QUESTIONS

1. Federal law requires each of the major credit agencies to provide, on request, a credit report as well as a process for correcting any errors (additional information can be seen at http://www.ftc.gov/bcp/edu/pubs/consumer/credit/cre34.shtm). What are the pros and cons for using this approach as a model to provide individuals on request a complete report on the data maintained in third-party aggregator databases?
2. Should third-party aggregators be required by law to delete all health-related personal data from their databases? Take a stand yes or no and justify your stand.
3. Could and should health-related data in third-party aggregator databases be used to target health-related messages to high risk individuals in the same way that ads are targeted? Explain why you think this would be an effective way to get the right message to the right person(s) or would not be an appropriate approach for health care providers. How can the different business models improve or hinder the quality and effectiveness of health-related media sites that are targeted to specific health providers such as nurses, and to specific individuals with health-related problems?

4. Identify three points learned in this chapter and how these points may help nursing or your agency offer services utilizing social media tools.
5. A professional colleague has expressed an interest in establishing a health related blog for young single moms. What business models would you consider and why?

EXERCISES

Exercise 1: Keeping Secrets

Purpose: *Third-party aggregators use a variety of analytic tools to tease out the information in large databases of personal data. The purpose of this exercise is to explore the impact or possible implications when these data are used by agencies, organizations or businesses.*

Objectives
At the completion of this exercise the reader will be prepared to:

1. Discuss the implications when personal information about specific individuals is identified from large databases of personal data maintained by third-party aggregators.
2. Explore how concepts about what is or is not private information are being changed by social media.

Directions
1. In February 2012, *The New York Times* reported that Target had inadvertently notified a father that his teenage daughter was pregnant when they mailed his daughter coupons that would be of interest to a pregnant women. A copy of this article was posted at http://www.nytimes.com/2012/02/19/magazine/shopping-habits. html?pagewanted=all (Duhigg, 2012). Retrieve and review the article.
2. Do a literature search including a review of the gray literature to determine what other information had been reported about this story. Watch for consistencies and inconsistencies in the different reports. The term gray literature refers to papers, reports, and other documents posted or published by governmental agencies, academic institutions, businesses, and other groups that are not usually peer reviewed or indexed in traditional literature databases such as Medline or CINAHL.
3. Write a paper no more than two pages in length describing the process that Target may have used to determine this woman was pregnant. For the purposes of this paper, begin with the assumption that the woman did not post information that she was pregnant on a social media website.
4. Conclude the paper by suggesting what role social media could have played in this story.

Exercise 2: Social Presence of Businesses in the Health Industry

Purpose: *Social media is not only changing personal relationships but is also changing the relationship between businesses and the customers who use their products. The purpose of this exercise is to introduce the reader to this changing relationship.*

Objectives

At the completion of this exercise the reader will be prepared to:

1. Compare and contrast the business website of a health-related company with their presence on a social media site.
2. Discuss the customer response and impression of the company as a result of viewing these two different types of websites.

Directions

1. During your next clinical visit, identify the brand or manufacturer of three products used in the clinical setting. These could be such things as the manufacturer of hospital beds, stethoscopes, and other equipment for measuring vital signs, health care information systems installed on the clinical units, materials for care of wounds, or medication given to patients.
2. Search for the Internet website of each company and answer the following questions for each of the three manufacturers:
    a. Is this a for-profit company? If yes, are they a private or publicly traded company? If they are publicly traded, what is their annual profit in the last year?
    b. Is the website completely a Web 1.0 site where the company provides information only, or is there any evidence of a Web 2.0 presence where patients or providers can interact with the company online? Describe your findings in terms of this question.
    c. Is there a link between the company's website and a social media site such as Twitter, Google+, Facebook, and so on?
    d. Review the Privacy Statement on the website and explain how this statement describes the company's use of personal information. Include a statement on how they define personal information.
3. Now search for the company on Facebook and answer the following questions for each of these same companies.
    a. Does the company have a Facebook page? If yes, proceed to questions b through e. If not, does the absence of a company webpage on Facebook impact your impression of this company? Explain your answer.
    b. How does the tone or feel of the Facebook site differ from the company's web page?
    c. While Facebook has its own privacy policy, are you able to determine how this company will use and protect privacy information posted on their Facebook page?
    d. Which of the two sites, the company website or the Facebook page, gives you a friendlier, more comfortable feel for each of the companies?
    e. Which of the two sites, the company website or the Facebook page, provides you with more specific information about the products offered by each company?
4. Prepare a PowerPoint-type slide presentation presenting what you learned about social media and its impact on marketing.

Exercise 3: Who Is Watching Me?

Purpose: *The purpose of this exercise is to examine the differences between first-and third-party cookies.*

Objectives

At the completion of this exercise the reader will be prepared to:

1. Control how first-and third-party cookies access their personal computers.
2. Identify individual companies providing third-party aggregator services on the Internet.
3. Analyze how these companies describe their services or products.

Directions

1. Open your Internet browser and locate the area where cookies that have been placed on your computer can be deleted or removed. You may need to look around or use the Help section for your specific browser.
2. Delete all of the cookies on your computer.
3. Set your browser to prompt you for first-party cookies. Again the specific procedure for completing this step varies depending on the specific browser being used but can be found in the Help file. As you reset your browser note the default settings.
4. Go to five different home pages on the Web including a .gov, .edu, .org, .com, and social media site.
5. At each site you will be prompted to save a cookie on your computer. Note the name of the site asking to leave a cookie. For example, if you visited the University of Pittsburgh, the website pitt.edu will ask to leave a cookie. Note what happens if you block the cookie and what happens if you accept the cookie.
6. Now reset your computer to accept first-party cookies but to prompt for third-party cookies.
7. Again visit five different homepages on the Web. Include a .gov, .edu, .org, and .com site as you move to the different home pages.
8. At each site you will be prompted to save one or more cookies on your computer. Note the name of the site asking to leave a cookie. Note what happens if you block the cookie and what happens if you accept the cookie.
9. Now search the Internet for information on the companies who wanted to leave a cookie on your device.
10. Write a two-page paper describing your experience and what you have learned. Include key points you would include in patient education materials from this experience.

Exercise 4: Identifying the Business Model and Related Patient Implications

Purpose: *The purpose of this activity is to explore business models used by health-related social media sites.*

Objectives

At the completion of this exercise the reader will be prepared to:

1. Determine if a health-related social media site is operated by a for-profit company or a not-for-profit organization.
2. Identify and describe business models used by specific health related social media sites.
3. Determine the amount of profit and the product(s) that are producing that profit for a publicly traded company offering a health-related social media site.

Directions

1. Using one or more of the following websites, select four health-related social media sites to explore:
   a. http://mastersinhospitaladministration.com/2011/top-25-health-and-medical-social-media-sites/
   b. http://nursingassistantguides.com/2009/25-excellent-social-media-sites-for-your-health/
   c. http://social-medicine-org.pressdoc.com/28681-social-networking-for-people-with-medical-conditions
   d. http://www.diet-blog.com/08/35_social_media_sites_for_the_health_conscious.php
2. Answer the following questions about each site:
   a. Is there a clear statement explaining who is managing the website?
   b. Do the users pay any fees? Does the site utilize third-party cookies?
   c. Is the site being managed by a for-profit or a not-for-profit company?
   d. Is the business model clearly stated?
   e. If this site is maintained by a for-profit company, is that company a private or publicly traded company?
   f. If the company is publicly traded, what was the profit in the last fiscal year and the source of that profit? The annual report, which can be found on the web, will be very helpful in answering these questions.
3. Create a brochure or podcast including key points that should be included in a patient-education document based on your learning from this activity.

Exercise 5: What Is in a Statement of Terms and Conditions?

Purpose: *The purpose of this activity is to understand the contents and implications of a statement of terms and conditions.*

Objectives

At the completion of this exercise the reader will be prepared to:

1. Assess a statement of terms and conditions for completeness, openness, and clarity.
2. Advise patients on how to read and analyze a statement of terms and conditions.

Directions

1. Using the URLs in the previous exercise, select two health-related social media sites.
2. Copy and paste the statement of Terms and Conditions from the selected sites into a word processing application.
3. Identify the length in either pages or total words and reading level of the document.
4. Complete the following table for each statement of terms and conditions. The first column lists the criteria for evaluating the document; the second column should be answered YES if the document includes content related to the criteria and NO if it is missing. The third column should explain if the criteria content is clearly stated or if there are limitations in the Privacy Statement in terms of that specific criterion.

Criteria for Content to Be Included:	Related Content Is Included?	Content Is Clearly Stated and Easy to Understand?
Scope of the document or overview of what information is included in the document		
Who is eligible to use the site		
A list of behaviors that are required		
A list of behaviors that are not permitted by all users		
A list of behaviors that are required and a list of behaviors that are not permitted by select groups. For example, if the account is established by a business as opposed to an individual, are there additional rules?		
Statement on ownership, copyright, and use of material you post on the site. For example, who holds the copyright to information, pictures, and other materials posted by users on the site?		
Relationships with third-party sites and developers are clearly explained		
Liability limits of the website company		
Rules and regulations specific to payments, refunds, and financial dealings between the user and the website company		
Description of the procedure(s) for resolving disputes		
Contact information for concerns and questions		

5. Write a summary conclusion describing the quality of the documents based on your analysis.

Exercise 6: What Is in a Privacy Policy?

Purpose: *The purpose of this activity is to understand the contents and implications of a privacy policy.*

Objectives
At the completion of this exercise the reader will be prepared to:

1. Assess a privacy statement for completeness, openness, and clarity.
2. Advise patients on how to read and analyze a privacy statement.

Directions
1. Using the URLs in the previous exercise, select two health-related social media sites.
2. Copy and paste the privacy statement from the selected sites into a word processing application.
3. Identify the length in either pages or total words and reading level of the document. Microsoft Word provides this information but you may need to check the Help section for additional directions on how to access this function.

4. Complete the following table for each privacy statement. The first column lists the criteria for evaluating the document; the second column should be answered YES if the document includes content related to the criteria and NO if it is missing. The third column should explain if the criteria content is clearly stated or if there are limitations in the privacy statement in terms of that specific criterion.

Criteria for Content to Be Included:	Related Content Is Included?	Content Is Clearly Stated and Easy to Understand?
Definition of terms including the definition of personal data		
List of types of data collected such as personal and/or technical		
List of personal identity data elements that are collected		
List of collected information that can be seen by the user		
Explanation of how data are being collected		
What third-party sharing of data is occurring and how are those data collected?		
What privacy agreements exist or do not exist with third-party companies?		
Are there other privacy statements that apply to the data collected by third-party companies?		
Options available for opting-in or opting-out of data collection and data sharing		
Description of how all data that are collected are used		
Provisions specific to collecting and using data from children		
Method and procedures for securing data		
Does the policy meet any recognized standards or have approval from any outside organization?		
Procedure for notification when changes are made		
Contact for questions and concerns		
Other comments		

5. Create a blog and write a summary and conclusion describing the quality of these documents based on your analysis.

REFERENCES

Amit, R., & Zott, C. (2001, June). Value creation in e-business. *Strategic Management Journal, 22,* 493–520.

Angie's List Inc. (2011, December 31). Annual Report. Retrieved from United States Securities and Exchange Commission: http://investor.angieslist.com/secfiling.cfm?filing ID=1193125-12-117450&CIK=1491778

Angie's List. (2012, April 12). Membership fees for our Pittsburgh Market. Retrieved from Angie's List: http://my.angieslist.com/angieslist/visitor/price.aspx?u=18

Angie's List. (n.d.). Angie's list overview. Retrieved from Angie's List: http://content.angieslist .com/company/images/SP/AngiesListHealthMediaKit.pdf

Bayley, E. (2009, November 16). The clicks that bind: Ways users "agree" to online terms of service. Retrieved from Electronic Frontier Foundation: https://www.eff.org/wp/clicks-bind-ways-users-agree-online-terms-service

Beales, H. (2010, March 3). The value of behavioral targeting. Retrieved from Network Advertising Initiative (NAI): http://www.networkadvertising.org/pdfs/Beales_NAI_Study.pdf

Bebinger, B. (2012, March 5). Castlight aims to turns patients into informed consumers. Retrieved from Healthcare Savvy: http://healthcaresavvy.wbur.org/2012/03/castlight-aims-to-turns-patients-into-informed-consumers

The Boston Globe. (2011, May 26). US Internet ad revenue hit $7.3B in 1st qtr. Retrieved from Boston.com: http://articles.boston.com/2011-05-26/business/29586807_1_interactive-advertising-bureau-ad-revenue-internet-advertising

Centers for Medicare and Medicaid Services, Office of the Actuary, National Health Statistics Group. (2012). Table 3 National Health Expenditures, Aggregate, and Average Annual Growth from Previous Year Shown, by Source of Funds, Selected Calendar Years 1960–2010. Retrieved from Centers for Medicare and Medicaid Services: https://www.cms.gov/NationalHealthExpendData/downloads/tables.pdf

Centers for Medicare and Medicaid Services. (2012). Expenditures Aggregate, Per Capita Amounts, Percent Distribution, and Average Annual Percent Change: Selected Calendar Years 1960–2010. Retrieved from Centers for Medicare and Medicaid Services: https://www.cms.gov/NationalHealthExpendData/downloads/tables.pdf

Daily Chart. (2012, February 12). Facebook by the Numbers: The social media giant is finally opening its doors to public investors. The Economist. New York, NY. Retrieved from http://www.economist.com/help/about-us#About_Economistcom

Dickler, J. (2012, March 29). Family health care costs to exceed $20,000 this year. Retrieved from CNN Money: http://money.cnn.com/2012/03/29/pf/healthcare-costs/index.htm?hpt=hp_t3

Duhigg, C. (2012, February 16). How companies learn your secrets. Retrieved from New York Times: http://www.nytimes.com/2012/02/19/magazine/shopping-habits.html?pagewanted=all

Federal Trade Commission, Bureau of Consumer Protection. (2000, June). Online profiling: A report to congress. Retrieved from Federal Trade Commission: http://www.ftc.gov/os/2000/06/onlineprofilingreportjune2000.pdf

The Gelman Library, George Washington University. (n.d.). National security archive. Retrieved from The Freedom of Information Act (FOIA): http://www.gwu.edu/~nsarchiv/nsa/foia.html

Hartman, M., Martin, A., Nuccio, O., Catlin, A., & The National Health Expenditure Accounts Team. (2010). Health spending growth at a historical low in 2008. *Health Affairs*, January 29(1), 147–155.

HealthGrades. (2011, November 2). HealthGrades and CPM to merge. Retrieved from Press Release: http://www.healthgrades.com/business/news/press-releases/healthgrades-cpm-merger-2011.aspx

HealthGrades. (n.d.). Physician relationship management. Retrieved from HealthGrades.Com: https://www.cpm.com/index.cfm/solutions/systems/prm-physician-relationship-management/

Hugo, K. (2011, February 28). Targeted advertising on social networking sites is not an invasion of privacy. Retrieved from The Daily Sundial: http://sundial.csun.edu/2011/02/targeted-advertising-on-social-networking-sites-is-not-an-invasion-of-privacy/

Krishnamurthy, B., & Craig, W. (2009, September 21). On the leakage of personally identifiable information via online social networks. Retrieved from Electronic Frontier Foundation (EFF): http://conferences.sigcomm.org/sigcomm/2009/workshops/wosn/papers/p7.pdf

Loayza, J. (2009, June 14). 5 Business models for social media startups. Retrieved from Mashable Inc: http://mashable.com/2009/07/14/social-media-business-models/

Mcdonald, A., & Cranor, L. (2008, March). The cost of reading privacy policies. *ACM Transactions on Computer-Human Interaction, 389*(3), 1–22.

NOLO Law For All. (n.d.). Suing the government for negligence: The federal tort claims act. Retrieved from NOLO Law For All: http://www.nolo.com/legal-encyclopedia/suing-government-negligence-FTCA-29705.html

P4 Healthcare. (n.d.). Privacy policy. Retrieved from Caring4Cancer: https://www.caring4cancer.com/go/home/policies/privacy-policy.htm

PatientsLikeMe. (n.d.). How does PatientsLikeMe make money? Retrieved from Corporate: http://www.patientslikeme.com/help/faq/Corporate#m_money

Purcell, K., Brenner, J., & Rainie, L. (2012, March 9). Search engine use 2012. Retrieved from Pew Research Center's Internet & American Life Project: http://www.pewinternet.org/Reports/2012/Search-Engine-Use-2012.aspx

Rappa, M. (2010, January 10). Business models on the web. Retrieved from Managing the digital Enterprise: http://digitalenterprise.org/models/models.html

Sermo. (n.d.). Get to know Sermo. Retrieved from Sermo: http://www.sermo.com/about/introduction

Teece, D. (2010, April). Business models, business strategy and innovation. *Long Range Planning, 43*, 172–194.

United Stated Department of Labor, Bureau of Labor Statistics. (2012, March 27). News release: Occupational employment and wages – May 2011. Retrieved from Bureau of Labor Statistics: http://www.bls.gov/news.release/archives/ocwage_03272012.pdf

United States Department of Labor, Bureau of Labor Statistics. (2010, March 25). Consumer out-of-pocket health care expenditures in 2008. Retrieved from TED: The Editor's Desk: http://www.bls.gov/opub/ted/2010/ted_20100325_data.htm

United States Department of Labor, Bureau of Labor Statistics. (2012, March 29). May 2011. National occupational employment and wage estimates. Retrieved from Bureau of Labor Statistics: http://www.bls.gov/oes/current/oes_nat.htm#29-0000

United States Department of Veterans Affairs. (2011, December 21). VA launches facebook pages for all 152 medical centers. Retrieved from Department of Public and Intergovernmental Affairs: Press Release: http://www.va.gov/opa/pressrel/pressrelease.cfm?id=2238

Web Ad Vantage. (n.d.). Types of online advertising. Retrieved from Web Ad Vantage: http://www.webadvantage.net/digital-marketing-services/online-media-buying-planning/types-of-online-advertising

Zott, C., Amit, R. H., & Massa, L. (2011, February 11). The business model: Recent developments and future research. Retrieved from Social Science Electronic Publishing, Inc.: http://ssrn.com/abstract=1674384 or http://dx.doi.org/10.2139/ssrn.1674384

CHAPTER 9

Professional Guidelines, Policies, Regulations, and Laws Impacting Health-Related Social Media Communication

Ramona Nelson

LEARNING OBJECTIVES

At the completion of this chapter the reader will be able to:

1. Apply ethical principles and professional guidelines when using social media for professional and personal purposes.
2. Discuss the role of selected federal and state agencies in regulating social media-related activities.
3. Create and implement a personal social media policy.

TERMS

Copyright
Federal Trade Commission (FTC)
Food and Drug Administration (FDA)
National Labor Relations Board (NLRB)

The Equal Employment Opportunity Commission (EEOC)
Trademark

*T*his chapter focuses on information and guiding principles that health-related institutions, professional associations, and health care workers can use in making decisions about appropriate social media-related health care activities. Health care workers include practicing professionals, administrators, faculty, and students. The chapter does not provide a list of do's and don'ts. The rapid development of Web 2.0 applications and the wide variety of approaches to utilizing these applications in the health care arena has made such a list an ineffective approach to guiding professional communication when using social media. The chapter does not cover all potential legal or professional risks that organizations or individuals may face when using social media, but rather provides a foundation for making appropriate decisions.

Social media is redesigning the information superhighway, but one soon discovers when driving on this new highway that the rules of the road are in flux as construction of the road itself is ongoing. On this redesigned information highway, well-positioned road signs do not indicate appropriate, legal, effective, and/or professional behavior. Rather, safe travel on this highway requires that health care professionals:

- Understand how social media applications actually function when a wide range of individuals and groups use them,
- Be aware of the ever changing online environment, and
- Be able to apply ethical principles to new and challenging situations when using social media.

This chapter presents relevant guidelines, laws, and regulations that select federal agencies and state governments enforce. The chapter begins with an analysis of professional guidelines and institutional policies. It concludes by reviewing current applicable laws and regulations.

PROFESSIONALISM AND SOCIAL MEDIA

Online social networks involve the building of connections and relationships by sharing information. The word network in combination with the word social indicates that a group of people are connected together. However, social networks vary in both format and purpose. The Privacy Rights Clearinghouse, in their *fact Sheet 35: Social Networking Privacy: How to be Safe, Secure and Social,* classified social networks into 5 different types (2011). This classification is summarized in Exhibit 9.1. While different social networking sites will emphasize one feature over another, any one site can include any combination of these classifications. In each of these cases, the kind of shared information determines the type of social network that is being utilized. This reality creates three fundamental challenges for health professionals. These are ensuring that the:

- Shared information does not violate the privacy of patients, colleagues, and/or institutions;
- Established connections and relationships with colleagues and patients are appropriate. Appropriate relations support the professional goal of maintaining and improving the health of individuals, families, communities, and other groups; and
- Shared information is professional in its nature, thereby encouraging public trust in the profession.

Protecting Privacy: Role of the Federal Government

At the federal level, the primary legislation protecting patient privacy is the Health Insurance Portability and Accountability Act (HIPAA), codified as amended in scattered sections of 42 USCS. The HIPAA Privacy Rule protects the privacy of health information by identifying who can look at and receive your health information. HIPAA also gives the patient specific rights over that information (Office for Civil Rights, n.d.). However, under the HIPAA Privacy Rule, covered entities may without restriction use or disclose health information that is de-identified. To de-identify data, a covered entity must remove each of the 18 elements listed in Exhibit 9.2. The covered entity also must

---

Exhibit 9.1 *Privacy Rights Clearinghouse: Types of Social Networks*

1. *Personal Networks:* Allow users to build online profiles to connect with other users with an emphasis on social relationships such as friendship. A well-recognized example is Facebook.
2. *Status Update Networks:* Allow users to post short messages in order to communicate with others quickly. A well-recognized example is Twitter.
3. *Location Networks:* Allow users to share their real-time location. Examples include Brightkite, Foursquare, and Loopt.
4. *Content Sharing Networks:* Allow users to share content such as music, slides, photographs, and videos. A well-recognized example is YouTube.
5. *Shared Interested Networks:* Allow users to build online profiles to connect with other users with an emphasis on shared interest. Examples include ANA:NurseSpace and PatientsLikeMe.

The Privacy Right Clearinghouse *Fact Sheet 35: Social Networking Privacy: How to be Safe, Secure and Social* (Privacy Rights Clearinghouse, 2011).

U.S. Department of Health & Human Services, National Institutes of Health (2004, July 13).

Exhibit 9.2 *HIPAA Private Health Information Data Elements*

1. Names.
2. All geographic subdivisions smaller than a state, including street address, city, county, precinct, ZIP Code, and their equivalent geographical codes, except for the initial three digits of a ZIP Code if, according to the current publicly available data from the Bureau of the Census:
   a. The geographic unit formed by combining all ZIP Codes with the same three initial digits contains more than 20,000 people.
   b. The initial three digits of a ZIP Code for all such geographic units containing 20,000 or fewer people are changed to 000.
3. All elements of dates (except year) for dates directly related to an individual, including birth date, admission date, discharge date, date of death; and all ages over 89 and all elements of dates (including year) indicative of such age, except that such ages and elements may be aggregated into a single category of age 90 or older.
4. Telephone numbers.
5. Facsimile numbers.
6. Electronic mail addresses.
7. Social security numbers.
8. Medical record numbers.
9. Health plan beneficiary numbers.
10. Account numbers.
11. Certificate/license numbers.
12. Vehicle identifiers and serial numbers, including license plate numbers.
13. Device identifiers and serial numbers.
14. Web universal resource locators (URLs).
15. Internet protocol (IP) address numbers.
16. Biometric identifiers, including fingerprints and voiceprints.
17. Full-face photographic images and any comparable images.
18. Any other unique identifying number, characteristic, or code, unless otherwise permitted by the Privacy Rule for re-identification.

---

have no actual knowledge that anyone could use the remaining information alone or in combination with other information to identify the individual who is the subject of the information (U.S. Department of Helath & Human Services, National Institutes of Health, 2004).

There are several social networking precautions one can take to avoid HIPAA Violations:

- *Do not expect anything to remain private on the Internet.* Treat all your comments as public publications. Always remember posted information on the Internet is information that someone saves somewhere on a computer.
- *Never talk about specific patients, even in general terms.* Even if you avoid all the PIH HIPAA elements, others can combine data from different sources, thereby making it possible for someone to recognize the specific patient you were discussing.

For example, you may have included on your Facebook wall your reaction to observing a colonoscopy for the first time that day. You may have been impressed that the doctor removed three potentially cancerous pulps from a middle-aged man and included this detail in order to stress the value of a colonoscopy. You are hoping that your father who is 60 will read this and schedule his first colonoscopy. One of your friends picks up on your comment and posts it on their blog with your name. Like you, they are trying to encourage their father to have a colonoscopy. However, the patient's employer happens to see this blog and searches the Internet for your name since he thinks he may know you.

In his search, he discovers in the local newspaper a few months prior an article about students in the area who are becoming health professionals. You are in the article with a comment that your next clinical will be at XYZ hospital. The employer realizes he has a middle-aged employee named Paul who took that same day off for a medical appointment at XYZ hospital. The employee never said why he would need a full day off for a medical appointment, but the employer now wonders. The employer is also in the process of making some difficult decisions about layoffs. Who knows how this will play out?

- *Don't be anonymous.* Many social media sites require people to use their real names. One of the primary reasons for this is that cyber-bullying has been associated with fake accounts (Pokin, 2007). More to the point for the health professional, posting anonymously gives a false sense of privacy. With that sense of privacy, one is more likely to say too much—leaving an information trail leading back to a specific patient. Dr. Robert Lindeman (aka Dr. Flea) demonstrates one of the best-known examples of this problem.

Dr. Lindeman opened a new practice and two months later was sued for malpractice. This was of course very stressful, and as Dr. Lindeman explained, "As the trial date approached, I felt increasingly isolated and anxious." His response was to develop a live blog about his experiences as a medical malpractice defendant under the name Flea: "I felt as though this story and the story of malpractice litigation in general, is one that ordinary folks have never heard and doctors are reluctant to tell. **I believed that the anonymity would shield me.**" The plaintiff's attorney discovered the blog and exposed Dr. Lindeman on the witness stand (Turkewitz, 2008). This cited source details the impact on Dr. Lindeman from both a personal and professional prospective.

- *Do not post in real time.* Put some time between preparing a post and actually posting your comments. When typing on a blank screen, the creative process of developing your ideas can distract you from effective editing. A day later—even a few hours later—you will see comments you do not want to publish on the web.

While it is important to avoid all HIPAA violations by exposing a patient's privacy, it is also important for nurses to share their perspective and insight on the Internet. While one should never talk about specific patients, you can talk about:

- Nursing,
- Health care and research, and
- Conditions, treatment options, and other health related topics in general terms.

Several examples of this careful balance can be seen at http://well.blogs.nytimes. com/author/theresa-brown-rn/, with titles such as:

A Hollywood Movie Takes on Cancer	October 5, 2011
Need Sleep? Stay Out of the Hospital	September 7, 2011
Feeling Strain When Violent Patients Need Care	January 30, 2012

Protecting Privacy: Role of Professional Organizations

Early in the development of the health care professional associations, measures to protect patient privacy became inherent in the concept of professional ethics. Social media has not changed that reality, but raises new challenges regarding what measures are necessary to protect that promise of privacy. In turn, professional associations have begun to develop guidelines for using social media in a safe and effective way. Table 9.1 includes several health-related professional organizations that have developed guidelines for using social media, along with links to those documents. In nursing within the United States, two key organizations that developed such guidelines are the American Nurses Association (American Nurses Association, 2011) and the National Council of State Boards of Nursing (National Council of State Boards of Nursing, 2011). The ANA lists six principles to guide nurses in the use of social media. The first principle reads as: "Nurses must not transmit or place online individually identifiable patient information." (p. 6) The NCSBN (2011) reinforces this principle with six specific steps for avoiding privacy problems:

1. First and foremost, nurses must recognize that they have an ethical and legal obligation to maintain patient privacy and confidentiality at all times.
2. Nurses are strictly prohibited from transmitting by way of any electronic media any patient-related image. In addition, nurses are restricted from transmitting any information that may be reasonably anticipated to violate patient rights to confidentiality or privacy, or otherwise degrade or embarrass the patient.
3. Do not share, post, or otherwise disseminate any information, including images, about a patient or information gained in the nurse-patient relationship with anyone unless there is a patient care-related need to disclose the information or other legal obligation to do so.
4. Do not identify patients by name or post, or publish information that may lead to the identification of a patient. Limiting access to postings through privacy settings is not sufficient to ensure privacy.
5. Do not refer to patients in a disparaging manner, even if the patient is not identified.
6. Do not take photos or videos of patients on personal devices, including cell phones. Follow employer policies for taking photographs or videos of patients for treatment or other legitimate purposes using employer-provided devices.

Table 9.1 *Health-Related Professional Organization Guidelines and Social Media*

Professional Association	Document Title	URL
American Medical Association (AMA)	Professionalism in the Use of Social Media	http://www.ama-assn.org/ama/pub/meeting/professionalism-social-media.shtml
American Nurses Association (ANA)	ANA's Principles for Social Networking and the Nurse	http://www.nursingworld.org/MainMenuCategories/ThePracticeofProfessionalNursing/NursingStandards/ANAPrinciples.aspx
National Council of State Boards of Nursing (NCSBN)	White Paper: A Nurse's Guide to the Use of Social Media	https://www.ncsbn.org/Social_Media.pdf
Royal College of Nursing (RCN)	Legal Advice For RCN Members Using the Internet	http://www.rcn.org.uk/__data/assets/pdf_file/0008/272195/003557.pdf
College of Nurses of Ontario (CNO)	Confidentiality and Privacy — Personal Health Information	http://www.cno.org/Global/docs/prac/41069_privacy.pdf
Nursing and Midwifery Council (NMC)	Social networking site guidance	http://www.nmc-uk.org/Nurses-and-midwives/Advice-by-topic/A/Advice/Social-networking-sites/
Australian Medical Association (AMA); New Zealand Medical Association; New Zealand Medical Student Associations (NZMSA) Australian Medical Student Association (AMSA)	Social Media and the Medical Professions: A Guide to Online Professionalism for Medical Practitioners and Medical Students	http://ama.com.au/socialmedia

Developing Appropriate Professional Relationships

Beginning early in their educational program, nurses learn to establish therapeutic relationships with patients and professional relationships with colleagues. Clear boundaries define each of these relationships as appropriate to the specific role in the relationship. These boundaries prescribe, for example, the type of clothing that would be appropriate, the titles professionals use, the amount of personal information that patients and professionals share, and topics that they could be expected to discuss. By prescribing the behaviors, boundaries provide a sense of security and comfort. Professionals and patients in their different roles know what to expect in that role. A number of documents clearly define these expectations. Exhibit 9.3 provides examples of how different professional organizations have described these boundaries. Behaviors that cross the defined boundaries are boundary violations.

There is a wide range of nurse-patient and professional colleague relationships. For example, a nurse may work briefly with a patient recovering from same-day surgery or spend months as the case manager of a patient dealing with a stage 4 cancer diagnosis. Nurses in small towns may care for a number of patients who they also know in a variety of other roles. Professional relationships also cover a wide range of connections. For example, colleagues may work together on committees with other members of a professional organization. The nurse may report to a manager or be responsible for supervising a health care team. Nursing faculty have a different relationship with undergraduates just beginning their education than a faculty member who chairs student doctoral committees has with those graduate students. In all of these examples, professional boundaries help to guide the relationship.

Exhibit 9.3 *Professional Boundaries Described by Profession Organizations*

American Nurses Association
When acting within one's role as a professional, the nurse recognizes and maintains boundaries that establish appropriate limits to relationships. While the nature of nursing work has an inherently personal component, nurse-patient relationships and nurse-colleague relationships have, as their foundation, the purpose of preventing illness; alleviating suffering; and protecting, promoting, and restoring the health of patients. In this way, nurse-patient and nurse-colleague relationships differ from those that are purely personal and unstructured, such as friendship. In the intimate nature of nursing care, the involvement of nurses is important and sometimes highly stressful life events and the mutual dependence of colleagues working in close concert all present the potential for blurring the limits to professional relationships. Maintaining authenticity and expressing oneself as an individual, while remaining within the boundaries established by the purpose of the relationship, can be especially difficult in long-term relationships. In all encounters, nurses are responsible for retaining professional boundaries (American Nurses Association, 2001).

National Council of State Boards of Nursing
Professional boundaries are the spaces between a nurse's power and the patient's vulnerability. The power of the nurse comes from the professional position, the access to private knowledge about the patient, and the patient's need for care. Establishing boundaries allows the nurse to control this power differential and allows for a safe interaction to best meet the patient's needs (National Council of State Boards of Nursing, 2011 p. 4 w).

College & Association of Registered Nurses of Alberta
Healthy boundaries keep the nurse-client relationship a safe one, where the client and registered nurse are both respected. The client's human dignity, autonomy, and privacy are safeguarded, and the registered nurse is recognized as a professional with certain obligations and rights (College & Association of Registered Nurses of Alberta, 2011 p. 3).

REFERENCES

American Nurses Association. (2001). *Code of ethics with interpretive statements.* Retrieved from http://nursingworld.org/MainMenuCategories/ThePracticeofProfessionalNursing/EthicsStandards/CodeofEthics.aspx

College & Association of Registered Nurses of Alberta. (2011, May). *Professional boundaries for registered nurses: Guidelines for the nurse-client relationship.* Retrieved from College & Association of Registered Nurses of Alberta: https://www.nurses.ab.ca/Carna-Admin/Uploads/professional_boundaries_May_%202011.pdf

National Council of State Boards of Nursing. (2011). *The nurses guide to professional boundaries.* Retrieved from https://www.ncsbn.org/2906.htm?iframe=true&width=500&height=270

However, the interactive communication inherent in the process of social networking can make the professional boundaries much more porous. As more information flows through these open boundaries, these relationships are changing. As more and more members of a profession become involved in the open world of online communities, one can anticipate that the culture of the profession will change. As a paradigm shift occurs, the emerging culture of social media use redefines and reestablishes these boundaries. For example, when this author began her nursing education, nurses addressed the head nurse as Miss, Mrs., or Mr. Both the head nurse and I would have been uncomfortable with any other title. We referred to all physicians with the title *doctor* at all times. Even physicians who had known each other since childhood called each other doctor when they were in the hospital. The titles reflected the culture of the profession; today, the first name is increasingly used in everyday conversations between physicians, nurses, and patients. The more informal approach changes the relationship and professional boundaries. In response to these challenges, professional organizations have provided guidelines to maintain professional boundaries with patients in a social media environment.

- Maintain professional boundaries in the use of electronic media. Like in-person relationships, the nurse has the obligation to establish, communicate and enforce professional boundaries with patients in the online environment. Use caution when having online social contact with patients or former patients. Online contact with patients or former patients blurs the distinction between a professional and personal relationship. The fact that a patient may initiate contact with the nurse does not permit the nurse to engage in a personal relationship with the patient (National Council of State Boards of Nursing, 2011 p. 3).
- Nurses who interact with patients on social media must observe ethically prescribed patient–nurse professional boundaries. The precepts guiding nurses in these matters are no different online than in person (American Nurses Association, 2011).
- When a client requests that a registered nurse be an online friend, the nurse must carefully examine the context of the situation, the therapeutic client-nurse relationship, the vulnerability of the client and the implications of the request for the nurse and the client. A number of potential problems can arise, such as inappropriate self-disclosure, client dependence on the nurse, the nurse meeting their own needs through the client and compromising patient privacy and confidentiality (College & Association of Registered Nurses of Alberta, 2011 p. 9).

Table 9.2 includes examples of warning signs that one is crossing professional boundaries when dealing with patients.

Professional boundaries with colleagues can be even more complex than patient relationships in a social media environment. Two areas are of specific concern. The first is inappropriate self-disclosure and the second deals with hostile behavior such as bullying.

Self-disclosure

Self-disclosure involves providing too much personal information about one's self and in turn damaging the professional relationship. Sometimes this can be obvious. Pictures that look funny at 20 years of age can be embarrassing for a 30-year-old professional who has just been promoted to his or her first significant management position. Even more complex is setting boundaries between professional and personal relationships with less obvious barriers.

Table 9.2 *Boundary Warning Signs*

From the Clinical Setting	From Facebook or Similar Social Media Sites
Sharing personal information	Including patient as a Facebook friend on a personal site
Changing dress style at work	Posting pictures in non-work clothing such as a swimming suit
Providing non-work-related contact information	
Spending free time with a patient	Reviewing patient's personal Facebook wall

One of the six principles from the ANA principles document states that:

"Nurses should take advantage of privacy settings available on many social networking sites in their personal online activities and seek to separate their online personal and professional sites and information. Use of privacy settings and separation of personal and professional information online does not guarantee, however, that information will not be repeated in less protected forums." (American Nurses Association, 2011 p. 6)

Implementing this principle can be difficult. One of the challenges is that relationships change over time. A close friend in college may become a distant professional relationship, or, over time, a professional colleague may become a close friend. In addition, professional and personal relationships tend to overlap. It is rare for a person to have no social relationships with people at work or from their professional association. Finally, in social media, as in real life, information flows across relationships. The main difference is that information in the social media environment can flow more quickly and further. With this reality in mind, one should consider information shared on social media sites as public information.

For example, imagine you are in a new management position for 6 months and are just beginning to feel comfortable giving directions and setting standards. During those 6 months, with a great deal of effort, you lost 20 pounds and are so pleased you look that good in your new swimsuit, especially since you now have a week of vacation planned. While on vacation you post several vacation pictures on Facebook, including a picture of yourself in your new swimsuit showing just how good you look. On your first day back from vacation you discover that your employees have a copy of your swimsuit picture. There are several mildly suggestive comments made and your sense of position and control is once again totally challenged. You can never be sure how this picture was distributed within hours of being posted, but you know a classmate from your master's program is a friend of a nurse who reports to you. Could the picture have moved through a "friends-of-friends" connection? Did you assume that a certain privacy setting would let friends look at your pictures but prevent friends-of-friends from seeing the pictures when this setting did not provide that level of privacy? The end result is that you waste professional time worrying about the picture and dealing with the fallout from its distribution.

Hostile Relationships

Hostile relationships in a professional environment also present significant problems for individuals that are involved as well as the associated institutions. The NCSBN included the following warning in their white paper: "Do not make disparaging remarks about employers or co-workers. Do not make threatening, harassing, profane, obscene, sexually explicit, racially derogatory, homophobic or other offensive comments (p. 3). " This guideline would seem to be obvious, but when one is angry, there is a tendency to vent these feelings. When typing on a computer screen, it is much easier to express these feelings than facing the person directly. In addition, if a friend or colleague reinforced your opinion, you can lack the necessary feedback to realize you are stepping over a professional boundary. The old saying "Think before you speak" is now translated in social media to "Think before you type, or at least before you push the post or send button."

Maintaining a Professional Image on the Internet

A nurse's professional image is tied to his or her own online reputation/image as a professional and to the online image of the profession as a whole. As a professional, you have responsibilities for both your professional image and the image of the profession. Exhibit 9.4 provides several clips from newspapers with examples of behaviors that impact the image of the profession as well as the professional reputation of the individuals involved. These news clips are only examples. In 2011, the Arizona State Board of Nursing reported that, in the past two years, approximately 10 cases of inappropriate use of social media resulted in discipline (Lee, 2011). A 2010 NCSBN survey of Boards of Nursing (BON) reported that a majority of these Boards (33 of the 46 respondents) reported receiving complaints of nurses who have violated patient privacy on social networking sites. These BONs responded with censure of nurses, issuing letters of concern, placing conditions on the nurses' license, or suspending the nurses' licenses (National Council of State Boards of Nursing, 2011).

One of the key ways you can exercise this responsibility is to be aware of unprofessional behavior and take action to stop such behavior. The NCSBN simply states

---

Exhibit 9.4 *Newspaper Headlines and Chips Demonstrating Unprofessional Behavior*

Los Angeles Times: When Facebook Goes to the Hospital, Patients May Suffer
William Wells arrived at the emergency room at St. Mary Medical Center in Long Beach on April 9 mortally wounded. The 60-year-old had been stabbed more than a dozen times by a fellow nursing home resident, his throat slashed so savagely he was almost decapitated.

Instead of focusing on treating him, an employee said, St. Mary nurses and other hospital staff did the unthinkable: They snapped photos of the dying man and posted them on Facebook... Employees should be reminded that anything they post online is public — no matter how many privacy settings they use — and that those posts related to their work must always remain professional. (Hennessy-Fiske, 2010)

San Diego News: Five Nurses Fired for Facebook Posting
Five nurses who work at Tri-City Medical Center in Oceanside were fired for allegedly discussing patient cases on Facebook.

"We recently identified an incident involving hospital employees who used social media to post their personal discussions concerning hospital patients," said Larry Anderson, Tri-City CEO. Anderson said that no patient names, photos or identifying information were posted. (Fink, 2010)

ABC-WISN.Com: Nurses Fired Over Cell Phone Photos of Patient
The patient was admitted to the emergency room with an object lodged in his rectum. Police said the nurse explained she and a co-worker snapped photos when they learned it was a sex device. Police said discussion about the incident was posted on her Facebook page, but they haven't found anyone who actually saw the pictures. (Nurses Fired over Cell Phone Photo of Patient, 2009)

The South East Texas Record: Nurse Accuses Hospital Employees of Posting Photos of Sedated Patients
TYLER-A former nurse is seeking more than $15 million from a Tyler hospital alleging she was fired after complaining about employees taking pictures of sedated patients and posting the pictures on Facebook.

Debbie Blevins filed suit against Tyler Cardiovascular Consultants on Dec. 22 in the Eastern District of Texas, Tyler Division.

She accuses the defendant of allowing staff, including doctors, to post pictures of sedated patients on social networking websites, such as Facebook, in violation of Health Insurance Portability and Accountability Act privacy laws, ethical standards and basic morals. (Massey, 2011)

"Promptly report any identified breach of confidentiality or privacy" (National Council of State Boards of Nursing, 2011 p. 3). In their six principles, the ANA also includes guidance for this problem. This document points out that nurses have an ethical obligation to take appropriate action regarding instances that reflect incompetent, unethical, illegal, or impaired practice. Nurses who view a colleague's social media content that violates ethical or legal standards should first bring the questionable content to the attention of the colleague. If the posting could threaten a patient's health, welfare, or right to privacy, the nurse has the obligation to followup, including reporting the problem to external authorities if necessary (American Nurses Association, 2011).

Nurses should also monitor their online image. This can be as simple as using several different search engines to search for your name on the Internet. Don't forget to search images and blogs. You can also use one of the free alert services. These services, such as Google Alerts, TweetBeep, or Social Media Firehouse will search and send you an email alert if it finds your name. If you are in a nursing field, such as a nurse practitioner in a local clinic, where you are subject to online reviews, you will also want to check these sites. For example, try searching for your name with the phrase (review OR rate) in the search string. You can better manage your online professional reputation if you use different social networking sites for professional and personal social networking, and in all cases use the security settings. If you do find information that is inaccurate and/or negative, you can contact the site and ask that they remove or correct the information. When maintaining your online image, you need to be sensitive to the image of others. Use great care in what you post on the Internet that reflects on others. For example, do not post embarrassing pictures of friends and colleagues.

Social Media Policies

Given the impact of social media, health care institutions, universities, and other educational institutions are developing or have developed social media policies. These documents also provide guidance for professional nurses. Different levels of social media policies to be developed at the university, school, and department level and even in course syllabi. As professionals, nurses should involve themselves in writing these policies. The ANA states in their Principles document, "Nurses are encouraged to participate in the development of policies and procedures in their institutions and organizations for handling reports of online conduct that may raise legal concerns or be professionally unethical" (American Nurses Association, 2011 p. 7). They should also seek involvement in writing policies that maximize the benefits social media offers to patient care and community health.

Writing and Implementing a Social Media Policy

There are several key points that a social media policy should include. These points are important whether you are writing the policy or following the policy.

- The policy should begin with an introduction that describes and defines the concept of social media for the purpose of the policy. The introduction should state the goals for the policy or why the policy exists. For example, does the policy exist to prevent potential employee legal problems such as HIPAA violations? Does the policy also exist to encourage employees to maximize the benefits of social media?

- The policy should clearly identify who is covered by the policy. For example, is this a policy for all employees, or is there a different policy for employees who have access to more sensitive information? Does the policy include guests in the institution, such as students and/or others with business relations such as physicians with staff privileges? Along with the policy, the institution should implement a process for informing individuals, who are covered by the policy that the policy exists and it applies to them. Those who might be subject to the policy should also take a proactive approach to determining if a policy exists. For example, if nursing students are going to a new setting for clinical, they should ask if there is a social media policy in place.
- The structure of the policy should be such that it clearly identifies and defines policies/rules and guidelines. For example, the policy might suggest guidelines for setting privacy settings, but *require* (rule) that all employees who indicated their place of employment also include a statement that they do not speak for the institution.
- The policy should unambiguously define and differentiate how the policy applies to employee-related social media and personal use of social media. For example, if a hospital maintains a blog where consumers, patients, and others might comment, what type of comments, if any, can employees make on this site? Does the institution permit access to personal social media sites from work? If yes, are there any restrictions?
- The policy should be explicit and comprehensive in identifying inappropriate behaviors. For example, a nurse who is acting as a preceptor may not realize that posting online, even positive comments on a student's performance, may be a Family Educational Rights and Privacy Act (FERPA) violation if the preceptor has any role in grading that student.
- The policy should be explicit in identifying appropriate behaviors. For example, the policy might encourage the sharing of certain intellectual property by establishing a process for sharing these materials. With this process in place, employees might develop a set of YouTube videos demonstrating healthy behaviors, thereby providing positive publicity for the institution.
- The policy should state how the institution will manage inappropriate behavior, including the level and type of discipline that one can expect.
- The policy should explain the responsibilities and expected action of employees that witness inappropriate use of social media.
- The policy should encourage employees to maximize the benefits of social media by identifying who they should inform at the institution about an opportunity or issue that needs to be address via social media. This would include questions or suggested changes to the social media policy.

When writing a policy, it is often helpful to look at policies developed by others. Table 9.3 includes links to several such policies as well as other resources for developing social media policies. The process of writing the policy should include input from employees who must follow the policy as well as employees who must implement the policy. In addition, the legal department should review the policy to ensure it is consistent with federal, state, and local laws. Several examples of employee policies that proved unenforceable are presented later in this chapter in the discussion related to the National Labor Relations Board.

Once the institution writes and approves the policy, there are two more steps before implementating the policy. First, other policies related to codes of conduct, discrimination, or harassment, and so forth, should be reviewed and modified for consistency across the policies. Once these policies are consistent, the institution can update employees' handbooks, orientation materials, and other related materials.

Table 9.3 *Resources for Developing a Social Media Policy*

Author	Title	Description	URL
Chris Boudreaux	Social Media Governance	A database of over 195 social media policies	http://socialmediagovernance.com/
Ed Bennett	Found in Cache	This site includes a number of social media policies as well as other information, statistics, and resources related to social media and health care.	http://ebennett.org/
Cecilia Backman, Susan Dolack, Denise Dunyak, Laurie Lutz, Anne Tegen, Diana Warner, and LaVonne Wieland	AHIMA: Social Media + Health care	A journal article that includes a sample media policy template.	http://library.ahima.org/xpedio/ groups/public/documents/ ahima/bok1_048693. hcsp?dDocName=bok1_048693
Dan Goldman	Legal Issues (Part, 1, 2, 3 & 4): Specific Suggestions When Drafting Your Policies	A series of four articles on legal and employee policy issues in social media for health care organizations.	http://socialmedia.mayoclinic.org/ category/legal/
Vanderbilt University Medical Center	Social Media Toolkit	An online resource including video developed for employees interested in having a social media presence on behalf of Vanderbilt University Medical Center.	http://www.mc.vanderbilt.edu/ root/vumc.php?site=socialmedia toolkit&doc=26923

Second, before the policy is effective, it is imperative that an employee education plan that ensures employees understand social media and the institution's related policies be developed and implemented. The social media policy will only be effective if the institution provides employee education to be sure employees understand the information. For example, if a group of employees have never used privacy settings on Facebook, a policy suggesting that they use a privacy setting will not in itself tell these employees how. The more inexperienced the employees are in using social media, the more likely that they will not understand the meaning of the policy and in turn make mistakes.

Statements from professional associations, institutional policies, and one's professional code of conduct provide a framework for guiding the professional nurses' use of social media. But social media is a phenomenon within the society as a whole. Federal and state laws and regulations provide formal societal guidelines in the use of social media. These guidelines not only guide the nurse and other health care professionals in making choices related to the use of social media, but also guide the individuals in what can be expected of others, including corporations and institutions.

FEDERAL AGENCIES AND SOCIAL MEDIA

As the use of social media has grown, several federal agencies are both applying current laws and regulations to social media activities and analyzing the need for new laws and regulations. In several cases, federal agencies are now developing new policies and regulations. As a result, draft regulations that this chapter discusses may be in final form when this book is published. Therefore, use the information here as a guide in searching for updated information from these agencies.

Federal Trade Commission (FTC)

The mission of the FTC is to prevent business practices that are monopolistic, deceptive, or unfair to consumers. In 1970, with the introduction of the Fair Trade Reporting Act, the charge to the FTC now includes protecting consumer privacy. The agency achieves its mission by:

1. Development of rules, regulations, and guidelines to support laws that it enforces,
2. Enforcement of laws as to monopolistic, deceptive, or unfair business practices,
3. Development and distribution of consumer education about these types of activities, and
4. Sharing its expertise with businesses as well as other areas and levels of government.

The FTC business practice regulations apply to the health industry as it does to all other industries. Table 9.4 includes examples of FTC-enforced health-related laws and regulations that are relevant to social media sites and networking activities.

Protecting Consumer Privacy—Domestic

In addition, social networking introduces a whole new range of business practices that may be perceived as monopolistic, deceptive, or unfair to consumers, including a number of practices that could threaten the privacy of consumers. For example, most sites provide a document outlining the terms and conditions for individuals who are considering using the site. The length of the document and the complexity of the language usually

Table 9.4 Sample U.S. Federal Trade Commission-Enforced Health Related Regulations

Name and URL for Actual Law	Description	URL for Description or Interpretation
The Children's Online Privacy Protection Act (COPPA): 15 USCS §§ 6501 et seq. http://www.ftc.gov/ogc/coppa1.htm	This act gives parents control over what information websites can collect from their children under age 13.	http://business.ftc.gov/privacy-and-security/children%E2%80%99s-privacy
The Health Breach Notification Rule: 16 CFR 318.1 et seq. http://www.ftc.gov/os/2009/08/R911002hbn.pdf	This rule requires certain businesses not covered by HIPAA to notify their customers and others if there's a breach of unsecured, individually identifiable electronic health information. For example, vendors of personal health records are covered by this rule.	http://business.ftc.gov/documents/bus56-complying-ftcs-health-breach-notification-rule
Fair Credit Reporting Act (FCRA) → Medical Identify Theft: 15 USCS §§ 1681 et seq. www.ftc.gov/os/statutes/031224fcra.pdf	This regulation outlines the patient's rights and business's responsibility when a patient experiences medical identity theft. HIPAA also gives the patient the right to correct errors in their medical records and billing information.	http://business.ftc.gov/documents/bus75-medical-identity-theft-faq-health-care-health-plan

discourages users from reading these documents. See Chapter 8, Terms and Conditions and Privacy Statements, for additional information related to this issue.

In response to these specific challenges, the FTC released a preliminary FTC staff report titled *Protecting Consumer Privacy in an Era of Rapid Change: A Proposed Framework for Business and Policymakers* for public comment (Federal Trade Commission, 2010). More than 450 comments were made in response to the preliminary report. The final report was released in March 2012. In this report, the FTC builds upon the previous models (1) notice-and-choice, which focus on giving consumers notice and offering a choice and (2) harm-based models, which focus on protecting consumers from specific harms. The report introduces a new framework—Privacy by Design (Center for Democracy & Technology, 2010, January 28).

Exhibit 9.5 provides an overview of the new framework. This new framework applies "… to all commercial entities that collect or use consumer data that can be reasonably linked to a specific consumer, computer, or other device, unless the entity collects only non-sensitive data from fewer than 5,000 consumers per year and does not share the data with third parties" (Federal Trade Commission, 2012, ES-vii).

In the final report, the FTC expressed strong concern about the current status of social media and the protection of consumer privacy—"consumers do not yet enjoy the privacy protections proposed in the preliminary staff report" (Federal Trade Commission, 2012, ES-i). To address these issues, the Commission called on Congress to enact baseline privacy legislation. They also recommended that Congress enact targeted

---

Exhibit 9.5 *Federal Trade Commission Framework for Protecting Consumer Privacy*

Scope of the Framework
The framework applies to all commercial entities that collect and use consumer data that can be linked to a specific consumer, computer, or other device. However, it does not apply to companies that collect only non-sensitive data from fewer than 5000 customers per year, provided they do not share the data with third parties.

Principles
1. **Privacy by Design:** Companies should promote consumer privacy throughout their organizations and at every stage of the development of their products.
  - Incorporate substantive privacy protections such as data security, reasonable collection limits, sound retention practices, and data accuracy.
  - Maintain comprehensive data management procedures throughout the life cycle of all products and services.
2. **Simplified Choice:** Companies should simplify consumer choice.
  - There is not a need to provide choice before collecting and using consumers' data for commonly accepted practices. For example, a company can request an address in order to ship an item. In these cases, permission is implied.
  - For practices requiring choice, companies should offer the choice at a time and in a context in which the consumer is making a decision about his or her data.
3. **Greater Transparency:** Companies should increase the transparency of their data practices.
  - Privacy notices should be clearer, shorter, and more standardized.
  - Companies should provide reasonable access to the consumer data they maintain.
  - Companies must provide prominent disclosures and obtain affirmative express consent before using consumer data in a different manner than claimed when the data was originally collected.
  - All stakeholders should work to educate consumers about commercial data privacy practices.

Source: Federal Trade Commission (2012).

legislation, providing greater transparency and consumer control of information brokers, pointing out that consumers are often unaware of these groups and their practices. Needless to say, health information is important data that is collected by these information brokers. Additional information on information brokers and their process for collecting these data can be found in the Process for Attracting Customers to the Product section of Chapter 8.

In lieu of any legislation, the FTC recommends that industries use self-regulation to implement the final privacy framework.

After issuance of this initial report, legal settlements with Twitter, Facebook, and Google demonstrated that the FTC is using the framework as a basis to protect consumer privacy in the world of social networking. In June 2010, the FTC finalized a settlement with Twitter, which resolved charges that Twitter deceived consumers and put their privacy at risk by failing to safeguard their personal information (Federal Trade Commission, 2011, March 3). In March 2011, Google Inc. agreed to settle FTC charges that it used deceptive tactics and violated its own privacy promises to consumers when it launched its social network, Google Buzz, in 2010. The settlement bars Google from future privacy misrepresentations, requires it to implement a comprehensive privacy program, and calls for independent privacy audits for the next 20 years. In addition, the settlement with Google is the first time the FTC alleged that a company violated privacy requirements of the U.S.-EU Safe Harbor Framework (Federal Trade Commission, 2011, March 30).

Protecting Consumer Privacy—Globally

The U.S.-EU Safe Harbor Framework provides a procedure for U.S. companies to transfer personal data lawfully between the European Union and the United States. The international agreement is important in the world of global health, where different countries have taken different approaches to protecting privacy. Exhibit 9.6 provides an overview of the U.S.-EU Safe Harbor Privacy Principles (Export.gov, 2011). There are several cases where the FTC enforced these principles.

In November of 2011, Facebook reached a settlement with the FTC on charges that it deceived Facebook users; Facebook told users that it kept their information private, but repeatedly shared that information. The FTC complaint record lists a number of instances in which Facebook allegedly made promises that it did not keep. For example:

- In December 2009, Facebook changed its website so certain information that users may have designated as private—such as their Friends List—was made public. They didn't warn users that this change was coming, or request their approval in advance.
- Facebook represented that third-party apps that users installed would have access only to user information that they needed to operate. In fact, the apps could access nearly all of users' personal data—data the apps didn't need.
- Facebook told users they could restrict sharing of data to limited audiences—for example, with "Friends Only." In fact, selecting "Friends Only" did not prevent the sharing of their information with third-party applications that their friends used.
- Facebook had a "Verified Apps" program and claimed it certified the security of participating apps. It didn't.
- Facebook promised users that it would not share their personal information with advertisers. It did.
- Facebook claimed that when users deactivated or deleted their accounts, their photos and videos would be inaccessible. But Facebook allowed access to the content, even after users had deactivated or deleted their accounts.

▪ Facebook claimed that it complied with the U.S.-EU Safe Harbor Framework that governs data transfer between the U.S. and the European Union. It didn't (Federal Trade Commission, 2011, November 29).

These settlements demonstrate that the FTC will continue to:

▪ Hold companies to their privacy promises and apply strong injunctive relief where the promises are false;
▪ Insist that a company must obtain affected consumers' affirmative consent to new privacy practices that apply retroactively;
▪ Look for and prosecute companies' failure to abide by the principles underlying their U.S.-EU Safe Harbor certifications;
▪ Utilize the new framework for privacy settlement agreements requiring a privacy by design approach (Delaney, Rubin, & Meister, 2012).

There is, of course, no way to know the number of health professionals who use these types of commercial social media sites and trust the privacy settings at these sites to provide privacy. The message here is "user beware" when using social media sites and trusting the privacy settings that these sites offer.

Exhibit 9.6 *United States-European Union Safe Harbor Privacy Principles*

Notice
Organizations must notify individuals about (1) the purposes for which they collect and use information; (2) how individuals can contact the organization; (3) the types of third parties to which it discloses information; and (4) the choices the organization offers for limiting information use and disclosure.

Choice
Organizations must give individuals the opportunity to opt out of whether their personal information will be disclosed. For sensitive information, individuals must be given an opt-in choice.

Onward Transfer (Transfers to Third Parties)
To transfer information to a third party, the third party organization must demonstrate that they have applied the notice and choice principles.

Access
Individuals must have access to personal information about them that an organization holds and be able to correct, amend, or delete that information.

Security
Organizations must take reasonable precautions to protect personal information.

Data Integrity
Reasonable steps should be taken to ensure that data are reliable for its intended use; accurate, complete, and current.

Enforcement
Organizations must provide (a) readily independent recourse mechanisms so that each individual's complaints and disputes can be resolved; (b) procedures for verifying that the commitments companies make to adhere to these principles have been implemented; and (c) sanctions sufficiently rigorous to ensure compliance by the organization. (Export.gov, 2011)

Copyright and Trademark

Most students are introduced to the concept of copyright and trademark protection long before they enter institutions of higher education. From the time they begin writing term papers, the professor tells them not to steal someone else's ideas and not to plagiarize. Following this golden rule is not as simple as it sounds, with cut and paste functionality available to students and a fire hose of content on the Internet.

Trademark

Trademark refers to a company's name, brand, or product names. The company owns these words, phrases, symbols, or designs, and another company cannot use them (Trademark, 2010). However, a reference to a product or company on a social network site does not constitute a trademark violation. Rather, the use of the trademarked materials or anything similar to the trademarked materials in a way that would confuse the public would constitute a trademark violation. For example, if one established a blog that focused on health care and used the name of the local hospital in the name of the blog, the public could assume that the local hospital sponsors the blog. In many cases, one could expect an attorney representing the local hospital to issue a "cease and desist" letter. The letter would require that the blogger change the name of the blog and identify the consequences if the blogger did not make this change.

Trademark infringement is not an issue if you reference a trademark when providing positive or negative comments about a product on a social media site. However, there are situations where these types of comments can produce legal problems for you. If you are an employee or have another material relationship with the company producing that product, federal advertising laws may apply to your posting. For example, if you are employed with a pharmacy company, FDA regulations may apply to your comments about specific medications on a social networking site. At times, you need to be proactive in avoiding problems. For example, if you are reviewing a health-related product with negative comments, avoid being charged by the company with disparagement and/or defamation by being factual and accurate in your comments.

Copyright

Copyright is different from trademark. Copyright is defined as the legal right to publish, create derivative works, reproduce, or distribute an original work. Essentially, the creator of an original work automatically owns the rights to that work once it is published in print or posted to a website (Beesley, 2011). However, copyright is not without limitation. The creator's rights are balanced with public interest in what is called "fair use." Fair use allows for limited and reasonable use of a copyrighted work as long as the use does not interfere with the owners' rights or impede their right to do with the work as they wish (Hawkins, 2011).

The copyright law lists the various purposes for which the reproduction of a particular work may be considered fair. These include, for example, criticism, comment, news reporting, teaching, scholarship, and research. Four factors to consider in determining whether or not a particular use is fair are:

1. The purpose and character of the use, such as whether the material is being used for a commercial project or used for nonprofit educational purposes,
2. The nature of the copyrighted work,

3. The amount and substantiality of the materials used in relation to the work as a whole, and

4. The effect of the use upon the potential market for, or value of, the copyrighted work (U.S. Copyright Office, n.d.).

The problem is that "the distinction between fair use and infringement may be unclear and not easily defined. There is no specific number of words, lines, or notes that may safely be taken without permission. Acknowledging the source of the copyrighted material does not substitute for obtaining permission" (U.S. Copyright Office, 2009, p. 1).

Computer technology and social media, by their very nature, can encourage users to copy and paste information, including copyrighted content. However, as the previous quote from the U.S. Copyright Office states, it is not always easy to determine what is fair use and what is copyright infringement. For example, one of your professional organizations has established a new local chapter in your area. The national association provides web space and a framework making it easy to populate the web page. The new president, who is a friend of yours, asked you to manage the web page. In searching the Internet looking for ideas, you discover that one of your local members won the best poster award at the last state conference for this association. She posted a picture of herself with the poster on Facebook. In the picture, the name of the organization is directly behind her. It is just the kind of material you are looking for, but if you copy the picture and post it on the web page for the local organization to announce her award, are you using copyrighted material without permission? She is the owner of the picture, but is this fair use? The safest approach to this question it to contact the individual and get permission to either link to her picture or to post the picture on your site.

Linking

Linking to another website is not a copyright violation, nor does it normally create the kind of confusion that generates a trademark infringement claim. However, one needs to be cautious about how the linking is done to avoid legal liability. "Different kinds of linking raise different legal issues, and the law is not entirely settled in all of these areas" (Citizen Media Law Project, 2008).

The safest approach is termed deep linking. Deep linking occurs when one places a link on their website that leads to a specific page within another site other than its homepage. Another similar approach is inline linking or embedding. With this approach, a line of HTML code is placed on one site so that the webpage will display content directly from another site. For example, many distance education faculty members will embed YouTube video in their course to illustrate a point.

Courts have ruled in the majority of copyright linking cases that linking, whether deep, or inline, does not give rise to liability for copyright infringement. However, one should avoid:

- Creating the impression that you are somehow affiliated with or endorsed by the site to which you are linking.
- Framing the linked content in such a way that the user might be confused about the source of the content on the webpage.
- Linking to a site that is clearly infringing on somebody's copyright, such as linking to pirated music files or commercially distributed movies.
- Linking to sites that offer technology, devices, or software that can be used to circumvent controls that are used to protect copyrighted work (Citizen Media Law Project, 2008).

The bottom line is to be transparent and honest in building links to other sites, and you are not likely to have any problems.

Food and Drug Administration (FDA)

The FDA is the agency within the federal government responsible for the regulation of medical products, such as drugs and medical equipment, including how these products are advertised. A key part of the approval process for over-the-counter and prescription drugs as well as medical devices are identifying the approved uses for these products. However, once a drug or medical device is FDA "approved," medical professionals can use these products as they deem appropriate in their professional judgment. Using products for other than the approved use is termed "off-label" use. FDA regulations make it illegal for a company to market a drug or encourage in any way off-label uses of drugs. However, a company may respond if they receive an unsolicited request for information concerning off-label use of a drug. Before the introduction of social media, most of these requests were private and professionals made the request. Social media changed that reality.

Since 2009, the FDA has been developing guidelines for companies that respond to unsolicited requests for off-label information about prescription drugs and medical devices. The FDA delayed the guidelines several times (Fisher, 2012). In December 2011, the FDA issued draft nonbinding "regulations for companies responding to unsolicited requests for off-label information about prescription drugs and medical devices" (Food & Drug Administration, 2011). The draft guidelines are posted at http://www.fda.gov/downloads/Drugs/GuidanceComplianceRegulatoryInformation/Guidances/UCM285145.pdf.

In developing these draft regulations, the FDA identified two types of unsolicited requests and two types of responses. These are non-public unsolicited requests and public unsolicited requests. Responses can also be non-public or public. Unsolicited requests for information are those that persons or entities initiate completely independent of the associated firm; solicited requests are those the firm initiates. For example, asking patients on an online discussion group to describe why they are using a drug could prompt questions about off-label use of that drug. Such questions would be considered solicited questions.

The draft guidelines provide recommendations about responding to public unsolicited requests for off-label information, including those that firms encounter through "emerging electronic media." For example, a patient participating in an online discussion forum may state that his physician had prescribed a new medication for his cluster headaches. This is a known off-label use of the drug. Since starting the drug he has experienced an intermittent burning pain on the outer aspect of his thigh. He asks if anyone else is taking this drug and if they have experienced a similar problem. Another patient posts a detailed and inaccurate explanation of how this drug would cause the intermittent burning pain and recommends that the patient cut the dose he is taking. If the company should become aware of this discussion, how should they respond, if at all? The nonbinding draft regulations for public comment include four recommendations:

1. If a firm chooses to respond to public unsolicited requests for off-label information, the firm should respond only when the request pertains specifically to its own named product.

2. A firm's *public* response to public unsolicited requests for off-label information about its product should be limited to providing the firm's contact information and should not include any off-label information except to convey that the question pertains to an unapproved use and who the individual can contact.
3. Representatives who provide public responses to unsolicited requests for off-label information should clearly disclose their involvement with the particular firm.
4. Public responses to public unsolicited requests for off-label information should not be promotional in nature or tone (Food & Drug Administration, 2011).

One can expect that the FDA will revise and edit these regulations after the public comment period and before approving them.

Nurses, as trusted health care advisors, are frequently asked about medication by patients who are currently receiving or considering the use of a particular drug. This is the case both online as well as off line. When responding to these requests for information, nurses should be sensitive to the reality that such communication can be regulated and should review the guidelines before participating in this type of communication.

The Equal Employment Opportunity Commission (EEOC)

"The U.S. Equal Employment Opportunity Commission (EEOC) is responsible for enforcing federal laws that make it illegal to discriminate against a job applicant or an employee because of the person's race, color, religion, sex (including pregnancy), national origin, age (40 or older), disability or genetic information" (Equal Employment Opportunity Commission, n.d.). These regulations can be important to nurses in their own career, whether they are participating in the hiring of a new employee, managing a group of employees, being hired, or are currently employed. These regulations can also be important when providing patients with eduation related to disability or genetic information.

The EEOC is the agency responsible for enforcement of the Genetic Information Non-Discrimination Act of 2008 (GINA). This act makes the acquisition of genetic information concerning an employee or applicant illegal. The Act broadly defines "genetic information" to include medical conditions of family members. However, there are a number of situations where the acquisition could be inadvertent. The use of social networking sites such as Facebook makes this even more likely. As a result, the regulations for enforcing this act include three exceptions.

1. When the firm has not obtained the information by "requesting, requiring, or purchasing" the genetic information.
2. When a manager or supervisor "inadvertently learns about the genetic information." This exception does not apply if the manager or supervisor learned the information when searching the Internet for information about the individual.
3. When the firm has obtained the genetic information via commercially and publicly available information resources. This third exception does not apply to media sources with "limited access." For example, a social media site where privacy settings have limited public access is not considered publicly available information (Equal Employment Opportunity Commission, 2010).

National Labor Relations Board (NLRB)

The NLRB is the federal agency charged with protecting the rights of most private-sector employees to join together to bargain collectively through representatives of their own choosing, or to refrain from such activities. Employees may join together to improve terms and conditions of employment with or without a union (National Labor Relations Board, n.d.).

In August 2011, the NLRB's Acting General Counsel released a report detailing 14 cases involving the use of social media and the employers' social and general media policies. Seven of these cases involve questions about employer social media policies. The court found five of those policies to be unlawfully broad, restricting protected concerted activities, such as discussing terms and conditions of employment with fellow employees. The court found one policy that restricted its employees' contact with the media. The final policy was lawful with revision.

The remaining seven cases involved discharging employees after they posted comments to Facebook. The court ruled these discharges to be unlawful if they flowed from unlawful employee policies. In one case, it upheld the discharge despite an unlawful policy because the employee's posting was not work-related (National Labor Relations Board, 2011).

Five months later, the Acting General Counsel issued a second report in which it stated that the 14 cases underscore two main points:

- Employer policies should not be so sweeping that they prohibit the kinds of activity that Federal labor law protects, such as the discussion of wages or working conditions among employees.
- An employee's comments on social media are generally not protected if they are mere gripes not made in relation to group activity among employees.

In addition, the Acting General Counsel asked that all regional offices send each meritorious social media related case to the NLRB Division of Advice in Washington D.C. The goal is to track these types of cases and develop a consistent approach to ruling on these cases. As of January 25th, 2012, regional offices had forwarded 75 cases (National labor Relations Board, 2012).

STATE LAWS, REGULATIONS, AND SOCIAL MEDIA

Each state has its own state laws that can have a direct impact on what the court can define as legal social networking behavior within that state. However, with the exception of cyber-bullying laws, very few states have passed legislation or taken other action dealing directly with social media. The Cyberbullying Research Center maintains a website at http://cyberbullying.us/aboutus.php that serves as a clearinghouse of information concerning the ways adolescents use and misuse technology. At this site, they maintain a list with the current status of all state laws that relate to cyberbullying (Hinduja & Patchin, 2012).

States are now examining other online relationships and the challenges these can present. One of the first to move in this direction was Missouri in 2011. The Amy Hestir Student Protection Act, which was to take effect on Aug. 28, 2011, prohibited teachers from having private online conversations with students under the age of 18. The law set strict limits on what it considered appropriate behavior when it comes to text messages and the use of social media sites like Facebook (Barkar, 2011).

The law, however, was controversial with groups such as the Missouri State Teachers Association, the Missouri School Boards Association, and the Missouri National Education Association speaking out in opposition. Shortly after passage of the bill, the courts issued an injunction blocking the law from taking effect because of concerns that it infringed on free-speech rights. In response, Missouri introduced a second bill requiring local school districts to develop their own social media policy by March 1, 2012 (Hancock, 2011).

Hawaii followed Missouri and took a more proactive approach. In December 2011, the Hawaii Senate, with the goal of providing guidance to users, both internally and in the public, adopted a social media policy. That policy "supports growing adoption of social media by its members and staff while providing guidance and standards of its use to ensure appropriate and effective use is consistent and in compliance with Federal and State rules and regulations" (Hawaii State Senate Adopts Social Media Use Policy, 2011). A copy of the policy is available at http://www.capitol.hawaii.gov/session2012/docs/SenateSocialMediaUsePolicy.htm.

While there are limited state laws that deal directly with social media, state laws that are not specific to social networking activities may have application to social networking activities. A case in New Jersey demonstrated this reality. In this case, a woman established a Facebook account for her ex-boyfriend. Her ex-boyfriend accused her of using this account to impersonate him and in turn harm his reputation: "The New Jersey Code of Criminal Justice defines the offense of impersonation/identity theft to include 'impersonating another or assuming a false identity and doing an act in such assumed character or false identity ... to injure or defraud another.' The woman asked the court to dismiss the case because the statute does not mention electronic communications. The judge found that fact irreverent and ruled that the case could go forward (Erickson, 2011). The judge's approach to this case clearly demonstrates that state privacy laws, for example, dealing with medical records, would not need to include electronic communication for these laws to apply when professionals are using social networking sites. This has very real implications for nurses' use of social media in their practice.

However, one cannot consider state laws independently of other legislation. Federal and local laws/regulations can apply to the same activity that state law regulates. In addition, social networking sites may include provisions in their Terms of Use that include certain restrictions for these same activities. Contests, sweepstakes, and other promotions, such as one might incorporate into a membership drive for a local professional group, provide an excellent example of this phenomenon. Federal laws related to contests fall under the jurisdiction of the Federal Trade Commission (Small Business Administration, 2011). California provides an example of a state law regulating contests and promotions (Department of Consumer Affairs, 2011). Rules and regulations for conducting contests and promotions are also included in the terms of use for Facebook, Twitter, and Google+ (Delaney, Rubin, & Meister, 2012). Their approaches and rules vary. What is acceptable on one site can be a violation of the terms on another site. In all of these cases, the restrictions, rules, and regulations change over time. This means that the procedures and rules for an organization's online membership drive from a previous year will need to be reviewed and possibly revised the following year.

SUMMARY

This chapter provided information and guiding principles that one can use in making decisions about appropriate social media-related activities by health-related institutions, professional associations, and individuals. However, one should always remember that social networking does not exist in isolation from the ethical codes and standards of practice inherent in the practice of professional health care. One cannot achieve effective, safe social networking by following a set of specific rules; it requires the application of professional judgment.

DISCUSISON QUESTIONS

1. It has been suggested that social media is changing society's concept of what is private information. For example, in most settings, one's name is not usually considered private information, but the balance in their bank account is often considered private information. In your opinion, is the concept of what is private information being impacted by social media? If yes, what implications does this have for the sharing of health-related information?
2. What impact does social media have on the concept of professional boundaries and what implications does this impact have on nursing roles and relationships?
3. Should university polices include guidelines, limits, or controls on what a student may post on their personal social networking site such as Facebook? Explain your answer.
4. The Federal Trade Commission recommended that Congress enact legislation protecting online privacy. What should be included in this legislation and how should it be enforced?
5. The Electronic Privacy Information Center, located at http://epic.org/, maintains a list of "Hot Topics" on their home page. Review this list and identify one topic of importance to health care professionals in terms of social media. Explain why and how that topic is important.
6. Compare and contrast the culture of participatory health care (http://participatorymedicine.org/) with the boundary concepts of professional organizations in health care.
7. In the fall term of 2010, four nursing students were expelled from Johnson County Community College for posting a picture of themselves with a human placenta. One of the four students elected to sue the college. A copy of her suit can be seen at http://www.courthousenews.com/2010/12/28/Placenta.pdf. Discuss the implications this suit has for the social media policy in your setting and for the professional image of nursing.
8. In February 2009, the University of Louisville expelled Nina Yoder for violating the nursing school's honor code with materials she posted on a blog. Ms. Yoder appealed the expulsion, but the appeal was denied. She then sued the University for reinstatement, alleging that it had violated her free-speech and due-process rights. She won this lawsuit in August 2009, when Judge Charles R. Simpson III of the U.S. District Court in Louisville ruled that Ms. Yoder could register for classes at the University as soon as she would like (Payne, 2009). The Judge's ruling is posted at http://www.nacua.org/documents/yoder.pdf. The document includes the blog as well as the Judge's rationale for the ruling. Discuss the implications this ruling has for the social media policy in your setting and for the professional image of nursing.

EXERCISES

Exercise 1: Implementing Policy by Design

Purpose: *The purpose of this exercise is to introduce the reader to the difference between security policies and security procedures.*

Objectives
1. Analyze security procedures for their adherence to a safe security policy.
2. Establish security settings on a social media website.

Directions
1. Reread the concept of Policy by Design, presented in this chapter.
2. Select a social media site and review the process for establishing your security settings.
3. Use the principle, Policy by Design, to evaluate the process offered by the social media site.
4. Based on your analysis, suggest changes you would make to improve the security effectiveness of the site.
5. Create or use the class blog. Share your findings and recommendations.

Exercise 2: Proactively Creating Effective Social Media Legislation

Purpose: *The purpose of this exercise is to encourage the reader to participate as a professional in the policy-making process.*

Objectives
1. Identify legislation with implications for the safe and effective use of social media.
2. Present data to support the legislative process to his or her community.

Directions
1. Search the Internet, including your state government website, to determine if your state of residence has experienced a lawsuit, new policy, or new legislation reflecting social media's impact on state laws and legislation. Make sure it is within the last five years. For example, does your state have a current cyber-bullying law?
2. Contact your local state representative to determine if his or her office is aware of any new policies or legislation being considered.
3. As a health professional, develop a position paper based on your research. This could be a position paper on the need for new legislation or a position paper on legislation currently being considered.
4. Share your position paper with your local representative.

Exercise 3: Professional Principles and Social Media Policies

Purpose: *The purpose of this exercise is to encourage the reader to evaluate social media policies based on professional principles.*

Objectives

1. Apply professional principles in analyzing social media policies.
2. Present recommendations based on this analysis.

Directions

1. Select a social media policy that currently applies to you. For example, if you are a nursing student, you might select the school of nursing's policy; if you are employed in a health setting, you could select your employer's policy.
2. Compare and contrast the selected policy with both the ANA's *Principles for Social Networking and the Nurse* and the NCSBN *White Paper: A Nurse's Guide to the Use of Social Media.*
3. Present your faculty or employer with a list of recommendations based on your analysis.

Exercise 4: Developing a Personal Social Media Policy

Purpose: *The purpose of this exercise is to introduce the reader to the process of creating a personal social media policy.*

Objectives

1. Develop an outline of the content that should be included in a personal social media policy.
2. Create a personal social media policy to guide personal decisions related to using social media.

Directions

1. Reread the section of this chapter titled Writing and Implementing a Social Media Policy.
2. Write a personal policy for using social media as a professional.
   - Include a statement for each of the points included in the section.
   - For each statement in the policy, document the resources used to write that statement and provide a rationale for your policy.
3. Share this policy on your blog site.

Exercise 5: Generational Differences

Purpose: *The purpose of this exercise is to introduce the reader to factors that influence how different individuals define privacy.*

Objective

1. Appreciate different viewpoints on what is private information.

Directions

1. Interview at least five professional nurses who vary in age by ten or more years.
2. Ask them what differences if any they see in values related to privacy between the different generations of nursing.

3. List at least five reasons you believe differences may or may not exist.

4. Discuss how individual concepts of privacy may influence how individuals use social networking as a professional.

REFERENCES

American Nurses Association. (2011). *ANA's principles for social networking and the nurse.* Washington, DC: NursesBooks.org

Barkar, T. (2011, August 4). *New Missouri law limits electronic contact between teachers, students.* Retrieved from STLtoday.com: http://www.stltoday.com/news/local/education/article_7430605a-f952-5583-bf68-db85a223b455.html

Beesley, C. (2011, September 7). *5 Tips for protecting your business intellectual property in a social media world.* Retrieved from U.S. Small Business Administration: Community Home Blogs: Business Law Advisor: http://community.sba.gov/community/blogs/community-blogs/business-law-advisor/5-tips-protecting-your-business-intellectual-property-social-media-world

Center for Democracy & Technology. (2010, January 28). *The role of privacy by design in protecting consumer privacy.* Retrieved from Center for Democracy & Technology: https://www.cdt.org/policy/role-privacy-design-protecting-consumer-privacy

Citizen Media Law Project. (2008, June). *Linking to copyright materials.* Retrieved from Citizen Media Law Project: http://www.citmedialaw.org/legal-guide/linking-copyrighted-materials

College & Association of Registered Nurses of Alberta. (2011, May). *Professional boundaries for registered nurses: guidelines for the nurse-client relationship.* Retrieved from College & Association of Registered Nurses of Alberta: https://www.nurses.ab.ca/Carna-Admin/Uploads/professional_boundaries_May_%202011.pdf

Contributor(s). (2012, January 27). *Wikipedia: Social media.* Retrieved from Wikipedia: http://en.wikipedia.org/wiki/Social_media

Delaney, J., Rubin, A., & Meister, G. (2012, January 12). *United States: Socially aware: The social media law update.* Retrieved from Mondaq.com: http://www.mondaq.com/unitedstates/x/160666/Social+Media/Socially+Aware+The+Social+Media+Law+Update

Department of Consumer Affairs, C. (2011). *Rules for operation of contests and sweepstakes: Legal guide U-3.* Retrieved from California Department of Consumer Affairs: http://www.dca.ca.gov/publications/legal_guides/u-3.shtml

Equal Employment Opportunity Commission. (2010, November 9). *Federal register. The daily journal of the United States Government.* Retrieved from Regulations Under the Genetic Information NondiscriminationActof2008:https://www.federalregister.gov/articles/2010/11/09/2010-28011/regulations-under-the-genetic-information-nondiscrimination-act-of-2008

Equal Employment Opportunity Commission. (n.d.). *About EEOC.* Retrieved from U.S. Equal Employment Opportunity Commission (EEOC): http://www.eeoc.gov/eeoc/index.cfm

Erickson, M. J. (2011, November 3). *Case against NJ woman charged with identity theft via Facebook will go forward.* Retrieved from Ekickson's Socialnetworkinglawblog.com: http://www.socialnetworkinglawblog.com/2011/11/case-against-nj-woman-charged-with.html

Export.gov. (2011, April 11). *U.S.-EU safe harbor overview.* Retrieved from Expert.gov: Helping US Companies Expert: http://export.gov/safeharbor/eu/eg_main_018476.asp

Federal Trade Commission. (2010, December 1). *Protecting consumer privacy in an era of rapid change: A proposed framework for business and policymakers.* Retrieved from Federal Trade Commission: http://www.ftc.gov/os/2010/12/101201privacyreport.pdf

Federal Trade Commission. (2011, November 29). *Facebook settles FTC charges that it deceived consumers by failing to keep privacy promises.* Retrieved from FTC News: http://www.ftc.gov/opa/2011/11/privacysettlement.shtm

Federal Trade Commission. (2011, March 3). *FTC accepts final settlement with Twitter for failure to safeguard personal information.* Retrieved from Federal trace commission: News: http://www.ftc.gov/opa/2011/03/twitter.shtm

Federal Trade Commission. (2011, March 30). *FTC charges deceptive privacy practices in Google's rollout of its Buzz social network.* Retrieved from Federal Trade Commission: News: http://ftc.gov/opa/2011/03/google.shtm

Federal Trade Commission. (2012, March). *Protecting consumer privacy in an era of rapid change: Recommendations for businesses and policymakers.* Retrieved from Federal Trade Commission: http://www.ftc.gov/os/2012/03/120326privacyreport.pdf, ESvii-viii

Fink, J. (2010, June 14). *Five Nurses Fired For Facebook Postings.* Retrieved Feb 10, 2012, from Scrubs Magazine: http://scrubsmag.com/five-nurses-fired-for-facebook-postings/

Fisher, T. (2012, January 13). *FDA guidance for pharma on social media and off-label use.* Retrieved, from Social Media Today: http://socialmediatoday.com/emoderation/431738/fda-guidance-pharma-social-media-and-label-use

Food & Drug Administration. (2011, December 1). *Guidance for industry responding to unsolicited requests for off-label information about prescription drugs and medical devices.* Retrieved from Food & Drug Administration: http://www.fda.gov/downloads/Drugs/GuidanceComplianceRegulatoryInformation/Guidances/UCM285145.pdf

Hancock, J. (2011, September 14). *Mo. Senate unanimously passes revised 'Facebook law'.* Retrieved from STLtoday.com: http://www.stltoday.com/news/local/govt-and-politics/political-fix/article_ff3c3aa4-dee7-11e0-8725-001a4bcf6878.html

Hawaii State Senate Majority Caucus. (2011, December 29). *Hawaii state senate adopts social media use policy.* Retrieved from Hawaii Senate Majority: http://www.hawaiisenatemajority.com/2011/12/hawaii-state-senate-adopts-social-media-use-policy/

Hawkins, S. (2011, November 23). *Copyright fair use and how it works for online images.* Retrieved, from Social media examiner: Your guide to the social media jungle: http://www.socialmediaexaminer.com/copyright-fair-use-and-how-it-works-for-online-images/

Hennessy-Fiske, M. (2010, August 08). *When Facebook goes to the hospital, patients may suffer.* Retrieved Feb 10, 2012, from Los Angeles Times: http://articles.latimes.com/2010/aug/08/local/la-me-facebook-20100809

Hinduja, S., & Patchin, J. (2012, February). *State cyberbullying laws.* Retrieved from CyberBullying Research Center: http://www.cyberbullying.us/Bullying_and_Cyberbullying_Laws.pdf

Lee, N. (2011, September, October, November). Are You on Facebook, Twitter, or Other Social Media Sites? *Alabama Nurse, 38*(3), 1. Retrieved from http://www.nursingald.com/Uploaded/NewsletterFiles/AL9_11.pdf

Massey, M. (2011, January 4). *Nurse accuses hospital employees of posting photos of sedated patients.* Retrieved Feb 10, 2012, from The South East Texas Record: http://www.setexasrecord.com/news/232304-nurse-accuses-hospital-employees-of-posting-photos-of-sedated-patients#

National Council of State Boards of Nursing. (2011, August). *White paper: A nurse's guide to the use of social media.* Retrieved from National Council of State Boards of Nursing: https://www.ncsbn.org/Social_Media.pdf

National Labor Relations Board. (2011, August 18). *Acting general counsel releases report on social media cases.* Retrieved from National Labor Relations Board (NLRB): https://www.nlrb.gov/news/acting-general-counsel-releases-report-social-media-cases

National labor Relations Board. (2012, January 25). *Acting general counsel issues second social media report.* Retrieved from National labor Relations Board: https://www.nlrb.gov/news/acting-general-counsel-issues-second-social-media-report

National Labor Relations Board. (n.d.). *Rights we protect.* Retrieved from National Labor Relations Board: https://www.nlrb.gov/rights-we-protect

Nurses Fired over Cell Phone Photo of Patient. (2009, February 26). Retrieved February 10, 2012, from ABC: WISN.Com: http://www.wisn.com/r/18796315/detail.html

Office for Civil Rights. (n.d.). Retrieved from U.S. Department of Health & Human Services: http://www.hhs.gov/ocr/office/index.html

Payne, J. (2009, March 12). *Explosive problem for the University of Louisville—nursing student expelled for MySpace blog.* Retrieved from Page One: http://pageonekentucky.com/2009/03/12/explosive-problem-for-the-university-of-louisville-nursing-student-expelled-for-myspace-blog/

Pokin, S. (2007, November 13). *Megan Meier's story.* Retrieved from Megan Meier Foundation: http://www.meganmeierfoundation.org/megansStory.php

Privacy Rights Clearinghouse. (2011, June). Fact Sheet 35' *Social networking privacy: How to be safe, secure and social.* Retrieved from https://www.privacyrights.org/social-networking-privacy

Small Business Administration, U. (2011, February 17). *How to use contests, sweepstakes, and give-aways as marketing tools - while staying within the law.* Retrieved from SBA.Gov: SBA Community: Business Law Advisor: http://community.sba.gov/community/blogs/expert-insight-and-news/business-law-advisor/how-use-contests-sweepstakes-and-giveaways-marketing-tools-while-st

Trademark, U. S. (2010). *Basic facts about trademarks.* Retrieved from the United States Patent and Trademark Office: http://www.uspto.gov/trademarks/basics/BasicFacts_with_correct_links.pdf

Turkewitz, E. (2008, January 15). *My interview with Robert (Dr. "Flea") Lindeman.* Retrieved from New York Personal Injury Law Blog: http://www.newyorkpersonalinjuryattorneyblog.com/2008/01/my-interview-with-robert-dr-flea-lindeman.html

U.S. Copyright Office. (2009, November). *Law and policy: Copyright law: Fair use.* Retrieved from Copyright: http://www.copyright.gov/fls/fl102.html

U.S. Department of Health & Human Services, National Institutes of Health. (2004, July 13). *How can covered entities use and disclose protected health information for research and comply with the privacy rule?* Retrieved from US Department of Health and Human Services National Institutes of Health: http://privacyruleandresearch.nih.gov/pr_08.asp#8d

CHAPTER 10

Social Media and Health Care—Tomorrow and Beyond

Irene Joos and Ramona Nelson

LEARNING OBJECTIVES

At the completion of this chapter the reader will be able to:

1. Examine selected developing technologies and their potential impact on social media, health care, and nursing.
2. Examine social media's impact on future health care delivery systems and nursing roles.
3. Analyze evolving definitions of Web 3.0, Web 4.0, Health 3.0, and Health 4.0.
4. Explore consumers' potential use of social media in future decades.

TERMS

Augmented reality	Nanobots
Consumer-centric commerce	Semantic web
Health 3.0 and 4.0	Syntax
Homo Zappiens	Web 3.0 and 4.0
Nanotechnology	

*I*n her editorial in the *Journal of the American Academy of Nurse Practitioners*, Dr. Loretta Ford (2010) challenged nurses to create a vision for the future. She went on to ask that nurses as a profession, act to advance nursing's mission to:

- Care for and about people,
- Prevent disease and disability, and
- Promote health and protect others in the public interest and for the public good. (p. 177).

In an editorial titled, "The Future of Nursing and Health Care: Through the Looking Glass 2030," Koeniger-Donohue and Hawkins (2010) predicted changes they see coming in health care delivery. These include:

- Health care will be a right and not a privilege accessible to all regardless of ability to pay. The system will be a single-payer system.
- Nurses will be the "glue" of the health care system and remain the caregivers closest to the patient.
- Nursing informatics will play an essential role in providing safe, cost-effective, quality care that is outcome based.
- Consumers will have a "smart" health care home and their own reliable personal electronic health records.
- Social media sites like Twitter, SMS (texting), social networking sites, wikis, interoperable consultations, and remote monitoring will enhance nursing care and communications.

Three of these five visions include some aspect of technology. The last one specifically addresses the enhancement of nursing care and communications by using social media. Questions generated by this prediction include:

- What will social media look like in the next 20 to 30 years?
- How will this technology be assimilated into every aspect of our day-to-day lives?
- What role will nurses have in fully developing and evaluating the utilization of these new technologies in the health care arena?
- How will technology change consumers and the practice of nursing?
- Will in-person patient encounters or office visits still exist?

Planning for the future and the changes likely to occur in nursing is difficult at best. What we do know is that the opportunities and challenges offered by changes in social media will happen with or without nursing's active involvement. If nursing is to proactively benefit from social media developments, nurse leaders must anticipate these changes and start preparing nurses now with the skill sets necessary for their future nursing roles. It is no longer acceptable to be computer and information illiterate; future nurses must be fluent in the use of social media. In light of this reality, this chapter focuses on developing technologies and their implications for nursing.

PREDICTIONS AND TRENDS

New medical discoveries, advances in treatments, new development in materials, growth in computer power along with miniaturized devices, increasing infrastructure speeds and advances in wireless technologies, and advances in communications systems will continue to drive health care innovation and the movement forward in promoting wellness (Task Force Members, 2006). The MBA Online website (http://www.mbaonline .com/a-day-in-the-internet/) documents the rapid growth of communication and social media applications. In one day:

- Users send 294 billion emails. The United States Postal Service would take 2 years to process that many pieces of postal mail.
- Bloggers write two million blog posts. This would fill *Time* magazine for 770 years.

- One hundred seventy-two million different people visit Facebook, 40 million people visit Twitter, and 22 million people visit LinkedIn daily.
- There are 1288 new apps to download and users have downloaded more than 35 million apps, and
- There are more iPhones sold than babies born throughout the world (Manning, 2012).

The April 2012 edition of *Health Management Technology* included a guide titled Mobile Devices Solutions Guide (Mobile Devices Solutions Guide, 2012). This guide listed products that are new to the market and included topics such as:

- "Mobile computing with a twist": This described the world's lightest convertible tablet PC with a multi-touch, digitizer screen.
- "Telehealth goes touch-tablet route": This is a touch-tablet that collects vital signs from patients and transmits them to a health care system suite. Health care providers then track and monitor these data.
- "Accountable care as a community effort": This described an integrated suite of programs that permits seamless connections between patients and their care team. Patients have access to their personal health records (PHRs) and can share information in real time.
- "Manage mobile devices through the cloud": This service secures and tracks a host of mobile devices like iPhone, iPad, Android, and Blackberry devices (pp. 28–29).

Mobile devices and social media are increasingly integrated into patient/health care interactions, thereby enhancing patient care and wellness initiatives. The following section of this chapter builds on these rapid changes in health care by describing 21st century predictions and health care trends. Current health care technology research is used as a basis to predicted future applications in health care. When reading this material, think about how these developing technologies and trends may change social media or social media may change them.

Twenty-First Century Predictions

There have been a number of published predictions describing life 50 years from now (Gilleo, n.d.; "2030–2039 Timeline Contents," n.d.). Selected predictions from these sources can be expected to significantly affect the nursing role and the daily activities of nurses.

- The global population is reaching a crisis point that's impacting availability of food, water, and energy and depleting basic building blocks like phosphorus. The aging population is stressing all resources. The daily stress levels for the average citizen continues to increase.
- AI (artificial intelligence) is wide spread with breakthroughs in computing, nano-technology, medicine, and neuroscience. Augmented reality glasses have customers interacting through them with others—both real and virtual.
- AIDS, cancer, and a number of other diseases are becoming curable with the advances in stem cell research, synthetic genomics, nanotechnology, and information technology growth that permit the ability to scan, analyze, and decode the human body.
- Web 4.0 is transforming the Internet landscape by using semantic analyzing programs that combine pattern recognition with speed and memory. Bloggers and other social media users outpace traditional news media in speed and accuracy of presenting events. The real world is augmented by the virtual world.

- Information management tools now control the massive growth of information that overwhelmed most health care providers at the turn of the century.
- Terabit Internet speeds are commonplace throughout the world with many connections through wearable or implantable devices.
- Holographic wall screens are not yet commonplace because of the cost but will soon drop in price. Images on these screens appear to jump out at the viewer.
- Bionic eyes surpass human vision with infrared nighttime vision and the teleportation of DNA and proteins.
- Full immersion virtual reality gives consumers the ability to actually be in a virtual world indistinguishable from the real world. Nanobots alter the real neuro signals to simulate the virtual world.

Health Care Trends

A number of current trends and pilot studies provide a basis for predicting future health care delivery and advances in nursing.

- Telehealth services are increasingly used as a means of keeping people home and healthy. Consumers are wired to their smart mobile devices, leading to health care cost savings. These devices permit daily self-monitoring and video check-in with the nurse using programs like Health Buddy (http://www.bosch-telehealth.com/en/us/products/health_buddy/health_buddy.html) and Trapollo's Independent Living Remote Health Monitoring System (http://www.trapollo.com/independent-living.php). Health Buddy combines a symptom review, vital sign monitoring, and education/health coaching by using a four-button interface to the Health Buddy Desktop. Health care providers use the desktop interface to monitor the patient. The idea is to intervene before conditions deteriorate. Trapollo's monitoring systems also provide in-home monitoring. The system includes monitoring of vital signs, daily health surveys, medication dispensers, motion tracking and fall alerts, triage services, and video consultations. This system attempts to provide continuous health and wellness services to keep the elderly independent longer.
- Early preemptive intervention and long-range preventive medicine are established strategies delivering cost-effective care and life-prolonging health maintenance (Gilleo, n.d.). This will be made possible by Bio-MEMS (Micro-Electro-Mechanical Systems) chips that can monitor an array of changes and deliver personalized medicine in minutes. These strategies will correct problems before the natural progression of disease and disability begins.
- Stem cell-derived tissue, biochemical-induced growth, and bioelectronics stimulation will lead to the manufacturing of organs such as eyes, kidneys, liver, and, by 2020, new teeth (Gilleo, n.d.). There may even be a "parts store" where body parts can be purchased.
- New delivery models will reshape health care. Two examples are mobile care such as WhiteGlove Health (http://www.whiteglove.com/) and hospitals without walls as in the Idaho case study (Chase, 2012a, 2012b). WhiteGlove is a health care service that comes to you at home or at work, 365 days a year, 8:00 am to 8:00 pm, within hours of your call. You can request an appointment, edit/view your health record, and view lab results from your mobile devices. Idaho's St. Luke's Center for Health

Care Innovation is working on changing the delivery model from the "do more, bill more" model of health care reimbursement to a collaborative care model that is patient centric, accountable, and coordinated. They are taking the care to the patients and using off-the-self software tools instead of expensive custom applications.

Research Developments and Studies

Some predicted changes in diagnosis and treatment that are currently in development include remote monitoring devices, nanotechnologies, augmented reality devices, robotics, and home-care laboratories. Several examples demonstrate how current developments and research can be used to predict future advances in health care.

Remote Monitoring Devices

BodyGuardian is developing a remote monitoring device that snaps onto an attachment similar to a Band-Aid. A high quality ECG is then sent via smartphones and wireless hubs to physicians. Transmission of these data can be initiated by the patient or by the device if cardiac changes are detected. The data are then sent to the patient's health care professional who may receive an SMS alert or message to review the data on tablet devices or computers. A more detailed description of this device may be seen at http://preventice.com/products/RemotePatientMonitoring.aspx and http://mhealthwatch.com/mayo-clinic-teams-with-preventice-for-body-guardian-remote-monitoring-device-19045/. Another example of monitoring devices is the Intelligence Toilet II from Toto that monitors weight, blood sugar levels, and other vital signs. These data are then wirelessly transferred to your computer for analysis (Saenz, 2009).

Currently, remote monitoring devices are being developed by individual teams and do not integrate well with each other. Future developments will include integration of the devices for gathering and interpreting the data. As patients become more literate in using these devices and in managing their health, the devices will increasingly provide decision support for patients to manage their own common health problems. In addition, futuristic patients will share with other non-medical personnel their aggregate and synthesized data on future social media platforms, thereby creating new and innovative approaches to health care research.

Nanotechnologies

Nanotechnologies refer to an approach of building things from the bottom up by manipulating individual atoms and molecules at the one-billionth of a meter level (Nanotechnology, n.d.). This technology holds promise for drug delivery systems to target specific cells. The drugs attach to a nanoscale delivery system like gold nanostars for transporting drugs directly to cancer cell nuclei (Dam et al., 2012; Paddock, 2012). While one might think this is "far out," the U.S. government is investing three-quarters of a billion dollars to enhance this new field through its National Nanotechnology Incentive (http://www.nano.gov/).

Nanotechnology will also have a major impact on the size and type of devices we now use for social media. For example, picture a device that rolls up like a piece of paper and can be placed in your pocket. While stored in your pocket the device could take dictation as you share your ideas while walking down the street or, if you prefer, could be unrolled to produce a full size keyboard.

Augmented Reality Contact Lenses and Glasses

The design of these lenses is to enhance vision, but could be expanded to include displaying text, translating speech into captions in real time, offering visual clues from a navigation system, and providing noninvasive monitoring of the wearer's biomarkers and health indicators using Natural User Interface or NUI (Halloway, 2012; Parviz, 2009). Imagine a time where technology can sense blood sugar, cholesterol, sodium, and potassium levels without piercing the skin and wirelessly transmit the results to health care professionals. Imagine all of this through the use of contact lenses. Now, imagine nano-sized projectors inserted into the iris and projecting onto the retina to enhance vision.

If one does not prefer contacts lenses, Google X labs and others are working on augmented reality glasses that will provide a wealth of information in real time on displays as well as an intelligent personal assistant. The wearer will also be able to carry on a phone conversation with a projected image of the person at the other end of the call. It will provide directions in accordance with your location, recognize faces as you walk around and look at others, and so forth. Check out the video of the glasses on YouTube (http://www.youtube.com/watch?v=Vb2uojqKvFM). All the basic technologies needed to make this happen are available today; work now needs to progress to make this a reality in terms of cost and mass production.

Just imagine nurses using these glasses to organize their day in caring for several patients. The glasses combine multiple tasks to be completed and a sensitive listening ability to project critical data the nurse needs to know in order to care for the patients. By wearing these glasses, the nurse can verbally pull data from a virtual electronic health record (EHR), document care using voice, receive reminders for tasks needing to be completed, and receive alerts on patients' conditions. A step further will have the computer system listening to the nurse-patient interaction and recording critical data on the EHR, with the nurse validating the data later.

The underlying value of current social media technologies is the ability to share information and to co-create. But the sharing of information and the creations produced by today's social media are limited to materials that can be shared on a screen. Yet what kind of home visit could be done if you could actually see the patient in their environment and not just the image that is projected on a monitor screen? What kind of sharing could occur if augmented reality glasses could produce the sense of presence that occurs in face-to-face meetings?

Robotics

In the last 20 years, robots have moved from the lab to the point of care. Examples of these advances span from robot-assisted surgery to robots assisting the elderly, disabled, and mentally challenged. Two such robots are Paro, the robot seal, being used to calm patients (http://www.parorobots.com/) and NurseBot (http://www.cs.cmu.edu/~flo/scope.html), an assistant robot that provides:

- Intelligent reminding,
- Tele-presence,
- Data collection and surveillance,
- Mobile manipulation, and
- Social interaction (Nursebot Project, n.d.).

But these robots are limited to preprogramed interactions. In the future, family members and caregivers will be able to interact together from remote sites to create new communication patterns with these robots. For example, NurseBot might remind an elderly person of their ever-expanding list of grandchildren and great-grandchildren including their names and current ages. Now imagine if NurseBot takes on the voice and image of a family member or loved one sharing calming thoughts, reminders, and so on.

With the use of sensors in one's home, independent living can be further supported with robotics and technology that give the elderly person a sense of family presence when in reality they are not physically present. A virtual presence that reminds elderly parents to take medicine, to eat breakfast, to tend to daily hygiene, or that shares gentle safety reminders to turn off the stove and to find out who is at the door before opening it could extend an elderly person's time in their own home and lead to a healthier, happier lifestyle for the older population.

Homecare Technologies

People of all ages want to stay in their homes as they age. Maintaining one's independence or living independently is a freedom no one wants to lose. While family members caring for the aged want to support their request, they also have a responsibility to keep their loved ones safe and secure. The following are examples of research programs and technologies that may assist people and their caregivers to support living independently in their home longer:

> *ORACATECH Living Labs Program*—The ORCATECH Living Laboratory (OLL) is a population of community-dwelling seniors who have agreed to participate on an ongoing basis in research on technology-based health monitoring, intervention, and support of independent aging. This Living Lab explores technologies to support independent living, to assess new behavioral markers, and to evaluate approaches for assessing neurological and other relevant health changes, all in the participant's home (LivingLaboratoryUsage, 2008). This resource is intended to promote examination of the effectiveness of various emerging technologies in a natural setting with the hope of reducing development-to-market times. Some of the pilot studies include:

> - Various sensors to estimate activity and speed of walking, social activity involvement, and movement around the home,
> - Medication tracking for medication compliance,
> - Bed mats and load cells (a transducer which converts force into a measurable electrical output) for assessing restlessness and activity in bed,
> - Robots in the home, and
> - A kiosk interface for administering short weekly cognitive tests.

> Some of the questions that this program is asking include: Do changes in mobility and walking speed predict cognitive decline? Is wiring pillboxes a better way to monitor medication compliance than counting pills? What impact does having a robot in the home have on the patient? The OLL is researching these and several other visionary ideas. For a listing of their many research projects see their website at http://www.orcatech.org/research/studies.

> *Healthy Aging and Independent Living (HAIL) Lab*—HAIL is a collaborative effort among the Robert and Arlene Kogod Center on Aging, Charter House, and the Mayo Clinic Center for Innovation. The project created the HAIL Lab to help seniors remain at home, healthy and independent (Healthy Aging and

Independent Living [HAIL] Lab, 2012). The three main objectives of the HAIL lab are to:

- Design tools and environments that promote health and safety, while sustaining independence and improving quality-of-life (The Living Environment).
- Prepare for and navigate major life transitions (Transitions).
- Target services and support that one can better integrate into the care delivery system (Caregiver Support and Education).

This project includes nanotechnology possibilities as well as technology developments. Two projects included the use of a tablet computer for tracking medications and health coaching, and sensors for real-time monitoring (Wang, 2011). Research questions included: Can a tablet computer effectively track how those with chronic diseases take their medications? Can that same computer provide health coaching? Will a Band-Aid-sized sensor for transmitting real-time data to health care professionals annoy those patients wearing it?

A key research question for the future is how will social media in conjunction with innovative technology be incorporated into the lives and social fabric of these individuals? Will this type of research result in creating a more humanistic life experience as opposed to the isolation of being house bound and living alone?

Mobile Devices

Mobile devices are forcing the development of apps that support a variety of health care initiatives for both the health care provider and the consumer. For example, fitness apps using virtual coaches seem to be more effective than apps that only monitor activity levels (Watson, Bickmore, Cange, Kulshreshtha, & Kvedar, 2012). Consumers can download apps for reminders to take medicine or drink water, monitor their heart rate, manage their carbohydrate intake, check their stress level, access a first aid guide, and the list goes on and on.

To date, long-term use of the apps is flat, with many people abandoning them when they no longer perceive them as relevant to their lives. For these devices to be effective, the individual must interact with the app instead of just having the app stimulate the individual to do something. At this time the benefit of these mobile devices remains dependent on the person using them. In the future, imagine health care settings that assist consumers in engineering/programming a platform of applications that will coach them on what they need. For example, a person needs to maintain a healthy lifestyle that, for this person, means 1500 calorie a day, exercise three times a week, medication reminders, a relaxation routine, 64 ounces of water per day, and so on. The health care provider selects the apps and adjusts the programs to monitor the consumer for these activities, selects coaches, and sets the alerts to notify the consumer when they are not following the routine.

Mobile device research is also being conducted in using a low tech solution—texting—to manage compliance to diabetes treatment. Initiatives such as txt4thealth (https://txt4health.com/txt4health/Display/display.aspx?CurrentXsltId=1) and Chartered Health's diabetes management texting program (http://www.chartered-health.com/index.php?option=com_content&task=view&id=220&Itemid=161) use texting to see if compliance with treatment increases. Since texting is a large portion of a person's phone use, is this a solution to compliance? Would these apps be more effective if they were combined with group support via social media? Could a weekly webinar have the same effect as attending a Weight Watchers or AA meeting?

WEB AND HEALTH DEVELOPMENTS

Web developments will continue to lead the way in innovative uses of technology. Health care will also continue to exploit these developments or be on the forefront of innovative use of these developing technologies to effectively improve the delivery of health care and health care outcomes.

Web 3.0 and 4.0

Chapter 1 introduced the concept of Web 1.0 and 2.0. Web 3.0, sometimes called the semantic or contextual web, is the next phase or generation of web technologies. In Figure 10.1, Web 1.0 is included in Web 2.0. In other words, Web 2.0 does NOT replace Web 1.0 but rather maintains all the features and function of Web 1.0 while adding a new range of features and functions that build on Web 1.0. An example of this can be seen with how one might contact the person(s) responsible for content on the website. In Web 1.0, one might have to email the webmaster with questions providing there was an email address posted on the website. With Web 2.0 one can post a comment or questions through a link to the blog or a social network site like Facebook, and so on. Today a majority of web pages contain numerous links one can use to convey your comment or concern. This same process will continue with the development of Web 3.0 and Web 4.0. One version does not replace the other but rather each version creates a whole new range of uses for the previous version and at the same time creates a whole new range of functions that are unique to the newly emerging version.

The focus with Web 3.0 is machine-facilitated understanding of information located on the web; about things and how they relate to each other; about context of the information; and about computers understanding the data. At present, computers don't understand the meaning behind the data on the web. The term *syntax* (demonstrated through Web 1.0 and 2.0) is how to display the data; *semantics* is the meaning behind the data

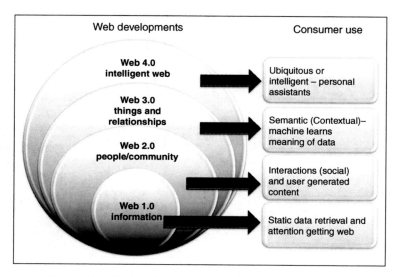

Figure 10.1 *Web 3.0 and 4.0 building on Web 1.0 and 2.0.*
Source: Concepts from Farber (2007) and Spivack (2009)

(Farber, 2007; Spivack, 2009; Strickland, n.d.). Web 3.0 will utilize logic to determine relationships to web objects (text, pictures, music, etc.) and interpret these data relationships to the needs of the consumer. Globally, companies are merging and collaborating in development of Web 3.0 products. For example, Radar Networks (product called Twine) was purchased by Evri, Inc. (http://www.evri.com/) and MetaWeb (product called Freebase) was purchased by Google. These products deal with creating semantic relationships with the data. Some experts believe this movement to Web 3.0 will be the building block for programming and interface development initiatives and not a new product development focus (Strickland, n.d.).

The key to understanding this movement is the context in which the objects—text, picture, painting, and so forth—relate to each other. Web 3.0 will see the development of semantic-based search engines and other tools that will make using the web easier. For example a search such as "I want to learn about diabetes, select a doctor, review treatment options, and read the views of doctors" will return usable results.

What role will nurses play with each advancement or elevation of web functionality? How will nursing impact patient outcomes with each level of web developments? In Web 1.0 nurses shared with patients and each other printed information found on static websites; for example, using a search engine to locate what immunizations are needed when traveling to Africa or what are the drug interactions for the medications the patient is taking. It was information retrieval. With Web 2.0, nurses created blogs or wikis for professional collaboration and interaction with communities of consumers, to assist consumers to achieve personal health and wellness goals. Nurses established nurse call centers to respond and interact with consumers. Moving to Web 3.0, nurses will work with companies that design software to synthesize data obtained from sensors and gleaned from objects on the Internet to provide value-added care to consumers. The nurse may advise patients on what medicines to take or insulin to administer that day based on custom information gleaned from the customer's personal and expert data that these systems will produce. The nurse may be using these tools to provide support and interpretation for their plan of care. See Figure 10.2 for an overlay of the nursing role.

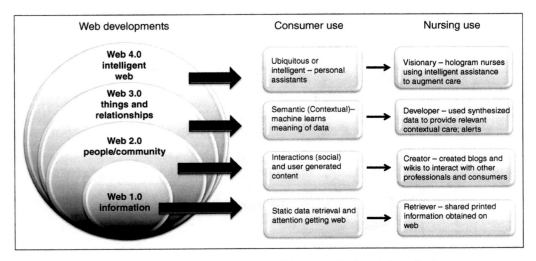

Figure 10.2 *Web 3.0 and 4.0 building on Web 1.0 and 2.0 and the role of nurses.*
Source: Concepts from Farber (2007) and Spivack (2009)

Web 4.0 (also called WebOS) predictions are not well defined; it is an idea in progress. The vision is an "intelligent" or "symbiotic" web with intelligent personal assistants who will anticipate the user's need. Current predictions of Web 4.0 include the following:

- The line between human and machine will blur; Web 4.0 will simulate the human brain,
- A pervasion of 3-D technologies like holographs,
- A web of things becomes a web of thoughts, and
- An increased use of Radio Frequency Identification Technology (RFIT) technologies where machine will communicate with other machines resulting in objects becoming interactive (Muller, n.d.).

What role will nurses take with Web 4.0? Will they rise to the occasion and be visionaries? Will we have a nurse robot that appears and speaks to patients using sensory data collected to advise or care for patients, or will it be a hologram image of the real nurse who interacts with the patient to make a decision? Will robots replace repetitive nursing activities? How will augmented reality influence the role of the nurse? How will Health 3.0 and 4.0 play off the Web 4.0 technology developments in furthering quality care and/or changing health care delivery models?

Health 3.0 and 4.0

The predictions for Health 3.0 and 4.0 build upon the predictions for Web 3.0 and 4.0 (see Figure 10.3). Health 3.0 will be characterized by consumer-centric commerce (Web 3.0). Consumer-centric commerce means "identifying, facilitating, and integrating online and offline communication and care delivery channels needed to reach and coordinate end goals (values) as defined by disparate customer segments such as the patient, provider, payer, policymaker, caretaker, etcetera" (Gorman & Braber, n.d. p. 1). Health 4.0 will be characterized by content, community, commerce and what we're currently missing—coherence (McCabe, 2008). What we may see for Health 3.0:

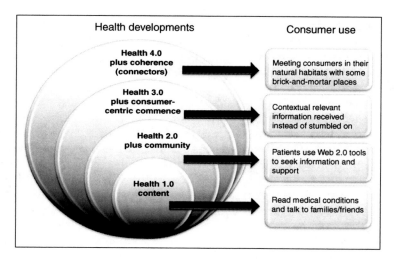

Figure 10.3 *Health 3.0 and 4.0 building on 1.0 and 2.0.*
Source: Concepts from McCabe (2008) and Nash (2008)

▪ The consumer will access health care information that they really want based on contextual meaning of the information. This means consumers will be able to search using plain language instead of medical terms and receive relevant results.

▪ Information will empower the consumer with action oriented information and resources that, at the consumer's request, can be incorporated into the consumer's personal plan of care (PPC) within their PHR. Compliance and adherence can be expected to improve.

▪ Health care provider communication will improve with more effective, culturally sensitive care that is customized. This means a health care provider can type a response to a patient that includes medical terms, at a post-graduate reading level, and the computer will suggest revisions to customize the response to the patient's individual health-literacy level in the same way word processing programs now offer spell check corrections.

▪ Ontologies (dictionaries of relationships between concepts) will be commonplace (Nash, 2008; Trzebucki, 2008). Once fully developed these ontologies will eliminate the need for standard nursing languages and the related codes. Watson, the IBM computer application, is an early version of this coming reality.

▪ Development of companies like American Well (http://www.americanwell.com/) founded in 2006, "to transform health care delivery through technology and improve access to quality care by removing traditional barriers to health care delivery such as distance, mobility, and time constraints" (American Well, n.d.), and Organized Wisdom (http://www.organizedwisdom.com/Home), designed to organize wisdom to help save doctors time, grow their practice and improve patient education through development of WisdomCards™ (Organized Wisdom, n.d.). These companies use a method of commerce and Web 3.0 technologies where both parties gain—the consumer and the company from the production of WisdomCards™ (Gorman, n.d.).

Health 3.0 will offer systems that add value for both consumers and companies by:

▪ Embedding feedback loops that include the patient as an equal partner interacting with the health care system,

▪ Requiring patients to share the responsibility for selecting appropriate options to meet their health care/wellness expectations,

▪ Mapping the interrelationships between the parts of the health care system,

▪ Using tools that provide the ability to communicate freely and openly, and

▪ Using frameworks that pull diverse information into consumer centric knowledge to improve health care decision making (H3PO, n.d.).

The prediction for Health 4.0 is that it will meet consumers in their natural habitats by integrating online services with traditional services that aggregate the total net benefit of consumptive capitalism (Gorman, n.d.; McCabe, 2008). Health 4.0 will see virtual house calls and health kiosks as the norm and robots to assist with care will abound. Electrode-packed skullcaps will read human thought and translate that into action. These may at some point be embedded in the skull. Imagine thinking about doing something and have the robot take that action based on your brain wave patterns wirelessly sent to the robot (Zammit, 2009). Imagine how this technology would change the treatment of a whole range of neuromuscular disorder and diseases.

With these intellectual visions and logical advancements, the critical questions are what skills will nurses need to work in this developing environment, and how will professional nurses embrace these developments to extend care to individuals outside a health care facility? Will nurses and other health care professionals be required to have a virtual license to ensure their competence in working with these technologies? What current skills will need to be further developed? What current skills will have "limited" use in this changing health care environment?

NURSING SKILLS/ROLE

Huston (2008) identified eight competencies for nurse leaders in 2020 (see Figure 10.4). These include:

- A global perspective or mindset regarding health care and nursing issues. Given the global nature of travel and the economy, one country's health threats become problems of the world.
- A working knowledge of technology. This means an ability to integrate technology and to examine what the potential may be for improving patient care and quality of life.
- Expert decision-making skills rooted in empirical science. Many health care problems require decisions of the ill-defined type. An ill-defined problem is one that addresses complex issues and one cannot easily describe them in a concise, complete manner. Because of the complexity of the ill-defined problem, there may be several approaches to solving the problem. This requires a careful analysis to determine the best approach to dealing with the problem.
- A creative organizational mindset that recognizes quality health care and patient/worker safety. This means setting standards for identifying errors and corrective actions when necessary. Nurses should be involved in the process of setting quality standards that include safety practices for both the patients and the health care workers.
- Political astuteness as to how things work in an organization. Nurses will use their power wisely to work toward organizational goals of quality care. It also means speaking up when there are health care issues to address at the state and national levels.

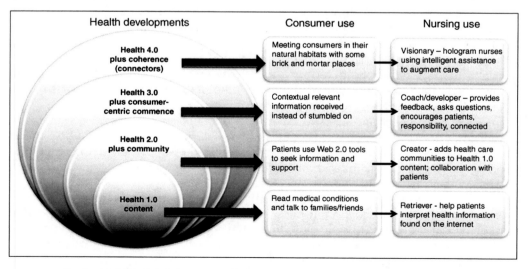

Figure 10.4 *Health 3.0 and 4.0 building on 1.0 and 2.0 and the role of nurses.*
Source: Concepts from McCabe (2008) and Nash (2008)

- A collaborative ability to work with others in building effective teams, where all are concerned with the quality of health care. Nurses will need to build positive and productive working relationships among team members and others in the organization in order to integrate quality goals with business goals.
- An ability to balance authenticity with performance expectations. Authenticity means being true to oneself and one's values while dealing with organizational performance expectations.
- An effective coping strategy to deal with change. Technology brings the need for nurses to be effective change agents.

These skills will advance patient care and, in turn, nursing, if we use them when evaluating technology and its potential for innovative approaches for delivering quality health care. Nurses will need:

- Involvement in assessing what consumers need to stay healthy, recover from illness, or cope with chronic conditions, and how technology can help. What applications might help the consumer deal with life-changing health care needs? This means working with app developers to assist in developing the right apps that effectively meet patient needs.
- Creative skills to look at devices like augmented glasses/lenses and envisioning how one might use that device to improve care or prevent health care problems. For example, nurses should be looking at these devices and working toward using them as virtual nursing coaches, monitoring systems, and so forth. The question to ask is can the patient use this device to effectively and efficiently improve their health care? In what ways? Is this just another technology fad that has no real long-term usefulness? What impact might these have in social media use and effectiveness? Will the device always be on, monitoring us and searching for information to give us? Will the device monitor, track, and report every move we or patients make? Will providing the consumer and health practitioner with data that neither had ever considered cause new problems or provide new solutions to old problems, or both?
- Research skills to effectively evaluate the outcomes from using new technologies in new situations and with new populations. How can this technology enhance social media use? What can all these data that sensors and remote monitoring collect tell us about effectiveness of treatments?
- Change skills to adapt to the changing location of health care delivery. While there will remain a need for hospital nursing, nursing will provide more nursing care in the home, in the community, and remotely. Nurses will need to be comfortable working with clients through technology and social media.
- Database and algorithm skills to develop and maintain databases? If nurses are collecting data through remote monitoring or sensors, they will need to help determine what conditions will trigger an alert or notification of a problem. Until the computer can learn to learn, individuals will still need to determine what data to collect, what triggers alerts, and so on.
- Questioning skills critical to working in this developing environment. With all these data and information floating around, how does one minimize the less important information while highlighting the important or critical information? People are in data overload...there are too many blogs, websites, tweets, and status updates to keep track of important information.
- Educational skills to bridge the gap in educating our consumers. The digital natives and digital immigrants have diverse ways of dealing with health issues, expectations

for health care, and technology. The coined words are homo sapiens versus the homo zappiens. They view the world, education, and health care, differently (Veen, n.d.).

▪ Ethical commitment to the appropriate use of information. This is a substantive concern when information can exist in cyberspace for years and years and when individuals are subject to monitoring and storage of that data in cyberspace or the "cloud." Use of public social media sites adds to this concern.

While some may see this as a frightening time in nursing, others see it as a time to be creative and make an impact on the future of health care delivery and the role of nurses in effectively and efficiently using the next generation of social media technologies.

SUMMARY

This chapter explored technology developments, health care trends, and the skills nursing will need to have in order to embrace these developments. Nurses are and will be involved in helping to design and select the appropriate technology for solving health related problems and challenges. A key issue in this process will be the appropriate use of technology to solve the appropriate human problems. This is an exciting time in nursing and health care, as nurses have an opportunity to influence how these technologies will be used to improve patient care and help meet Health 3.0 and 4.0 goals.

DISCUSSION QUESTIONS

1. What role will nurses have in fully developing and evaluating the capabilities of new technologies in health care? What research projects do you envision doing to evaluate the effectiveness of new technologies?

2. What do you see as major issues with augmented contact lenses or glasses? What impact might these have on health care? On the nurses role?

3. Your patient expresses concern about the sensors being placed in her home including a smart toilet, a bed sensor to detect movement in bed, and a robot. The patient doesn't want anyone "watching" what she is doing; she believes these interventions are an invasion of her privacy. She agreed to this because she wants to stay at home and not go to an assistive living arrangement. Describe how you would approach her concerns and what information you would provide her.

4. How do you believe these technologies will impact the cost of health care delivery? Support your answer with at least two resources.

5. Some people believe that all the information being shared through social media and collected through remote sensing and monitoring with and without our knowledge may be used against them (as it is currently being used by potential employers and schools) far into the future. Some are especially concerned with health care data and the archiving of our every thought and activity. Explain how the information you obtained from this chapter will influence you personally or professionally.

6. Read the article located at http://www.newrulesofmedicine.com/blog/virtual-medicine/. Discuss what you believe this may mean to nursing practice and nurses use of social media.

7. Describe a practical social media application that could be built on the functionality of Web 3.0 or Web 4.0.

EXERCISES

Exercise 1: ORACTECH Living Lab Program

Purpose: *The purpose of this exercise is to explore a website dedicated to helping consumers age successfully and to reduce the cost of health care through development of key independent living technologies, creation of research infrastructure to support aging-in-place research, partnerships with industry and academic leaders, and establishing the evidence-base for technologies supporting aging.*

Objectives
1. Explore the research currently being conducted that melds technology with successful aging.
2. Reflect on how this impacts nurses and consumers use of social media.

Directions
1. Access http://www.orcatech.org/.
2. Look around the site for research being conducted on various aspects of this project. Find one that is a study and not just an abstract.
3. Select one of the studies. What were they studying? What was the study design? Who was the population? What are the results?
4. Use your blog to write a short summary on this study and how these results might impact nurses and consumers. Include a link to the study on your blog. NOTE: If you didn't create a blog in Chapter 2, do so now.

Exercise 2: A Physicist's View of Our Changing World

Purpose: *This exercise has you looking into the future via the eyes of a physicist and relating that vision to social media's use in delivering health care. The purpose of this exercise is to encourage you to consider the perspective of other disciplines when evaluating the potential uses of different technologies.*

Objectives
1. Explore another disciplines contributions to innovations in social media and health care technologies.
2. Increase awareness of how developments in other disciplines impact health care delivery.

Directions
1. View the video *The World in 2030* with Dr. Michio Kaku located at http://www.youtube.com/watch?v=219YybX66MY. Please note it is about 1 hour in length.
2. Select one of the developments presented. Provide a 150 word or less description of this development.
3. Incorporate into your description the answer to the following two questions:
   - What implications will the development have on health care delivery and social media usage?
   - What impact will the development have on nursing's role?

Exercise 3: Sci-Fi and Reality

Purpose: *The purpose of this exercise is to distinguish what is possible and what is not, given our current state of technological innovations.*

Objectives

1. Summarize the technologies used in an older film and whether those predictions of that technology are now a reality.
2. Envision how those technologies can be used to further health care delivery, nursing care, and social media use.
3. Create a podcast.

Directions

1. Review the 1966 science fiction movie *Fantastic Voyage* (available through Netflix, Amazon Instant Movie, and other sites).
2. Summarize the technologies from the file, their impact on health care if developed, their use in nursing, their impact on social media, and how you may envision social media tools of the future.
3. Develop a podcast summarizing your thoughts.
4. Upload the podcast to YouTube (create an account if you don't have one and make your post private if you prefer; invite your classmates to view your podcast).

Exercise 4: The Year 2030

Purpose: *The purpose of this exercise is to learn what others predict will be happening in the year 2030 and how these predicted happenings could alter the directions for health care delivery and social media tools.*

Objectives

1. Research predictions for the years 2030 and 2040.
2. Develop a paper of nursing's future role in delivering care in the years 2030 and 2040.
3. Use the class wiki to merge everyone's ideas and produce one document.

Directions

1. Review the websites A Picture of Health 2030 (http://www.iae.ie/site_media/ pressroom/documents/2009/Jun/09/A_Picture_of_Health_.pdf) and FutureTimeline .net (http://www.futuretimeline.net/21stcentury/2030-2039.htm).
2. Find another "future" predictions document, video, blog, or so on, and review it.
3. Select one prediction or development from objectives 1 and 2 above and answer the following questions:
   a. How do you see these developments impacting consumers' and health care professionals' use of social media?
   b. How might that technology development change the media itself?
   c. Provide examples to support your ideas.
4. If no class wiki was created in Chapter 2, create one now and invite your classmates to the wiki. Post your thoughts to the class wiki. Edit and refine others' comments so that ONE document is developed with everyone's input and refinements.

Exercise 5: Homo Zappiens—The New Generation

Purpose: *The purpose of this exercise is to learn what others are expecting of our next generation and how that expectation may impact the nursing role when interacting with future health care consumers in providing for their health care needs.*

Objectives
1. Create a description of our new health care consumer using what was learned throughout this book and specifically in this chapter.
2. Examine what this new consumer might mean to the future role of nurses using social media.

Directions
1. Review these two documents:
   - Homo Zappiens and the Need for New Education Systems which can be accessed at http://www.oecd.org/dataoecd/0/5/38360892.pdf. This is a brief article looking at the changing student population.
   - Homo Zappiens Learning and Knowledge: The Digital Mindset. This document is a PowerPoint PDF file located at http://www.oecd.org/dataoecd/14/25/38337941.pdf.
2. Create a similar document or PowerPoint presentation but predict the characteristics of the homo zappien health care consumer in the year 2030 or 2040. Make sure you include factors driving this changing health care consumer and what health care and nurses need to do in 2030 or 2040 to accommodate this changing scene.

Exercise 6: Web 3.0 and 4.0

Purpose: *The purpose of this exercise is to examine what changes are predicted for the Internet (Web 3.0 and 4.0) and what impact that has on social media, health care, and nurses. In addition to keeping current on health care changes, technology-literate nurses must keep abreast of what is coming down the road. In this case, the example will be Web 3.0 and 4.0.*

Objectives
1. Keep yourself abreast of the changing technology scene and how this may impact health care delivery and nursing practice.
2. Subscribe to a blog, RSS feed, or magazine that looks at trends, technology developments, and/or future predictions.

Directions
1. Search for a blog, RSS feeds from technology news sites, or a magazine that looks at trends, technology developments, and/or future predictions regarding the Internet and Web 3.0 and 4.0. These are generally not research journals or scholarly publications.
2. Select one and add the blog, RSS feed, or hyperlink to your blog so when you read/add to your blog you can easily be updated. Do this for one month.
3. Write a short post to your blog about what you learned from this experience. What new developments did you learn about and how might that impact the practice of nursing and the use of social media? How might that influence the movement to Health 3.0 and 4.0?

Exercise 7: A Day in the Life of Nurse Pat

Purpose: *The purpose of this exercise is to provide an opportunity to create a vision of what nursing might be like in the years 2030–2040.*

Objectives
1. Research new technology developments and their possible application in health care.
2. Write a **creative** piece describing the life of Nurse Pat in the years 2030–2040.

Directions
1. Research current technology developments described in technology and engineering journals.
2. Write a two page document describing the Day in the Life of Nurse Pat. This is to be FIRST person as if you are Nurse Pat. Alternatively, you could do this as a podcast.
3. Provide a reference page with a brief description of resources used.
4. Be creative and have fun with this.

REFERENCES

American Well (n.d.). About Us. Retrieved from http://www.americanwell.com/aboutus.htm

Chase, D. (2012a). *Healthcare field of dreams in Idaho: Health system opens innovation center.* Retrieved from http://techcrunch.com/2012/01/04/healthcare-field-of-dreams-in-idaho-health-system-opens-innovation-center/

Chase, D. (2012b). *Nimble medicine set to reshape healthcare.* Retrieved from http://www.forbes.com/sites/davechase/2012/03/02/nimble-medicine-set-to-reshape-healthcare/

Dam, D., Lee, J., Sisco, P., Co, D., Zhang, M., Wasielewski, M., & Odom, T. (2012). Direct observation of nanoparticle – cancer cell nucleus interactions. *ACS Nano, A-I.* Retrieved from http://pubs.acs.org/doi/pdfplus/10.1021/nn300296p

Farber, D. (2007, February 14). *From semantic web (3.0) to the webos (4.0).* Retrieved from http://computer.howstuffworks.com/web-30.htm

Ford, L. (2010). Celebrate the past and create a vision for the future. *Journal of the American Academy of Nurse Practitioners, 22,* 177.

Gilleo, K. (n.d.). *The sci-fi future of medicine...the next 50 years.* Retrieved from http://www.allflexinc.com/PDF/Future%20of%20Medicine.pdf

Gorman, J., & Braber, M. (n.d.). *Semantic web sparks evolution of health 2.0 – A road map to consumer-centric healthcare.* Retrieved from http://nguyendangbinh.org/Proceedings/IPCV08/Papers/SWW3923.pdf

Halloway, J. (2012). *Microsoft developing electronic contact lens to monitor blood sugar.* Retrieved from http://www.gizmag.com/microsoft-electronic-diabetic-contact-lens/20987/

Healthy Aging and Independent Living Lab. (2012). Retrieved from http://www.mayo.edu/center-for-innovation/what-we-do/healthy-aging-and-independent-living-lab

H3PO. (n.d.). *People centered design principles.* Retrieved from https://sites.google.com/site/health30wiki/design-principles

Huston, C. (2008). Preparing nurse leaders for 2020. *Journal of Nursing Management, 16,* 905–911.

Koeniger-Donohue, R., & Hawkins, J. (2010). The future of nursing and healthcare: Through the looking glass 2030. *Journal of Nursing Management, 22,* 233–235.

LivingLaboratoryUsage. (2008). *The ORCATECH Living Lab Program (OLL).* Retrieved from http://www.orcatech.org/LivingLaboratoryUsage.pdf

Manning, K. (2012). *A day in the Internet.* Retrieved from http://www.mbaonline.com/a-day-in-the-internet/

McCabe, J. (2008). *So has health 3.0 arrived?* Retrieved from http://healthmgmtrx.blogspot.com/search/label/Health%204.0

Mobile Devices Solutions Guide. (2012). *Health management technology.* Retrieved from http://www.healthmgttech.com/ebook/HMT201204/resources/32.htm

Muller, N. (n.d.). *The future is now.* Retrieved from http://www.heg-fr.ch/files/recherche/entrepreneuriat/presentation_muller.pdf

Nanotechnology. (n.d.). *Britannica academic edition.* Retrieved from http://www.britannica.com/EBchecked/topic/962484/nanotechnology

Nash, D. (2008). Health 3.0. *P&T, 33*(2), 69, 75. Retrieved from http://www.ncbi.nlm.nih.gov/pmc/articles/PMC2730068/

Nursebot Project. (n.d.). Retrieved from http://www.cs.cmu.edu/~nursebot/web/scope.html

Organized Wisdom (n.d.). Saving Doctors Time While Creating Healthier, Happier Patients. Retrieved from http://www.organizedwisdom.com/Home

Paddock, C. (2012, April 8). Nanostars deliver cancer drugs direct to nucleus. *Medical News Today.* Retrieved from http://www.medicalnewstoday.com/articles/243856.php

Parviz, B. (2009). *Augmented reality in a contact lens.* Retrieved from http://spectrum.ieee.org/biomedical/bionics/augmented-reality-in-a-contact-lens/0

Saenz, A. (2009). *Smart toilets: Doctors in your bathroom.* Retrieved from http://singularityhub.com/2009/05/12/smart-toilets-doctors-in-your-bathroom/

Spivack, N. (2009). *The evolution of the web: Past, present, and future.* Retrieved from http://www.novaspivack.com/uncategorized/the-evolution-of-the-web-past-present-future

Strickland, J. (n.d.). *How Web 3.0 will work.* Retrieved from http://computer.howstuffworks.com/web-30.htm

Task Force Members, Engineers Ireland and The Irish Academy of Engineering. (2006). *A picture of health 2030: Engineering the future of health and medicine.* Retrieved from http://www.iae.ie/site_media/pressroom/documents/2009/Jun/09/A_Picture_of_Health_.pdf

2030–2039 Timeline contents. (n.d.). Retrieved from http://www.futuretimeline.net/21stcentury/2030-039.htm

Trzebucki, A. (2008, June 13). E-health 3.0: How can the semantic web change the world of Internet health information? *Medical News Today.* Retrieved from http://www.meedicalnewstoday.com/articles/111201.php

Veen, W. (n.d.). *Homo Zappiens and the Need for new education systems.* Retrieved from http://www.oecd.org/dataoecd/0/5/38360892.pdf

Wang, S. (2011, October 18). Living lab sets up at a seniors residence: Scientists are getting some real-life lesson on how to stave off the effects of old age. *The Wall Street Journal.* Retrieved from http://online.wsj.com/article/SB10001424052970203658804576636911479895894.html

Watson, A., Bickmore, T., Cange, A., Kulshreshtha, A., & Kvedar, J. (2012). An Internet-based virtual health coach to promote physical activity adherence in overweigh adults: A randomized controlled trial. *Journal of Medical Internet Research, 14*(1), e1. Retrieved from http://www.imir.org/2012/1/e1/

Zammit, D. (2009). *Work in progress: iHealth.* Retrieved from http://www.jwtintelligence.com/production/JWT_iHealth.pdf

Appendix: Additional Online Resources

This section of the Appendix provides additional online social media resources that were not included in the body of the text. The reader is encouraged to explore the sites listed here and to create their own set of online resources.

CHAPTER 1: AN INTRODUCTION

- A university-level course on social media and medicine offered free on the Internet is located at http://med20course.wordpress.com/
- A broad list of resources related to nursing in social media can be accessed at http://www.webicina.com/nursing/

CHAPTER 2: SOFTWARE APPLICATIONS SUPPORTING SOCIAL MEDIA

- Examples of blogs include: KevinMD.com;
  http://smartermedicalcare.org/;
  http://news.consumerreports.org/health/healthy_living/;
  http://laughingatmynightmare.1000notes.com/;
  individual blog of a young person dying and
  Monitor Your Own health (http://www.virtualhealth.com/).
- This is a classic book on Virtual Communities: Rheingold, H. (2000). *The virtual community: Homesteading on the electronic frontier* (rev ed.). Cambridge, MA: The MIT Press.
- Lists of social media software: http://www.best-practice.com/best-practice-software/healthcare-software/recommended-software-for-healthcare-on-social-media/ and http://dochunterdiary.com/20-best-healthcare-social-media-resources/2010/06/30/.
  Meaningful use blog site that also includes social media: http://www.meaningful usenetwork.com/
- Turkle, S. (2011). *Alone together: Why we expect more from technology and less from each other.* New York: Basic Books.

CHAPTER 3: SELECTING DEVICES AND RELATED HARDWARE TO SUPPORT SOCIAL MEDIA

▦ A significant list of resources supporting mHealth provided by the eHealth Initiative is located at http://www.ehealthinitiative.org/resources/viewcategory/39-general.html

CHAPTER 4: APPLICATIONS AND TOOLS PROMOTING HEALTH 2.0 VIA SOCIAL MEDIA

▦ An extensive collection of health-related social media resources can be found at http://www.webicina.com/?select=null

CHAPTER 5: CONSUMER-CENTERED VIRTUAL HEALTH COMMUNITIES

▦ An excellent example of rules for participating in online health-related communities can be seen at http://www2.acor.org/pages/rules
▦ Ten Simple Rules for Getting Help from Online Scientific Communities, located at http://www.ncbi.nlm.nih.gov/pmc/articles/PMC3182872/pdf/pcbi.1002202.pdf
▦ An example of organizations supporting engaged patients can be found at http://cfah.org/about/letter.cfm

CHAPTER 6: PERSONAL HEALTH RECORDS (PHRs)

▦ A quick guide to personal health records designed for clinicians along with other related resources can be accessed at http://www.bcbs.com/healthcare-partners/personal-health-records/Clinician-Quick-Reference-Guide.pdf
▦ An interesting vision of how health care providers would really have access to the patient's health history. What if the patient was included? http://www.youtube.com/watch?v=mJ2kMtRH9NY&feature=youtu.be

CHAPTER 7: TELEHEALTH

▦ Free Webinar Series, providing timely information and demonstrations by experienced telehealth professionals from the HRSA-designated Telehealth Resource Centers (TRCs) can be accessed at http://www.telehealthresourcecenter.org/post/national-webinar-series

CHAPTER 8: BUSINESS MODELS AND HEALTH-RELATED SOCIAL MEDIA

▦ An example of a business philosophy (*Ten things we know to be true*) within a business model can be seen at http://www.google.com/about/company/philosophy/

CHAPTER 9: PROFESSIONAL GUIDELINES, POLICIES, REGULATIONS, AND LAWS IMPACTING HEALTH-RELATED SOCIAL MEDIA COMMUNICATION

- An interesting analysis of privacy and social media: Barnes, S. B. (2006, September 4). A privacy paradox: Social networking in the United States. *First Monday* [Online], *11*(9). Retrieved from http://firstmonday.org/htbin/cgiwrap/bin/ojs/index.php/fm/article/view/1394/1312
- A research study discussing Ensuring Trust, Privacy, and Etiquette in Web 2.0 Applications can be reviewed at http://sintef.academia.edu/PetterBaeBrandtzæg/Papers/814035/Ensuring_Trust_Privacy_and_Etiquette_in_Web_2.0_Applications

CHAPTER 10: SOCIAL MEDIA AND HEALTHCARE—TOMORROW AND BEYOND

- Futures research is the study of the future. An overview of methods used to conduct futures research can be accessed at http://crab.rutgers.edu/~goertzel/futuristmethods.htm

JOURNALS FOCUSED ON HEALTH 2.0 ISSUES

- *Journal of Medical Internet Research* (JMIR). Additional information can be found at http://www.jmir.org/index
- *Journal of Participatory Medicine*. Additional information can be found at http://www.jopm.org/
- *Bulletin of the World Health Organization*. The May 2012 issue is focused on eHealth and can be viewed at http://www.who.int/bulletin/en/
- *WORLDview ON EVIDENCE BASED-BASED PRACTICE*. The April 2012 issue focuses on the role of technology with several Health 2.0 related articles. Additional information is located at http://onlinelibrary.wiley.com/doi/10.1111/wvn.2012.9.issue-2/issuetoc

GROUPS WITHIN ESTABLISHED SOCIAL NETWORKING SITES

The groups selected for this section of the appendix are formally established professional groups who have established a group page on a social networking site and are OPEN to non-members.

LinkedIn

- **American Nurses Association:** This is the LinkedIn professional group created by the American Nurses Association. ANA is a national professional association that advocates for all registered nurses and the patients they serve by establishing and promoting high standards in nursing, advancing the rights of nurses in the workplace, and lobbying Congress and regulatory agencies.

- **Health Informatics Technology** is a remarkable fusion of clinical care and technology. In HIT we strive to keep healthcare providers' base values and move into a broader realm of helping the patient and our fellow providers through the adoption of technology in healthcare.
- **American Nursing Informatics Association:** CNIOs and Nurses (RNs) involved in the Nursing IT World, using computers and technology gathering Clinical Information involved in Administrative Decision Support to Improve Patient Care and Safety and address Workflow issues (RN).

Facebook

- **National Student Nurses Association** (NSNA) and the Foundation of the NSNA (FNSNA) maintain an OFFICIAL Facebook page. NSNA's mission is to mentor students preparing for initial licensure as registered nurses.
- The **National League for Nursing** also maintains a Facebook page. The NLN is dedicated to excellence in nursing education and is a preferred membership organization for nurse faculty and leaders in nursing education.

Twitter

- FutureofNursing @FutureofNursing. The campaign, coordinated through @ChampionNursing, initiative of @AARP, @RWJF, envisions health system where nurses contribute to full extent of their capabilities. http://www.thefutureofnursing.org
- NSNA @NSNAinc maintains an official Twitter page for the National Student Nurses Association.

Glossary

Aggregator An aggregator is a website, company, software program, or individual who combines data from a variety of sources to create a data set related to a specific topic, individual, or group (Chapter 8).

Alexa rankings Alexa rankings are traffic rankings of web usage compiled by Alexa, a web-based information company. The rankings are based on three months of aggregated historical traffic data from millions of users (Chapter 2).

Apps The term apps is an abbreviation for applications that run on mobile devices (Chapters 2 and 3). Also see mobile application.

Augmented reality Augmented reality is the integration of digital information with the users' real world in real time (Chapter 10).

Behavior targeting Behavior targeting is the process of carefully selecting a potential customer to receive a specific advertisement or information based on their current or previous activities such as searching for information on the Internet (Chapter 8).

Blog Blogs or web logs are online journals, posts, or entries in chronological order that one updates frequently (Chapter 2).

Blog archive Blog archive is an area of the blog page where the site places old posts. The visitor can access these generally by date (Chapter 2).

Blogger The person who creates and maintains the blog site is the blogger. This is also the name of one of the most well known blogging sites (Chapter 2).

Blogosphere Blogosphere is a term used to describe the collective community of all bloggers and their blogs (Chapter 2).

Blogs Blogs is plural for blog (Chapter 2).

Browsewrap Browsewrap is an online contract signing process that binds the user by passive conduct, such as continuing to use the website or proceeding past its homepage (Chapter 8).

Business model A business model is a conceptual framework used to describe the process by which an organization generates income (Chapter 8).

Business strategy Business strategy is the process used to design and implement a business model (Chapter 8).

Camcorder A camcorder is a free-standing electronic device capable of recording video and audio as its primary function (Chapter 3).

Cellular phone A cellular phone is a portable, usually cordless, telephone for use in a cellular system (Cell phone, n.d.; Chapter 3).

Clickthrough agreement Clickthrough agreement is an online contract that requires the user to click or perform another specific activity to indicate they agree with the terms of the contract. This is also referred to as a clickwrap agreement (Chapter 8).

Clickwrap agreement Clickwrap agreement is an online contract that requires the user to click or perform another specific activity to indicate they agree with the terms of the contract. This is also referred to as a clickthrough agreement (Chapter 8).

Cloud The term cloud refers to a service model in which data are maintained, managed, and backed up remotely and made available to users over a network (typically the Internet). The cloud serves as a safe and more secure site to share information and is a way of sharing services over the Internet. There are three types of cloud models; public, private, and hybrid (Cloud Computing, 2007) (Chapter 4).

Collective intelligence Collective intelligence is a phenomenon where a shared or group intelligence emerges from the collaboration and competition of many individuals (Collective Intelligence, n.d.; Chapter 5).

Computer literacy/fluency Computer fluency is a level of computer knowledge and skill that goes beyond proficiency to being able to express creatively, reformulate knowledge, and synthesize new information using a wide range of information technology (Chapter 1).

Consumer health informatics "Consumer health informatics is the branch of medical informatics that analyses consumers' needs for information; studies and implements methods of making information accessible to consumers; and models and integrates consumers' preferences into medical information systems" (Eysenbach, 2000, p. 1713). Consumer health informatics is also referred to as consumer informatics (Chapter 1).

Consumer informatics See consumer health informatics (Chapter 1).

Consumer-centric commerce Consumer-centric commerce means "identifying, facilitating, and integrating online and offline communication and care delivery channels needed to reach and coordinate end goals (values) as defined by disparate customer segments such as the patient, provider, payer, policymaker, caretaker, etcetera" (Gorman & Braber, n.d.; Chapter 10).

Contacts Also called Friends. Term that most often describes relationships in a social network site (Chapter 2).

Contextual targeting Contextual targeting is the process of displaying a specific ad or ads based on related content a user is currently viewing online (Chapter 8).

Copyright Copyright is the legal right to publish, create derivative works, reproduce, or distribute an original work (Chapter 9).

Criteria Criteria are the standards or yardstick against which you measure the quality of information (Chapter 1).

Crowdsourcing Crowdsourcing refers to the process of using the collective intelligence or skills of a group or of the public at large to complete tasks that a company would normally either perform itself or outsource to a third-party provider. The labor is provided for free or at minimum cost (Chapter 1).

Cyberbullying Cyberbullying is defined as the online posting of mean-spirited, hostile messages about a person with malicious intent to harm that person emotionally or physically (Chapter 2).

Data mining Data mining is the analysis of data for relationships, correlations, or patterns that have not previously been discovered among dozens of fields in large databases (Chapter 2).

Desktop computer A desktop computer is a combination of individual interconnected wired or wireless devices such as a monitor, keyboard, tower, speakers, camcorder, and mouse that is usually stationary for daily use atop a desk or office table (Chapter 3).

Digital games Digital games are a form of technology that stimulate human interactivities through virtual experiences (Yengin, 2011) (Chapter 4).

Digital literacy Digital literacy includes competency with digital devices of all types; the technical skills to operate these devices as well as a the conceptual knowledge to understand their functionality; the ability to creatively and critically use these devices to access, manipulate, evaluate, and apply data, information, knowledge, and wisdom in activities of daily living; the ability to apply basic emotional intelligence in collaborating and communicating with others, and the ethical values and sense of community responsibility to use digital devices for the enjoyment and benefit of society (Chapter 1).

Digital native A digital native is a person who was born sometime after 1980, after the general introduction of computer-related technology to the general public, and through interacting with digital technology from an early age is believed to have a greater comfort and understanding of its concepts. The term was coined by Marc Prensky (2001; Chapter 1).

EEOC See The Equal Employment Opportunity Commission (Chapter 8).

eHealth eHealth is "the ability to seek, find, understand, and appraise health information from electronic sources and apply the knowledge gained to addressing or solving a health problem" (Norman & Skinner, 2006, p. e9; Chapter 1).

EHR See electronic health record (Chapter 6).

Electronic health record (EHR) Electronic health record refers to aggregate electronic data from multiple sources for one individual that is used to manage one's overall state of health. The EHR is considered more powerful than an EMR because information is security-shared across a variety of health care settings, and the data in an EHR go beyond the clinical data in an EMR to focus on the full health status of the individual (DHHS: Office of the National Coordinator, 2011; Chapter 6).

Electronic medical records (EMR) Electronic medical records refer to the electronic storage of health information by a licensed health provider who created, gathered, and manages a patient's data. An EMR is the digital version of a patient chart designed for a specific setting (DHHS: Office of the National Coordinator, 2011; Chapters 4 and 6).

EMR See electronic medical record (Chapter 6).

Engaged consumer An engaged consumer is an actively involved health care consumer seeking an ongoing dialog with health care providers and others concerning their health and health care options (Chapter 1).

eReaders An eReader is an electronic, portable, flat, thin device used for reading books and other text materials that have been downloaded from the Internet or computer (Chapter 3).

Exergame An exergame is a video game that requires the user to participate in physical activity to play the game (Healthgamers, n.d.; Chapter 4).

FDA See Federal and Drug Administration (Chapter 9).

Federal Trade Commission (FTC) The Federal Trade Commission is the federal agency charged with preventing business practices that are monopolistic, deceptive, or unfair to consumers and with protecting consumer privacy (Chapter 9).

First party tracking First party tracking occurs when the website a user is visiting places a cookie on the user's computer to collect information about that user's activities as well as statistics about how the website is being used. The data usually facilitates the user's experience on the site, however, the amount and type of data can be extensive (Chapter 8).

FOIA See Freedom of Information Act (Chapter 8).

Food and Drug Administration (FDA) The Food and Drug Administration is the agency within the federal government responsible for the regulation of medical products, such as drugs and medical equipment, including how these products are advertised (Chapter 9).

Freedom of Information Act (FOIA) The Freedom of Information Act is the federal law ensuring public access to U.S. government records, unless those records are covered by an exception in the law (Chapter 8).

Friending Friending is the act of adding someone to your list of friends on a social networking site (Chapter 2).

Friends Friends and Contacts are the terms that most often describe relationships in a social networking site (Chapter 2).

FTC See Federal Trade Commission (Chapter 9).

Geo-targeting Geo-targeting is the process of displaying on the user's screen a specific ad or ads based on a user's geographical location (Chapter 8).

GNP See Gross National Product (Chapter 8).

Gray literature Gray literature refers to papers, reports, and other documents posted or published by governmental agencies, academic institutions, businesses, and other groups that are not usually peer reviewed or indexed in traditional literature databases such as Medline or CINAHL (Chapter 8).

Gross National Product (GNP) Gross National Product is the value in dollars of all goods and services produced in the country, plus the value of goods and services that are imported, less the value of goods and services that are exported (Chapter 8).

Health 2.0 Health 2.0 is the use of social media and mobile applications to promote collaboration among stakeholders, including empowered patients/consumers within the health care system with the goal of improving the health and quality of life for individuals, families, and communities (Chapter 1 and 4).

Health 3.0 Health 3.0 is a health-related extension of the concept of Web 3.0. Users interface with personalized information on the web to gain help in health-related issues. Health 3.0 is characterized by content, consumers, and commerce. Health 3.0 is influenced by one's ability to adapt to self-management or self-care (Chapter 10).

Health 4.0 Health 4.0 builds on Health 3.0 and adds coherence or connectors. Health 4.0 will rely strongly on self-management of disease or one's health promotion efforts (Chapter 10).

Health care consumer A health care consumer is defined as anyone who receives or has the potential to receive health care services, regardless of whether the individual pays for those services directly or indirectly (Guo, 2010; Chapter 1).

Health information exchange (HIE) A health information exchange provides for the electronic movement of health-related information among organizations utilizing nationally recognized standards and policies (HIMSS, 2009; Chapter 4).

Health literacy Health literacy is the ability to access, evaluate, and apply information to health-related decisions. See Exhibit 1.2 for additional definitions of this term (Chapter 1).

HIE See health information exchange (Chapter 4).

Homo Zappiens Homo Zappiens refers to the generation of children who were born after 1990 and have never known a world without the Internet. They are used to learning through collaboration, explorations, and experimentation, thereby making many traditional teaching approaches ineffective (Veen &Vrakking, 2007; Chapter 10).

ICH See Informatics for consumer health (Chapter 1).

Informatics for consumer health (ICH) See consumer health informatics (Chapter 1).

Information literacy Information literacy is a set of abilities requiring individuals to recognize when information is needed and have the ability to locate, evaluate, and effectively use the needed information (American Library Association, 2000; Chapter 1).

Initial Public Offering (IPO) Initial Public Offering refers to the first sale of a company's stock to the public. In selling the stock to the general public, the company moves from being a privately owned company to a publicly traded company (Chapter 8).

IPO See Initial Public Offering (Chapter 8).

Laptop computer A laptop computer is similar to a desktop computer, but includes all the items in one device and is typically smaller and more convenient to move and transport (Chapter 3).

Leakage Leakage occurs when an individual logs in to a social networking site and the social network includes their advertising and tracking code in such a way that the third party aggregator can see and record the contents of the profile page for that individual (Chapter 8).

Microblog Microblog is a term to describe a subset of blogging that limits posts to brief updates (Chapter 2).

Microblogging Microblogging is the process of posting to microblogs (Chapter 2).

MMS See multimedia message service (Chapter 3).

Mobile applications Mobile applications are software programs developed for small handheld devices such as mobile phones, tablets, or PDAs. Mobile applications are frequently referred to as "apps" (Viswanathan, n.d.). Caution: The terms application and app are not used consistently, and are often interpreted by the context in which they are used. At times they have overlapping definitions. At other times the term application refers to a software program with multiple functions running on a computer, while app refers to a limited-purpose program running on a mobile device (Chapters 3 and 4).

Multimedia message service (MMS) Multimedia message service is the ability to send and receive different forms of media such as pictures, videos, or graphics from one cellular device to another, or to another mobile electronic device (Chapter 3).

Nanobot A nanobot is a microscopic, self-propelled robot used in nanotechnologies (Chapter 10).

Nanotechnology Nanotechnologies refer to an approach of building things from the bottom up by manipulating individual atoms and molecules at the one billionth of a meter level (Nanotechnology, n.d.; Chapter 10).

National Labor Relations Board (NLRB) The National Labor Relations Board is the federal agency charged with protecting the rights of most private-sector employees to join together to bargain collectively through representatives of their own choosing, or to refrain from such activities (Chapter 9).

Netbook computer A netbook computer is smaller than a notebook computer and is typically used for accessing Internet-based applications (Chapter 3).

NLRB See National Labor Relations Board (Chapter 3).

Notebook computer A notebook computer is comparable to a laptop computer but is typically lighter in weight and smaller in size (Chapter 3).

Object-centered sociality Object-centered sociality is an interest in connecting with other people who have an object of common interest. That object may be, for example, a job, a hobby, or a medical record (Steward, 2009; Chapter 6).

Participatory engagement Participatory engagement is a cooperative health care model that actively involves the patient and/or patient caregiver as an integral part of the full range of care continuum (Chapter 5).

Patient empowerment 2.0 Patient empowerment 2.0 refers to an engaged patient who is actively involved in their health care through the use of social media and other Web 2.0 tools (Chapter 1).

PC video camera A PC video camera is an input device that the operator uses to capture video. It may be used to send video images as email attachments, to make video telephone calls (video conferencing), and to post live, real-time images to a web server (Joos, Nelson, & Smith, 2010; Chapter 3).

Personal health information (PHI) Personal health information refers to any information that can be used to identify an individual's health status (Chapter 6).

Personal health records (PHR) Personal health records are consumer-centric tools designed for individuals to maintain their own health information. These are also known as patient health records.

Personal identifiable information (PII) Personal identifiable information are data that can be used to distinguish or trace a specific individual's identity either alone or when combined with other information (Krishnamurthy & Craig, 2009; Chapter 8).

PHI See personal health information (Chapter 6).

PHR See personal health records (Chapter 6).

Portable media player Portable media player refers to any portable mobile device that plays music and video, stores images, and/or has hardware that supports Internet connectivity. Examples include an MP3 or MP4 player (Chapter 3).

Profile Profile is what the user tells others about himself or herself in accordance with a completed form (Chapter 2). On Facebook, the term was replaced with Timeline.

Publicly traded Company A publicly traded company is a company whose stock is traded publicly on at least one stock exchange or in the over-the-counter market (Chapter 8).

Regional health information organization (RHIO) A regional health information organization is a health information organization that brings together health care stakeholders within a defined geographic area and governs health information exchange among them for the purpose of improving health and care in that community (DHHS: Office of the National Coordinator: The National Alliance for Health Information Technology, 2008; Chapter 4).

RHIO See Regional Health Information Organizations (Chapter 4).

Semantic web Semantic web, also called Web 3.0, refers to a framework that allows data to be shared and reused across application and community boundaries by emphasizing the meaning of the data rather than the syntax (Chapter 10). See Web 3.0 for additional information.

Short message service (SMS) Short message service is a method of communicating using short messages from one cellular mobile device to another. SMS is also known as "text messaging" (Chapter 3).

Simple Markup Language Simple Markup Language is the code that permits the writing and publishing of a wiki page through a web browser (Chapter 2).

SNS SNS is an abbreviation that refers to social network sites (Chapter 2).

Social network sites Virtual communities where users establish and maintain relationships with others through sharing life events.

SMS See short message service (Chapter 3).

Social media Social media are web-based and mobile technologies such as social networking and microblogging sites that are used to turn the one-way communication of Web 1.0 into interactive dialogue where users create online communities to share information, ideas, personal messages, and other content (Chapters 1 and 2).

Software programs Software programs are step-by-step instructions that direct the computer hardware to perform specific tasks. Caution: This term can be confused with mobile applications, for at times they have overlapping definitions. The terms are not used consistently and are often interpreted by the context in which they are used (Joos, Nelson, & Smith, 2010) (Chapter 3).

Status update Status update is the term for the updates in the member's life that are shared on a social network site such as Facebook (Chapter 2).

Super-cookies There is not a generally accepted definition for super-cookies. However, these types of cookies cannot be blocked with browser settings, are stored deep in the computer files where it is difficult to delete them, and are not deleted by most applications designed to delete cookies. If manually deleted, these cookies may recreate themselves. Other names for these cookies include flash-cookies, zombie-cookies, and ever-cookies (Chapter 8).

Syntax Syntax refers to how words are configured within a sentence or how data are displayed (Chapter 10).

Tablet A tablet is a thin, flat, lightweight electronic device that is usually smaller than a laptop computer screen, in which one touches the screen to interact with the device. This device supports the use of mobile applications and has the capability of connecting to the Internet. It generally relies on the touch screen and virtual keyboard with no physical keyboard, and has less built-in storage. Caution: This term can be confused with tablet computers. These terms can have overlapping definitions and are not used consistently. The terms are often interpreted by the context in which they are used (Chapter 3).

Tablet computer Tablet computer is a mobile computer similar to a notebook, but with the effect of a tablet surface. The screen part of a laptop can be swiveled and collapsed to take the form of a tablet. The primary input device is the keyboard and pen, with larger built in storage. Caution: This term can be confused with tablet. The terms are not used consistently and at times have overlapping definitions. The terms are often interpreted by the context in which they are used (Chapter 3).

Tags Tags are keywords added to the blog in the tag field for easier searches and aggregation (Chapter 2).

Telecommunications "Telecommunications is the use of the telephone, Internet, interactive video, remote sensory devices, or robotics to transmit information from one site to another" (American Academy of Ambulatory Care Nursing, 2011, p. 42; Chapter 7).

Teleconferencing Teleconferencing involves "interactive electronic communication between two or more people at two or more sites, which make use of voice, video, and/or data transmission systems" (National Research Council, 1996, p. 248; Chapter 7).

Telehealth Telehealth is the use of technology to address the health needs of others across a geographical area. It is also "an umbrella term used to describe the services delivered across distances by all health-related disciplines" (Academy of Ambulatory Care Nursing, 2011, p. 42; Chapter 7).

Telehealth nursing practice Telehealth nursing practice is "the delivery, management, and coordination of care and services provided via telecommunications technology within the domain of ambulatory care nursing. Telehealth nursing incorporates a vast array of telecommunications technologies (e.g., telephone, fax, email, Internet, video monitoring, and interactive videos) to remove time and distance barriers" (Espensen, 2009, p. 5; Chapter 7).

Telemedicine Telemedicine is "the use of electronic and telecommunications technologies to provide and support medical care when distance separates the participants" (National Research Council, 1996, p. 248; Chapter 7).

Telemonitoring Telemonitoring is "the use of audio, video, and other telecommunications and electronic information processing technologies to monitor patient status at a distance" (National Research Council, 1996, p. 248; Chapter 7).

Telenursing Telenursing refers to a nurse's use of technology to address the health needs of others across a geographical area (Chapter 7).

Telepresence Telepresence is the use of robotic and other devices that allow a person to perform a task at a remote site. This may include manipulation of instruments and receiving sensory information or feedback that creates a sense of being present at the remote site (National Research Council, 1996; Chapter 7).

Teleradiology Teleradiology is "the electronic transmission of radiological patient images, such as x-rays, CTs, and MRIs, from one location to another for the purposes of interpretation and/or consultation (Webster's Online Dictionary, n.d.; Chapter 7).

Telerehabilitation Telerehabilitation is "the application of evaluation, preventative, diagnostic, and therapeutic rehabilitation services via two-way or multi-point interactive telecommunication technology" (American Occupational Therapy Association, 2010, p. 1; Chapter 7).

The Equal Employment Opportunity Commission (EEOC) The U.S. Equal Employment Opportunity Commission is responsible for enforcing federal laws that make it illegal to discriminate against a job applicant or an employee because of the person's race, color, religion, sex (including pregnancy), national origin, age (40 or older), disability, or genetic information (Equal Employment Opportunity Commission, n.d.; Chapter 9).

Third-party tracking Third-party tracking is the process used to tract a user across multiple websites, thereby building an extensive browsing history for that user. See third-party tracking cookies (Chapter 8).

Third-party tracking cookies Third-party tracking cookies are cookies placed on a user's computer by a site other than the site that is being viewed by that user. These cookies are used to track behavior across different websites, providing third parties with information about the web browsing habits of the user (Chapter 8).

Timeline A Facebook feature introduced in September 2011 and available to all users in February 2012. Timeline combines a user's Facebook Wall and Profile into one page. It includes a user's Facebook history with key life points.

Trademark Trademark refers to a company's name, brand, or product names. The company owns these words, phrases, symbols, or designs, or a combination thereof, such as logos, symbols, or names, and another company cannot use them without permission (Trademark, 2010; Chapter 9).

Typology Topology is a schematic description of the arrangement of a community and the components of importance to studying it (Chapter 5).

User-generated content Information found on the Internet that is created by a user or consumer is referred to as user-generated content (Chapter 5).

Virtual communities A virtual community is a gathering of individuals who share a common interest, focus, or need, who use an Internet platform to frequently interact with each other, and who identify with the predefined community, which provides a sense of belonging or ownership (Chapter 5).

Virtual worlds Virtual worlds are Internet-simulated environments where inhabitants interact with other inhabitants (Chapter 2).

Wall Wall is the term that describes a place where others can leave a message on someone else's profile on social networking sites (Chapter 2). Facebook has now replaced the term with, Timeline.

Web 1.0 Web 1.0 refers to static websites that are viewed by users but without interactive involvement between the user and the website or others who visit the web site (Chapter 1).

Web 2.0 Web 2.0 refers to a set of economic, social, and technology trends characterized by user participation, openness, and networking through the use of social media and other online collaborative tools. The term was coined by Tim O'Reilly (2005; Chapter 1).

Web 3.0 Web 3.0 is machine-facilitated understanding of information found on the web: About things and how they relate to each other; about context of the information; and about computers understanding the data (Chapter 10). See Semantic web for additional information.

Web 4.0 Web 4.0 is a term used to define a generation of web technologies; also called WebOS, symbiotic, and intelligent web (Chapter 10).

Web conferencing Web conferencing is an interactive meeting conducted over the Internet, generally in real time with 50 or less attendees (Chapter 5).

Webcam Webcam is a video camera that interfaces to a desktop computer and feeds real-time images to a computer or network using a Wi-Fi, USB, or cable connection (Chapter 3).

Webcast Webcast is a media presentation, broadcast as a live video feed over the Internet to a large number of users and a small number of presenters using streaming technology (Chapter 5).

Wikis Wikis are applications or websites that permit people to quickly comment on, edit for the purpose of improving, and collaborate in sharing their expertise for the benefit of the web page content contained on the wiki website (Chapter 2).

Wisdom of crowds Wisdom of crowds refers to the ability of a group of people to function creatively in making decisions as opposed to the ability of individuals to perform these same activities (Chapter 1).

REFERENCES

American Academy of Ambulatory Care Nursing. (2011). *Scope and standards of practice for professional telehealth nursing* (5th ed.). Pitman, NJ: Author.

American Occupational Therapy Association. (2010). Telerehabilitation. *American Journal of Occupational Therapy, 64*(6), S92–S102. Retrieved from http://dx.doi.org/10.5014/ajot.2010.64S92

Cell Phone. (n.d.). *Merriam-Webster dictionary.* Retrieved from http://www.merriam-bster.com/dictionary/cell%20phone

Cloud Computing. (2007). *Search cloud computing.* Retrieved from http://searchcloudcomputing.techtarget.com/definition/cloud-computing

Collective Intelligence. (n.d.). In *Dictionary.com.* Retrieved from http://dictionary.reference.com/browse/collective+intelligence.

DHHS: Office of the National Coordinator. (2011, January 4). *EMR vs EHR – What is the Difference?* Retrieved from Health ITBizz: http://www.healthit.gov/buzz-blog/electronic-health-and-medical-records/emr-vs-ehr-difference/

DHHS: Office of the National Coordinator: The National Alliance for Health Information Technology. (2008). *Defining key health information technology terms.* Retrieved from http://www.healthit.hhs.gov/defining_key_hit_terms

Equal Employment Opportunity Commission. (n.d.). *About EEOC.* Retrieved from U.S. Equal Employment Opportunity Commission (EEOC): http://www.eeoc.gov/eeoc/index.cfm

Espensen, M. (Ed.). (2009). *Telehealth nursing practice essentials.* Pitman, NJ: American Academy of Ambulatory Care Nursing.

Eysenbach, G. (2000, June). Consumer health informatics. *British Medical Journal, 320*(24), 1713–1716.

Gorman, J., & Braber, M. (n.d.). *Semantic web sparks evolution of health 2.0 – A road map to consumer-centric healthcare.* Retrieved from http://nguyendangbinh.org/Proceedings/IPCV08/Papers/SWW3923.pdf

Guo, K. (2010, January/March). Consumer-directed health care understanding its value in health care reform. *The Health Care Manager, 29*(1), 29–33.

Healthgamers. (n.d.). *Glossary.* Retrieved from http://www.healthgamers.com/glossary/

HIMSS. (2009). *2009: Health information exchanges in the United States.* Retrieved from http://www.himss.org/content/files/HIETopicSeries_Fact%20Sheet%20071709.pdf

Joos, I., Nelson, R., & Smith, M. (2010). *Introduction to computers for healthcare professionals.* Sudbury, MA: Jones and Bartlett Publishers.

Krishnamurthy, B., & Craig, W. (2009, September 21). *On the leakage of personally identifiable information via online social networks.* Retrieved from Electronic Frontier Foundation (EFF): http://conferences.sigcomm.org/sigcomm/2009/workshops/wosn/papers/p7.pdf

Mediaplatform. (2010). *Webcasting vs. web conferencing white paper: Sorting out the difference between two related but different technologies.* Retrieved from http://info.mediaplatform.com/site/Webcastingvs.Webconferencing.html and then you have to sign in to get the paper located at the URL provided in the entry listed on p 260.

Nanotechnology. (n.d.). *Britannica academic edition.* Retrieved from http://www.britannica.com/EBchecked/topic/962484/nanotechnology

National Research Council. (1996). *Telemedicine: A guide to assessing telecommunication for healthcare.* Washington, DC: The National Academies Press. Retrieved from http://www.nap.edu/openbook.php?record_id=5296&page=R1

Norman, C., & Skinner, H. (2006, June 16). eHealth literacy: Essential skills for consumer health in a networked world. *Journal of Medical Internet Research, 8*(2), e9.

O'Reilly, T. (2005, March 30). *What is web 2.0?* Retrieved from O'Reilly Media, Inc.: http://oreilly.com/web2/archive/what-is-web-20.html

Prensky, M. (2001). Digital natives, digital immigrants. *On the Horizon* (Vol. 9, No. 5). MCB University Press. Retrieved from http://www.marcprensky.com/writing/prensky%20-%20digital%20natives,%20digital%20immigrants%20-%20part1.pdf

Social Media. (n.d.). *In merriam-webster: An encyclopedia britannica company online.* Retrieved from http://www.merriam-webster.com/dictionary/social%20media

Stewart, D. (2009). *Socialized medicine: How personal health records and social networks are changing healthcare*. Retrieved from http://www.econtentmag.com/Articles/ArticleReader.aspx?Article ID=56166&PageNum=3

Trademark, U. S. (2010). *Basic facts about trademarks*. Retrieved from The United States Patent and Trademark Office: http://www.uspto.gov/trademarks/basics/BasicFacts_with_correct_links.pdf

Veen, B., & Vrakking, B. (2007). *Homo Zappiens: Growing up in a digital age*. New York, NY: Network Continuum Education.

Viswanathan, P. (n. d.). *What is a mobile application?* Retrieved from http://mobiledevices.about.com/od/glossary/g/What-Is-A-Mobile-Application.htm

Webster's Online Dictionary. (n.d.). *Teleradiology*. Retrieved from http://www.websters-online-dictionary.org/definitions/Teleradiology#Wikipedia

Yengin, D. (2011). Digital game as a new media and use of digital game in education. *The Turkish Online Journal of Design, Art and Communication, 1*(1), 20–25. Retrieved from http://www.tojdac.org/tojdac/HOME_files/v01i103.pdf

Index